Ambulatory EEG Monitoring

Ambulatory EEG Monitoring

Editor

John S. Ebersole, M.D.
Associate Professor of Neurology
Yale University School of Medicine;
Director, Clinical Neurophysiology Laboratory
Yale–New Haven Hospital
New Haven, Connecticut; and
Chief, Clinical Neurophysiology
Veterans Administration Medical Center
West Haven, Connecticut

Raven Press 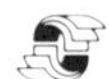 New York

Raven Press, 1185 Avenue of the Americas, New York, New York 10036

Made in the United States of America

Library of Congress Cataloging-in-Publication Data

Ambulatory EEG monitoring / editor, John S. Ebersole.
p. cm.
Includes bibliographies and index.
ISBN 0-88167-505-9
1. Ambulatory electroencephalography. 2. Patient monitoring.
I. Ebersole, John S.
[DNLM: 1. Ambulatory Care. 2. Electroencephalography.
3. Monitoring, Physiologic—methods. WL 150 A497]
RC386.6.A45A42 1989
616.8'047547—dc19
DNLM/DLC
for Library of Congress 87-43192
CIP

The material contained in this volume was submitted as previously unpublished material, except in the instances in which credit has been given to the source from which some of the illustrative material was derived.

Great care has been taken to maintain the accuracy of the information contained in the volume. However, neither Raven Press nor the editors can be held responsible for errors or for any consequences arising from the use of the information contained herein.

9 8 7 6 5 4 3 2 1

Preface

Fifteen years ago, recording EEG on cassette tape with a portable device was an experimental procedure. Ten years ago, ambulatory EEG systems with four data channels were commercially introduced. Today, cassette EEG monitoring, using eight or more channels for data, is a well-established diagnostic tool. This evolution has come about not only because of technological advances that have improved recording and analysis systems, but also because of a growing appreciation for the clinical utility of long-term EEG and polygraphic monitoring in a variety of disorders with paroxysmal or intermittent symptoms. Ambulatory EEG has filled the gap that existed between routine laboratory EEG and intensive inpatient monitoring at specialized epilepsy or sleep centers. The diagnostic benefits of long-term recordings, such as improved diagnosis, characterization, and quantification of these disorders and their electrographic markers, are now conveniently available to a growing population of ambulatory outpatients.

Before the publication of this volume, only individual research articles or review chapters were available to those interested in ambulatory cassette EEG. Our goal is to provide a comprehensive and up-to-date review of the subject that covers topics from theoretical to the very practical. This book will be of interest to clinical specialists in neurology, sleep-disorders medicine, and psychiatry, as well as to electroencephalographers, polysomnographers, and technologists in both specialties. The reader will find in-depth discussions of available instrumentation and techniques for recording and analyzing EEG and polygraphic data. Clinical indications for the use of cassette recordings in the evaluation of both epilepsy and sleep disorders are reviewed in the context of the published literature and personal experiences. Experts in particular applications of cassette EEG or polygraphy recount their own clinical series.

It is my expectation as editor that this compendium of ambulatory monitoring experience will serve well both the neophyte, who wishes to learn about cassette EEG, and the experienced practitioner of the technique, who wishes to have a complete and convenient reference source.

John S. Ebersole

Acknowledgments

The assistance of many individuals has been invaluable during the past eight years of clinical ambulatory cassette EEG research. First and foremost, I wish to thank my two former fellows, Sam Bridgers and Rob Leroy, who worked with me to establish the clinical utility of cassette EEG in the evaluation of seizure disorders. Now as academic colleagues, both have continued their efforts in this regard, as evidenced by their contributions to this volume. EEG data for our various comparative studies could not have been obtained without the diligent assistance of the Epilepsy Unit nurses at the West Haven Veterans Administration Medical Center in addition to the cooperation of my colleagues, Dick Mattson, Peter Williamson, and Susan Spencer. The quality and thus the ultimate potential value of an ambulatory EEG is dependent upon the expertise and commitment of the cassette EEG technologist. Many of the EEGs depicted in this volume attest to the skills of two such individuals, Cloe Silva of Yale–New Haven Hospital and Doris Kelly of Lawrence and Memorial Hospital. In an environment where industry and medicine work closely together, medical instrumentation evolves with clinical utility a foremost consideration. It has been my pleasure to work with Oxford Medical, Inc., and in particular with Terry Murphy, the national sales manager. Last on the scene, but in no way least deserving of my thanks, is my present fellow, Peter Wade, whose organizational skills helped get me through the last weeks of editing.

To Ellen,
who waited patiently for the spring and summer that never were

Contents

Ambulatory EEG Monitoring in Seizure Disorders

Clinical Series

Contributors

Sonia Ancoli-Israel, Ph.D., A.C.P.
Associate Adjunct Professor
Department of Psychiatry
University of California, San Diego 92110; and
Veterans Administration Medical Center
3350 La Jolla Village Dr.
San Diego, California 92161

Nicolette Bergel
University of Oxford
Special Centre for Children with Epilepsy
Regional Paediatric EEG Unit
Park Hospital for Children
Headington, Oxford OX3 7LQ
England

Howard W. Blume, M.D., Ph.D.
Chief, Division of Neurosurgery
Department of Surgery
Beth Israel Hospital
Harvard University
330 Brookline Avenue
Boston, Massachusetts 02215

Andrew C. Bragdon, M.D.
Assistant Professor of Medicine (Neurology)
Duke University Medical Center; and
Neurodiagnostic Center
Veterans Administration Medical Center
Durham, North Carolina 27705

Samuel L. Bridgers, M.D.
Assistant Professor
Department of Neurology
Yale University School of Medicine
333 Cedar Street
New Haven, Connecticut 06510; and
Neurology Service
Veterans Administration Medical Center
West Haven, Connecticut 06516

Roger J. Broughton, M.D., Ph.D., F.R.C.P.(C)
Professor of Medicine and Neurology
Division of Neurology
University of Ottawa
Ottawa, Ontario K1H 816
Canada

Sandra L. Clenney, R.EEG. T.
EEG Product Manager (USA)
Oxford Medical, Inc.
11526 53rd St. North
Clearwater, Florida 33520

John S. Ebersole, M.D.
Associate Professor of Neurology
Director, Clinical Neurophysiology Laboratory
Yale University School of Medicine
333 Cedar Street
New Haven, Connecticut 06510; and
Chief, Clinical Neurophysiology
Neurology Service and Epilepsy Center
Veterans Administration Medical Center
West Haven, Connecticut 06516

Jack D. Edinger, Ph.D.
Staff Psychologist
Veterans Administration Medical Center
Durham, North Carolina 27710; and
Associate Clinical Professor of Psychiatry
Ambulatory Sleep Laboratory
Duke University Medical Center
Durham, North Carolina 27710

C. William Erwin, M.D.
Professor of Psychiatry
Ambulatory Sleep Laboratory
Duke University Medical Center
Durham, North Carolina 27710

Janet Eyre, D.Phil., MRCP.
First Assistant in Child Health
Department of Child Health
The Medical School
Framlington Place
Newcastle Upon Tyne NE2 4HH
England

Jean Gotman, Ph.D.
Montreal Neurological Institute; and
Department of Neurology and Neurosurgery
McGill University
3801 University Street
Montreal, Quebec H3A 2B4
Canada

Timothy J. Hoelscher, Ph.D.
Assistant Clinical Professor of Medical Psychology
Duke Sleep Disorders Center
Duke University Medical Center
Durham, North Carolina 27710

John R. Ives, B.Sc.
Director of Neuroelectronics
Department of Neurology
Beth Israel Hospital
Harvard University
330 Brookline Avenue
Boston, Massachusetts 02215

Marshall J. Keilson, M.D.
Associate Director
Division of Neurology
Maimonides Medical Center
4802 10th Avenue
Brooklyn, New York 11219

Robert F. Leroy, M.D.
Assistant Professor
Department of Neurology
University of Texas
Southwestern Medical Center at Dallas
5323 Harry Hines Blvd.
Dallas, Texas 75235

Jason P. Magrill
Neuro-Monitoring Inc.
55 Atlantic Avenue
Lynbrook, New York 11563

Gail R. Marsh, Ph.D.
Associate Professor of Medical Psychology
Department of Psychiatry
Duke University Medical Center
Durham, North Carolina 27710

W. Vaughn McCall, M.D.
Assistant Professor of Psychiatry
Ambulatory Sleep Laboratory
Duke University Medical Center
Durham, North Carolina 27710

Rodney A. Radtke, M.D.
Assistant Professor of Medicine (Neurology)
Duke Sleep Disorders Center
Duke University Medical Center
Durham, North Carolina 27710

Kalpana K. Rao, M.D.
Department of Neurology
University of Texas
Southwestern Medical Center at Dallas
5323 Harry Hines Blvd.
Dallas, Texas 75235

Moshe Reitman, R.PSG. T.
Director, University Sleep Center
Department of Medicine
New York Medical College
Valhalla, New York 10595

Marvin W. Sams, R.EEG. T., CRET
Bio-Scan Inc.
1717 S. Ervay St.
Dallas, Texas 75215

Donald L. Schomer, M.D.
Director, Laboratory of Clinical Neurophysiology
Department of Neurology
Beth Israel Hospital
Harvard University
330 Brookline Avenue
Boston, Massachusetts 02215

Gregory Stores, M.D., F.R.C.P., F.R.C.Psych.
Consultant in Neuropsychiatry and Clinical Lecturer
Department of Psychiatry
University of Oxford; and
Section of Child and Adolescent Psychiatry
Park Hospital for Children
Headington, Oxford OX3 7LQ
England

Barbara J. Voth, R.EEG. T.
Department of Neurology
University of Texas
Southwestern Medical Center at Dallas
5323 Harry Hines Blvd.
Dallas, Texas 75235

Ambulatory EEG Monitoring,
edited by John S. Ebersole.
Raven Press, Ltd., New York © 1989

1

Evolution of Ambulatory Cassette EEG

John R. Ives

Department of Neurology, Beth Israel Hospital, Harvard University,
Boston, Massachusetts 02215

The long-term ambulatory monitoring of an outpatient's EEG is a considerable technological challenge. It is compounded by several factors such as noise level, power consumptions, weight, and size. These are multiplied because of the desire to record from as many channels as possible. The simplest solution for this engineering problem is illustrated humorously in Fig. 1,[1] illustrating "our first attempt at ambulatory monitoring at the Montreal Neurological Institute (MNI) using conventional equipment." On a more serious note, it was in late 1973 that the first patient with epilepsy was sent home wearing a continuous 4-channel, 24-hr ambulatory EEG cassette recorder (1,2).

Recently, at Boston's Beth Israel Hospital, an outpatient with intractable epilepsy, who was under consideration for the surgical treatment of his problem, was sent home wearing a 24-channel event type ambulatory EEG cassette recorder. The recording incorporated a combination of surface and chronic sphenoidal electrodes, but more significantly, the patient also carried with him a small portable (6 lb, 5 × 7 × 10 in.) computer/hard disk EEG data-acquisition unit that was capable of automatically detecting and recording spikes, sharp waves, and electrographic seizures. The convenience and simplicity of this home monitoring unit are illustrated in Fig. 1 of Chapter 12 (*this volume*).

During the past 14 years, there has been a major evolution in the field of ambulatory EEG monitoring, which will be covered in this historical review. More important, the routine use of ambulatory EEG monitoring for the diagnosis of seizures and sleep disorders is leading to more appropriate treatment for those afflicted.

---

[1]The credit for this photo goes to the magic camera of Mr. Charles Hodge of the Photographic Department at the Montreal Neurological Institute.

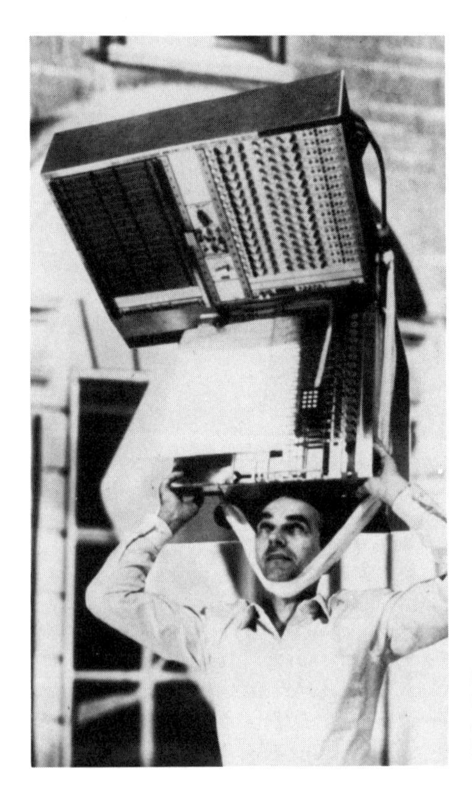

FIG. 1. The complexity and the engineering magnitude of the problem of performing outpatient ambulatory EEG monitoring can be seen in this tongue-in-cheek picture.

BASIC RATIONALE FOR AMBULATORY MONITORING

Long-term ambulatory monitoring of the EEG is an ideal means of investigating patients with epilepsy or those in whom a differential diagnosis includes epilepsy. This is exemplified in several recent publications (3–5). The main complaint of these patients (e.g., blackouts, smells, tastes, seizures), and thus the most important and significant symptom, comes from the actual ictal event experienced by them. Recording spontaneous events with as many channels as possible provides the physician with significant physiological information concerning the nature of the problem. These findings aid in the diagnosis of the event and, therefore, can contribute to a successful treatment program.

Routine, conventional EEG contributes to the documentation of the patient's normal background in a controlled state. Routine EEG, by the limited nature of its temporal sample, is not very successful in documenting ictal events, even when coupled with light sleep. In pre–long-term monitoring days at the MNI, a survey of a large group of patients with focal epileptic disorders under investigation for surgery revealed that fewer than 25% had a seizure while connected to a conventional EEG machine (3,6). Although detailed review was not done, it is reasonable to believe that some of the seizures were recorded with inappropriate montages designed for sleep, hyperventilation, or photic stimulation and, therefore, were not ideally designed for epileptic localization purposes. A significant number of the seizures were obliterated by movement artifact because of long leads (e.g., 25 ft between electrode and amplifier). Others were obscured by muscle artifact due to the open band width of 0.5 to 70 Hz that is routine during standard recording. A conservative estimate would be that fewer than 10% of the patients had a documented seizure that was technically intact and legible. As a result, the majority of patients prior to 1970 were diagnosed and had surgery recommended for their disorder based on interictal localization.

During the 1970s, there was an increase in the use of in-hospital long-term intensive EEG and video monitoring as outlined in a number of summary articles from various centers (7–14). With the development of video technology, the patient's clinical activity during the seizure could now also be captured. The in-hospital intensive monitoring units with 16-channel EEG or higher and simultaneous video/audio became the ideal way to document ictal events. This concept is very expensive and labor-intensive, thus limiting the number of such facilities and the number of patients that could be evaluated.

Ambulatory monitoring is not easily amenable to continuous video monitoring in the home environment (see Chapter 10, *this volume*). One can argue, however, that the EEG is the more essential element. If preliminary long-term EEG data have been obtained during ictal events, a more rational decision can be reached in terms of the necessity to investigate the patient further in a hospital-based intensive EEG/video recording unit. Having the ability to do either inpatient or outpatient monitoring in a given patient provides the best of both worlds. An initial outpatient examination provides preliminary data on which triage decisions can be based. The decision to bring the patient into the hospital for intensive EEG/video monitoring can be based on hard evidence and thus provide a higher yield of relevant diagnostic information. Another advantage of outpatient ambulatory monitoring is that it does not affect the occurrence of spontaneous seizures. The decreased frequency of spontaneous seizures is a frustrating phenomenon seen in a high percentage of epileptic patients when they are hospitalized (15).

Ambulatory outpatient monitoring is an extremely efficient procedure in terms of direct medical costs and use of limited resources and equipment and is more convenient for the patient.

CONTINUOUS VERSUS EVENT/INTERMITTENT RECORDING

There are two distinct concepts of ambulatory cassette recording systems. The methodologies for each have evolved along parallel but separate lines. The first concept is that of a continuous recorder, while the second is that of an intermittent or event/seizure recorder (noncontinuous).

Continuous Ambulatory Cassette Recording (16,17)

The continuous recorder had its beginnings in 1947 in the field of cardiology when Norman Holter demonstrated his single-channel radiotelemetry system, that was used to transmit the EKG and then also the EEG (18). Since a single channel of EEG is not very useful clinically, we had to wait until the early 70s for the technical development of a 4-channel cassette recorder. This technology was later expanded to 8 channels in the early 80s.

The continuous ambulatory recorder essentially is a temporal extension of the routine EEG. It is similar in concept to that type of intensive inpatient monitoring in which all EEG activity is recorded for later review. Complete review of a 24-hr EEG has been made feasible by newer technology that permits a fast video pagination of the EEG along with an auditory signal that is created by the high-speed replay of the EEG.

The main advantage is that the EEG is recorded continuously for the entire 24-hr period of monitoring. This is useful in generalized seizure disorders in which the patient has no aura and particularly in absence seizures in which clinical manifestations are minimal even to observers. Subclinical electrographic seizures during sleep can also be identified. In those patients who did not have an attack during monitoring, continuous EEG recording during sleep allows interictal transients to be detected routinely, which can help support a clinical diagnosis. This technique is also more appropriate for quantitating the number or duration of spike-wave paroxysms over a period of time, as might be useful in adjusting a drug regimen. The lesser number of EEG channels permits a more socially acceptable appearance for the patient. Patients may be willing to go about their normal activities at home, work, or school. In these situations, ambulatory monitoring has been shown to provide more realistic information (17). Beyond utility in epilepsy, continuous recording is necessary for most evaluations of sleep disorders, particularly if characterizing sleep stage architecture is important. Finally, the video and audio replay technology permits the relatively fast location and identification of relevant EEG wave forms and the rejection of artifact.

The main disadvantages of continuous ambulatory monitoring include the limited number of channels (4 or 8), which precludes detailed characterization of abnormalities, the need for experienced reviewers to extract relevant information during rapid playback of data, the necessity of reviewing all the data, and the expense.

Event Type Ambulatory Cassette Recording

In the early 70s, with the use of chronically placed depth electrodes at the MNI, it became obvious that weeks of continuous paper recording were unmanageable and overwhelming. In response to the situation, we created a 2-

min delay of the 16 channels of EEG by means of programming a digital computer with a large hard disk. We did this in order to have in computer memory the patient's EEG of the immediate past 2 min and thereby we hoped to capture the onset of a clinical event even after the fact. Over the past few years, as technology has advanced, equipment has been miniaturized to a point where an ambulatory recorder featuring 16 or 24 channels of EEG with a variable delay up to 2 min and periodic sleep sampling can now be worn home by a patient.

There are several advantages of a periodic/event system. These include greater number of channels for simultaneous recording and thus greater spatial resolution. Patient/observer selection of areas of greatest interest by pushing the event button when symptoms are experienced or observed means that less data must be reviewed. The expense is considerably less than for continuous recorders, and an accessory computer for the automatic detection of relevant electrographic events can augment the ambulatory study. Presently, the disadvantages of intermittent ambulatory recordings include the need for patient or independent-observer cooperation in pushing the event button and the fact that not all the EEG activity generated has been recorded.

MILESTONES: CONTINUOUS RECORDING

The beginnings of ambulatory EEG monitoring can be traced to some original work in the early 40s. At that time, the radio transmission of a single channel of EEG and EKG was demonstrated. Because cardiac monitoring needed only single-channel recording, this discovery led to the development of the "Holter" EKG monitors (18). The single-channel coverage precluded its use for EEG. It was not until the introduction of a 24-hr, 4-channel cardiac recorder that it was feasible to attempt EEG monitoring (19). The initial EEG systems were used by the British navy for sleep recordings on subjects in the Antarctic (Oxford Medical Systems, *personal communications*). The MNI purchased a recorder to test under more normal circumstances. With the addition of neck-mounted miniature EEG preamplifiers, a clinical ambulatory EEG system was developed (1,2).

The playback, recovery, analysis, and extraction of relevant EEG data from the 24-hr recorder evolved as technology allowed. Initially, the 24-hr tapes could be re-recorded and then replayed at a slower speed to permit the EEG to be transcribed through a conventional EEG machine (20).

A Mingograph ink-jet EEG machine at the MNI had a high frequency response of 700 Hz, which enabled the entire EEG to be written out in 24 min in a highly compressed fashion (e.g., 20 min per standard EEG page). Any electrographic ictal event could be identified relatively easily by its amplitude, which was significantly different when compared to baseline activity. This section could be selectively replayed at a more normal speed to permit traditional review of the EEG (3). At the same time, the EEG was "listened to," since electrographic discharges, background EEG, muscle artifact, etc., when replayed at high speed, seem to produce very distinct and identifiable sounds (3,17,21).

With the introduction of small individual preamplifiers that could be placed on the head (22), the commercialization of a 4-channel ambulatory EEG system by Oxford Medilog Inc. was realized. This soon became a readily available unit for use in the EEG field. Video display of the rapid pagination of 4-channel EEG led to a new era of more efficient 24-hr EEG analysis (23).

In the mid-80s, a continuous 8-channel ambulatory system was introduced. A number of new analysis features were incorporated, including digital real time on a separate ninth channel, automatic search capabilities to a specific time or to event marks, over a minute of memory so that the approximately 30 sec before or after the present video screen of EEG could be reviewed without tape movement, gain and filter adjustments on the screen without tape movement, continuous or epoch printout of EEG, and stereo audio output using any combination of channels. This new system also allows for the recording of other forms of polygraphic data, such as eye movement, muscle activity, cardiogram, and respiration, and has opened the way for investigation of sleep-related as well as epileptic problems.

The main disadvantage of the continuous forms of ambulatory EEG remains its limited channel coverage of 4 or 8. Several studies of ambulatory EEG montage design have demonstrated that, with careful selection of the montage, sufficient information can be obtained for diagnosis in most situations (16,17). This is not true for detailed characterization of the abnormality, particularly if surgical intervention is a consideration. Probably the main limitation of having only 4 or 8 channels of EEG recording is in distinguishing artifact from significant EEG activity. When questionable events are recorded with greater numbers of channels, the likelihood is greater that the experienced reader can distinguish between the two. If the past is predictive, technology will be developed that will permit an expansion of the continuous recorder to 16 channels, thus obviating its major disadvantages.

MILESTONES: EVENT/PERIODIC

With the introduction of a chronic depth-electrode investigation program at the MNI in 1972, the problem created by vast quantities of paper recordings quickly overwhelmed the system's capabilities. Obviously, some data-reduction technique was necessary. The EEG prerequisite in these patients with intractable epilepsy was to record the EEG during their habitual seizures. A cabled telemetry system was developed that allowed the patient to have some degree of freedom of movement during the monitoring session, which lasted, on average, 21 days. The cable telemetry permitted on-head amplification of EEG, which significantly reduced artifact due to long electrode leads. Since the signal was multiplexed, 16 channels of EEG could be transmitted by wire up to a DEC PDP-12 computer. A computer program was written (24) that allowed us to delay the EEG on the computer's hard disk by 2 min and thus store the entire event, if the patient's seizure push button was activated. The events were reviewed directly on a Tektronix screen and serially photographed for reading by the electroencephalographer. Thus, the era of data reduction began. Eventually, the loop was closed by including output software that reassembled the delayed EEG into the multiplexed format for transmission to another demultiplexing unit coupled with a Mingograph EEG machine. If a clinical event occurred, the activation of the seizure button caused the event to be stored permanently on the computer tape and activated the EEG machine to write out the 2 min of delayed EEG. Periodically, the EEG machine was timed to obtain samples of the EEG during the natural sleep of the patient (25).

This system proved not only essential for the diagnostic management of patients being investigated with long-term chronic depth electrodes but also proved to be reasonable for the investigation of patients with intractable epilepsy who had standard surface/sphenoidal electrodes and were being investigated as possible surgical candidates. In the late 70s, a new computer was purchased that was capable of monitoring two patients simultaneously. Even this capacity was soon overwhelmed by the demand for long-term monitoring.

As smaller microcomputers became available, along with larger and less expensive memory systems, a stand-alone system was developed that could be moved to the patient's bedside. This was the "F4-P4" unit (26). It consisted of an Intel 8085 computer with 1 Mbyte of RAM, an A/D-D/A input/output board, and a standard cassette tape deck for record storage. This unit emulated the larger computer in terms of delay and channel capacity. A time-code generator allowed independent video recording to be synchronized to the EEG (27). An EEG sample control unit automatically saved timed EEG samples.

In the early 80s, further electronic miniaturization enabled the functions of the F4-P4 to be placed in a completely ambulatory cassette recorder called the A1-A2 (28), which incorporated the existing technology of the Walkman audio cassette recorder to store the multiplexed EEG signals, as well as the time of day. Initially, technology issues, such as size, capacity, and power consumption limitations of static RAM, allowed only a 5-sec delay of the EEG. However, each year, electronic advancements in the field of SRAM memory circuits have allowed us to archive 2 or more min of delay on the present ambulatory unit.

With the increase in delay time, it was possible to increase the channel capacity from 16 to 24 (29). Thus, when used on a patient with sphenoidal electrodes (30–32), all major head regions could be covered simultaneously.

Once a seizure has been recorded, high-frequency muscle artifact is frequently present that can at times completely obscure the underlying EEG. Various filtering techniques have been developed in digital (33) and analog (34) formats. Recent technical developments in the field of charge-coupled capacitive filters have provided us with a simple and inexpensive means of replaying high-frequency muscle-contaminated events with a 6-pole filter that has variable frequency settings ranging from 9 to 70 Hz (35).

In order to aid the time-locking of EEG with video, computer, or observation, a "time-scribe" digital clock capable of both displaying replay time and writing it out in a readable fashion on the EEG paper was developed (36,37).

MILESTONES: AUTOMATIC EEG DETECTION AND THE AMBULATORY EEG

In the early 70s, it was demonstrated that temporal-lobe seizures recorded from patients with implanted depth electrodes could be automatically detected and recorded using analog filters and a digital computer (38). In the mid- to late 70s, the automatic detection of epileptic spikes and sharp waves was accomplished using a Digital Equipment Corporation PDP-12 computer (39,40). Later, using a more powerful computer (DEC PDP11/60), the simultaneous automatic detection of electrographic seizures was possible (41). Still later, it was also possible to detect automatically spike and wave activity (42).

With the introduction of the micro PDP 11/23 series of computers, dedicated spike and seizure detection systems for up to 16 channels of EEG could be mounted in the F4-P4 cart (7,26). This unit then became a total recording system that was portable but not ambulatory.

In the mid-80s, with continued technological advancements in the area of personal computers of the IBM PC type, the feasibility of having on-line detection software installed in a portable computer (Corona portable 286) was investigated (43). This system was developed and tested in highly selected patients. It was placed at the bedside for on-line monitoring during the night. It was capable of automatic identification and storage of morphologically significant events that occurred during the recording session.

After successfully demonstrating the feasibility of this concept, this rather heavy computer (>25 lb) was redesigned into a dedicated stand-alone unit, which we called the "ELB" (EEG Lunch Box) (44). It weighed about 6 lb and could accept 16 or 24 channels of EEG. It would store 3 hr of EEG data on its 40-Mbyte hard disk. When the patient returned the next day, the frequency, quality, and time histogram of the detections were assessed on a host computer system. The EEGs could be viewed on a computer screen before selective paper recordings of confirmed events were transcribed on the more standard paper format.

About the same time, an arrangement between the Telefactor Corporation and Dr. Gotman in transcribing the on-line detection software from the DEC/Fortran world to the IBM/C world was accomplished, which resulted in the "SzAC" on-line computer system for in-hospital use.

The next logical step has now been taken, and this software has been installed in the portable take-home computer "Micro SzAC," which can be taken home or used in the hospital environment by patients wearing a 16- or 24-channel ambulatory recorder.

Thus far, computer analysis of continuous EEG record obtained from ambulatory cassette recorders has been done off-line and has been limited to spike-wave paroxysms (3,42,45). Future technological advances likely will allow automated review of these records at rapid replay rates or will further shrink the size of an on-line system, so that it can be affixed to an ambulatory patient.

CLINICAL APPLICATION

The continuous 4- and 8-channel systems and the event/periodic 16- and 24-channel systems have been used extensively in various clinical settings as eloquently outlined by Ebersole (16,17). Their utility is being defined and expanded as the use of ambulatory monitoring matures. An example of this expanding role is the use of the 8-channel continuous system in polysomnography (46,47). The technological expansion from 4 to 8 channels did not necessarily mean that the 4-channel system was obsolete, however. In specific applications, it remains an ideal 24-hr monitoring system. Patients with spike and wave, absence-type discharges are evaluated quite adequately with this system when one wants to determine the number or length of discharges over a specific period of time before, after, or during treatment. The 8-channel system has advantages in some areas over the 4-channel system, particularly in the area of the differential diagnosis of epilepsy. With its increased coverage capacity, the 16- or 24-channel event-recording system would appear to have more applications in the area of the preliminary investigation of seizure disorders, particularly when surgery is being contemplated (see Chapter 12, *this volume*).

In our own situation, *all* long-term monitoring is performed with an ambulatory cassette system. The degree of freedom of the patient varies depending on the clinical applications. In the outpatient environment, the patient may be sent home wearing the 16- or 24-channel ambulatory recorder and also may be given the ELB to place at the bedside to be connected only through the night.

With a hospitalized patient, there are three options depending on the clinical situation. The first option is to have the patient wear just the 16- or 24-channel recorder and be restricted only by the usual nursing or medical orders. At the next level, we may have the patient plug himself into a telephone-type jack only on going to bed at night. This would be interconnected with either one or both of the video systems, if the clinical documentation of nocturnal seizures is required, or the ELB, for on-line detection of EEG morphology during the night. At the next restrictive level, the patient wearing the 16- or 24-channel event recorder is interconnected either to the video or to the video and the ELB all the time.

Other prolonged examinations incorporating the continuous monitoring of the EEG, such as Wada speech and memory tests, endarterectomies, etc., are also performed using a 16- or 24-channel cassette as a convenient source of high-quality multiplexed telemetered EEG that can be written out continuously on any EEG machine. In this situation, the tape-recording section may not be used unless an interesting event occurs.

SUMMARY

As ambulatory EEG technology has become more routine and clinically established, its applications are expanding and its integration into the clinical EEG departments has significantly improved the accuracy and efficiency of arriving at a diagnosis. In our institution, this has progressed to the point that we now perform about 30% of our total EEG activity using ambulatory monitoring.

It seems likely that eventually a system will evolve that will combine the best qualities of the continuous recorders and the event recorders. Ideally, this system would be capable of continuously recording from many channels of a variety of parameters and operate for at least 24 hr. There would also be automatic on-line EEG classification computer programs that would catalog the entire record as designed for a specific clinical situation. The entire 24-hr record would be available but automatically classified to a variety of levels of significance and relevance to permit reasonably fast review and turnaround.

REFERENCES

1. Ives JR, Woods JF. Four-channel 24-hour cassette recorder for long term EEG monitoring of ambulatory patients. *Electroencephalogr Clin Neurophysiol* 1975;39:88–92.
2. Ives JR. Electroencephalogram monitoring of ambulatory epileptic patients. *Postgrad Med J* 1976;52(suppl 7):86–91.
3. Ives JR, Woods JF. The contribution of ambulatory EEG to the management of epileptic patients. In: WA Littler, ed. *Clinical ambulatory monitoring,* London: Chapman and Hall, 1980;122–147.
4. Gotman J, Ives JR, Gloor P, eds. *Long-term monitoring in epilepsy* (EEG suppl 37). Amsterdam: Elsevier Science Publishers BV, Biomedical Division, 1985.
5. Gumnit RJ, ed. *Intensive neurodiagnostic monitoring, advances in neurology,* vol 46. New York: Raven Press, 1987.
6. Rasmussen T. Localization aspects of epileptic seizure phenomena. In: Thompson RA, Green JR, eds. *New perspectives in cerebral localization.* New York: Raven Press, 1982;177–203.
7. Gotman J, Ives JR, Gloor P, et al. Monitoring at the Montreal Neurological Institute. In: Gotman J, Ives JR, Gloor P, eds. *Long-term monitoring in epilepsy* (EEG suppl 37). Amsterdam: Elsevier Science Publishers BV, Biomedical Division, 1985;327–340.
8. Binnie CD, Aarts JHP, Van-Bentum-De Boer PTE, et al. Monitoring at the Instituut voor Epilepsiebestrijding Meer en Bosch. In: Gotman J, Ives JR, Gloor P, eds. *Long-term monitoring in epilepsy* (EEG suppl 37). Amsterdam: Elsevier Science Publishers BV, Biomedical Division, 1985;341–356.
9. Ebersole JS, Mattson RH, Williamson PD, et al. Monitoring at the West Haven VA/Yale University School of Medicine Epilepsy Center. In: Gotman J, Ives JR, Gloor P, eds. *Long-term monitoring in epilepsy* (EEG suppl 37). Amsterdam: Elsevier Science Publishers BV, Biomedical Division, 1985;357–370.

10. Egli M, O'Kane M, Mothersill I, et al. Monitoring at the Swiss Epilepsy Center. In: Gotman J, Ives JR, Gloor P, eds. *Long-term monitoring in epilepsy* (EEG suppl 37). Amsterdam: Elsevier Science Publishers BV, Biomedical Division, 1985;371–384.
11. Nuwer MR, Engel J Jr, Sutherling WW, et al. Monitoring at the University of California, Los Angeles. In: Gotman J, Ives JR, Gloor P, eds. *Long-term monitoring in epilepsy* (EEG suppl 37). Amsterdam: Elsevier Science Publishers BV, Biomedical Division, 1985;371–384.
12. Kellaway P, Frost JD Jr. Monitoring at the Baylor College of Medicine, Houston. In: Gotman J, Ives JR, Gloor P, eds. *Long-term monitoring in epilepsy* (EEG suppl 37). Amsterdam: Elsevier Science Publishers BV, Biomedical Division, 1985;403–414.
13. Sato S, Long RL, Porter RJ. Monitoring at the National Institute of Neurological Communicative Disorders and Stroke. In: Gotman J, Ives JR, Gloor P, eds. *Long-term monitoring in epilepsy* (EEG suppl 37). Amsterdam: Elsevier Science Publishers BV, Biomedical Division, 1985;415–422.
14. Roberts R, Fitch P. Monitoring at the National Hospital, Queen Square, London. In: Gotman J, Ives JR, Gloor P, eds. *Long-term monitoring in epilepsy* (EEG Suppl 37). Amsterdam: Elsevier Science Publishers BV, Biomedical Division, 1985;423–436.
15. Riley TL, Porter RJ, White BG, et al. The hospital experience and seizure control. *Neurology* (Cleveland) 1981;31:912–915.
16. Ebersole JS, Ambulatory cassette EEG. *J Clin Neurophysiol* 1985;2(4):397–418.
17. Ebersole JS, Bridgers SL. Ambulatory EEG monitoring. In: Pedley TA, Meldrum BS, eds. *Recent advances in epilepsy no. 3.* Edinburgh: Churchill Livingstone, 1986;111–135.
18. Holter NJ. New method for heart studies. *Science* 1961;134:1214–1220.
19. Marson GB, McKinnon JB. A miniature tape recorder for many applications. *Control Instrumentation* 1972;4:46–47.
20. Wilkinson RT, Mullaney D. Electroencephalogram recording of sleep in the home. *Postgrad Med J* 1987; 52(suppl 7):92–96.
21. Stalberg E. Experience with long-term telemetry in routine diagnostic work. In: Kellaway P, Petersen I, eds. *Quantitative analytic studies in epilepsy.* New York: Raven Press, 1976;269–278.
22. Quy RJ. A miniature preamplifier for ambulatory monitoring of the electroencephalogram. *J Physiol* (Lond) 1978;284:23–24.
23. Stores G, Hennion T, Quy RJ. EEG ambulatory monitoring system with visual playback display. In: Woods JA, Penry JK, eds. *Advances in epileptology,* The Xth Epilepsy International Symposium. New York: Raven Press, 1980;89–94.
24. Ives JR, Thompson CJ, Gloor P. Seizure monitoring: a new tool in electroencephalography. *Electroencephalogr Clin Neurophysiol* 1976;41:422–427.
25. Ives JR, Gloor P. Automatic nocturnal sleep sampling: a useful method in clinical electroencephalography. *Electroencephalogr Clin Neurophysiol* 1977;43:880–884.
26. Ives JR. "F4-P4": a self-contained mobile 16-channel EEG data acquisition system for recording seizures. *Electroencephalogr Clin Neurophysiol* 1982;54:37P.
27. Ives, JR, Gloor P. A long-term time-lapse video system to document the patient's spontaneous clinical seizures synchronized with the EEG. *Electroencephalogr Clin Neurophysiol* 1978;45:412–416 [short article].
28. Ives JR. A completely ambulatory 16-channel recording system. In: Stefan H, Burr W, eds. *Mobile long-term EEG monitoring.* Stuttgard: Gustav Fischer, 1982;205–217.
29. Ives JR, Schomer DL. Recent technical advances in long-term ambulatory outpatient monitoring. *Electroencephalogr Clin Neurophysiol* 1986;64:37P.
30. Ives JR, Gloor P. New sphenoidal electrode assembly to permit long-term monitoring of the patient's ictal or interictal EEG. *Electroencephalogr Clin Neurophysiol* 1977;46:575–580.
31. Ives JR, Gloor P. Update: chronic sphenoidal electrode. *Electroencephalogr Clin Neurophysiol* 1978;44:789–790.
32. Ives JR, Schomer DL. The significance of using chronic sphenoidal electrodes during the recording of spontaneous ictal events in patients suspected of having temporal lobe seizures. *Electroencephalogr Clin Neurophysiol* 1986;64:23P.
33. Gotman J, Ives JR, Gloor P. Frequency content of EEG and EMG at seizure onset: possibility of removal of EMG artifact by digital filtering. *Electroencephalogr Clin Neurophysiol* 1981;52:626–639.
34. Barlow JS. EMG artifact minimization during clinical EEG recordings by special analog filters. *Electroencephalogr Clin Neurophysiol* 1984;58:161–174.

35. Ives JR, Schomer DL. A 6-pole filter for improving the readability of muscle contaminated EEG. *Electroencephalogr Clin Neurophysiol* 1988; 69:486–490.
36. Ives JR. "Time-scribe": a universal time writer for any EEG/polygraph chart recorder. *Electroencephalogr Clin Neurophysiol* 1984;57:388–391.
37. Ives, JR. Recording the time of day. In: Gotman J, Ives JR, Gloor P, eds. *Long-term monitoring in epilepsy* (EEG suppl 37). Amsterdam: Elsevier Science Publishers BV, Biomedical Division, 1985;83–89.
38. Ives JR, Thompson CJ, Gloor P, et al. The on-line computer detection and recording of temporal lobe seizures from implanted depth electrodes via a radio telemetry link. *Electroencephalogr Clin Neurophysiol* 1974;37:205P.
39. Gotman J, Gloor P. Automatic recognition and quantification of interictal epileptic activity in the human scalp EEG. *Electroencephalogr Clin Neurophysiol* 1976;41:513–529.
40. Gotman J, Ives JR, Gloor P. Automatic recognition of interictal epileptic activity in prolonged EEG recordings. *Electroencephalogr Clin Neurophysiol* 1979;46:510–520.
41. Gotman J. Automatic recognition of epileptic seizures in the EEG. *Electroencephalogr Clin Neurophysiol* 1982;54:530–540.
42. Koffler D, Gotman J. Automatic detection of spike and wave bursts in ambulatory EEG recordings. *Electroencephalogr Clin Neurophysiol* 1985;61:165–180.
43. Ives JR, Schomer DL. Preliminary technical experience using a portable computer (PC-AT) for on-line data analysis of epileptic spike activity on 16 channels of telemetric EEG data. *Epilepsia* 1986;27(5):626.
44. Ives JR, Mainwaring NR, Gruber LJ, et al. Home computing: a remote intelligent EEG data acquisition unit for monitoring epileptic patients in the home environment. *Electroencephalogr Clin Neurophysiol* 1988;69:49P.
45. Quy RJ, Fitch P, Willison RG. High speed automatic analysis of EEG spike and wave activity using an analog detection and microcomputer plotting system. *Electroencephalogr Clin Neurophysiol* 1980;49:187–189.
46. Wilkinson RT, Mullaney D. Electroencephalogram recording of sleep in the home. *Postgrad Med J* 1976;52(7):92–96.
47. Hoelscher TJ, Erwin CW, Marsh GR, et al. Ambulatory sleep monitoring with the Oxford-Medilog 9000: technical acceptability, patient acceptance, and clinical indications. *Sleep* 1987;10:606–607.

Ambulatory EEG Monitoring,
edited by John S. Ebersole.
Raven Press, Ltd., New York © 1989

2

Recording and Playback Instrumentation for Ambulatory Monitoring

Marvin W. Sams

Bio-Scan Inc., Dallas, Texas 75229

Some 40 years ago, as brand-new 8-channel Grass Model IIIs were being delivered to the nation's largest hospitals, Holter and Generelli (1) were recording the EEG of a subject as he rode about on a bicycle. If it were not for the equipment weighing 80 lb and its having to be carried in a large pack on the patient's back, the history of clinical EEG might well have been dramatically different, that is, equipment for EEG testing would likely have been designed to record patients for long periods where their "spells" occurred—at home, at play, and in the workplace. Instead, the clinical EEG examination was, and continues to be, performed as the patient lies quietly in an unfamiliar, darkened room for a recording period that usually only lasts about 20 to 30 min.

Brief recording times and unfamiliar surroundings are less than optimal for several reasons. First, the chances of recording a spontaneous seizure or clinical event are remote because of their relatively rare occurrence, their distribution in the circadian cycle, and the patient's distance from the precipitating environment or circumstance. Second, the EEG is recorded in a strange and stressful environment. Third, brief EEGs run on different occasions cannot be reliably compared to determine if the patient is improving clinically. Long-term EEG recording, by comparison, minimizes these problems and allows more useful information to be collected.

LONG-TERM EEG RECORDING

The first practical long-term EEG recordings on active ambulatory patients were done with radiotelemetry (2,3). In 1971, for example, Porter, Wolf, and Penry reported on the ambulatory EEGs recorded from football players, pilots, astronauts, and epileptic patients. While radiotelemetry is still popular for inpatient monitoring, there are marked disadvantages to its use for outpatients, namely, the transmitting/receiving range of the data is short, and the necessary equipment must be set up and maintained in very specific, circumscribed ways. Additionally, the patient is confined to home or hospital ward or, if outdoors, to a carefully delineated space. In either case, it cannot be said that the patient is going about his or her "usual activities" when radiotelemetry is employed.

In contrast, ambulatory cassette recording allows multiparameter physiologic activity to be monitored over hours, days, or even weeks in the patient's usual environment. EEG activity can be recorded, for example, during all phases of the wake/sleep cycle, as a means to determine physiologic reactions to environmental conditions and to establish the efficacy of anticonvulsant and other types of medication.

HISTORY

In 1972, Marson and McKinnon (4) reported a portable, 1½ lb, 4-channel, industrial recorder that used analog recording technology and a standard C-type cassette tape. With improvements (5,6), the device became capable of recording high-voltage physiologic data and, with a C-120 tape, could record continuously for up to 24 hr.

When Ives and Woods began their work in 1975, the cassette recorder had been modified by Oxford Medical and was being sold for use as a "Holter" (long-term EKG) recorder. Played-back noise level with a shorted input was on the order of 50 μV/pp, which approximates the amplitude of normal background EEG activity. Therefore, only large EEG signals such as high-voltage, generalized spike-and-wave activity could be recorded for later identification. Ives and Woods' first task was to develop suitable preamplifiers to reduce the noise levels so that EEG could be recorded in the patient's everyday world.

The next major obstacle confronting early investigators was how to review quickly 24 hr of physiologic data. Ives and Woods' solution (7,8) was to use an Elema Schonander Mingograf ink-jet EEG instrument to print the data onto chart paper in a compressed form. With a high-frequency response of 700 Hz and the ability to print data at up to 600 mm/sec paper speed, 24 hr of EEG could be quickly played back at various speeds with reasonable fidelity. Replay at 20 or 60 times the recorded speed yielded an equivalent upper-frequency response of 35 Hz and 12 Hz, respectively. While spikes or sharp waves would not be apparent, high-voltage discharges such as 3/sec spike-and-wave easily stood out from background activity. The usual technique was to replay the tape at 60 times the recorded speed. The EEG was written onto chart paper in a compressed format at either 2 or 20 min of data per 30-cm page. Discharges of interest could be studied by printing out the activity at the more familiar paper-speed equivalent of 15 or 30 mm/sec.

Ambulatory EEG monitoring became a practical reality for clinical facilities in 1979 when Oxford Medical introduced a commercial system. The new technology addressed and satisfactorily resolved many of the recording and replay problems. The system included head-mounted EEG preamplifiers (HDX-82) (Fig. 1), the Medilog 4-channel, 24-hour cassette recorder (4-24) (Fig. 2), and an audiovisual playback system (PMD-12) (Fig. 3) (9). The playback unit represented a breakthrough in EEG analysis in that it presented video "pages" of the data with concomitant audio output. The pages are electronically "turned" to present the data at speeds 20 or 60 times real time, which are displayed on a CRT at the equivalent of 15 or 30 mm/sec paper speed. DelMar Avionics followed suit with a similar recording and playback system in 1981.

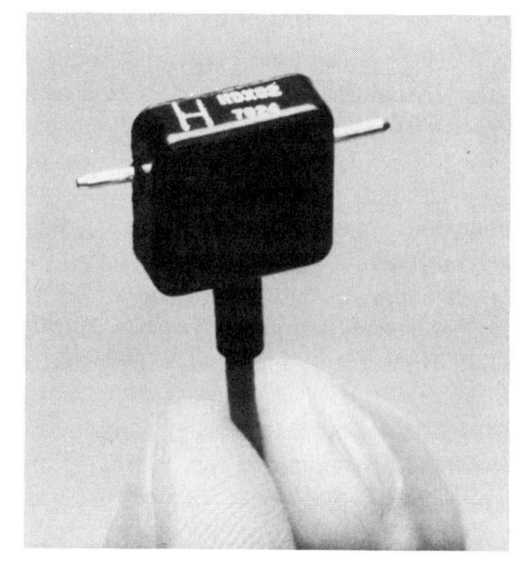

FIG. 1. The small size of the HDX-82 on-head EEG preamplifier chip is evident in this photo.

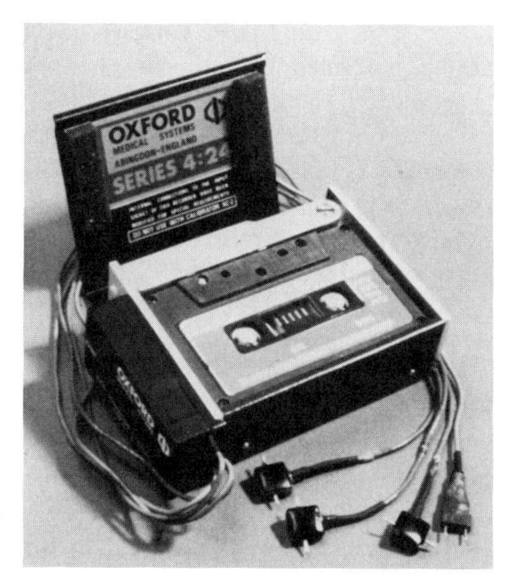

FIG. 2. The Oxford Medilog 4-24 pictured here was the first commercial ambulatory cassette EEG recorder.

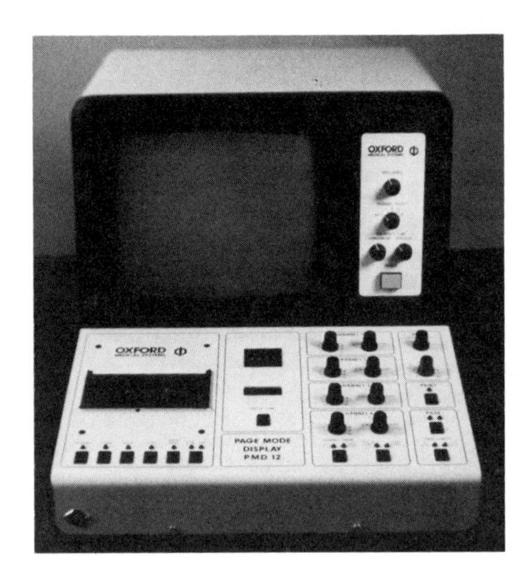

FIG. 3. The Oxford Medilog page mode display unit (PMD-12) was the first commercial device to provide rapid EEG replay in a video and audio format.

In 1982, Ives (10) introduced a 16-channel "epoch" or "event" recording system. The recorder was of the commercial Walkman type. A standard cassette tape speed of $1\frac{7}{8}$ in./sec is used, as the signal multiplexing rate of 200 samples/sec/channel necessitates a high-frequency response. Using a C-120 tape, 45 min of recording time is available. High-quality metal tapes are used to ensure maximum fidelity.

As the first version recorded only in response to someone pressing a button on the recorder, data were principally recorded in response to the patient or an observer responding to an aura or a spell. Therefore, the onset of a seizure was often missed. In a subsequent version, advances in computer-memory technology were employed to sample continuously the 2 min of background activity that preceded the button push. Onset in now recorded on all noted seizures. Data can also be collected by periodic sampling. For example, the recorder can be programmed to record 20-sec samples of EEG every 5 min. Data can be collected until the tape runs out or it is felt that an adequate sample has been obtained.

The EEG and time code from such epoch recorders are written out with a standard polygraph in real time. The polygraph's filter controls allow appropriate or desired sensitivity and high and low filtering of the data. A stand-alone, 6-pole, switched-capacitor, high-frequency filtering system is also available to help reduce muscle artifact.

Recently, a 24-channel epoch recorder using similar technology was introduced by Ives. The epileptiform discharges are stored on a 40-Mbyte hard disk, which has the capacity of 3.5 hr of EEG. The computer add-on is the size of a lunch box and is usually placed at the patient's bedside at night. (A detailed discussion of epoch recorders and their advantages and disadvantages relative to continuous recorders is provided in Chapters 1 and 12.) Optionally, a small, portable computer using detection programs to identify spikes and seizures can be added to monitor the ongoing EEG.

It took only a few years before the second generation of continuous-recording ambulatory monitoring systems were developed. The Oxford Medilog 9000 8-channel physiologic recorder and visual replay unit was offered commercially in 1983 (Figs. 4 and 5). In addition to the expanded number of channels, accomplished by a recording technology termed blocked analog (see Cassette Recorders, below), many features were able to be added. These are reviewed in detail in a later section in this chapter.

An 8-channel system using different technology was introduced by DelMar Avionics in 1984. Analog recording, as is used in the 4-channel system, was maintained, but in order to do so, a special ¼ in. cassette tape was used to accommodate the nine recording tracks. Many of the playback features of this system are similar to those of the Oxford Medical device. Since the number of DelMar units in clinical use is small, a detailed discussion is not provided.

Cadwell Laboratories' version appeared in 1988. This version also uses block analog technology (Fig. 6). The playback unit's features are similar to the Oxford Medical system. Two major differences are the use of a mouse instead of a keyboard control and of a separate video display unit for the system and filter controls.

PREAMPLIFIER SYSTEMS

The preamplifier pack developed by Ives and Woods is small (1 × 2 × 2 cm) and light (10 g); the pack is taped with waterproof adhesive to the patient's neck just below the collar. The gain is a factor of 20, which reduces the noise level to a

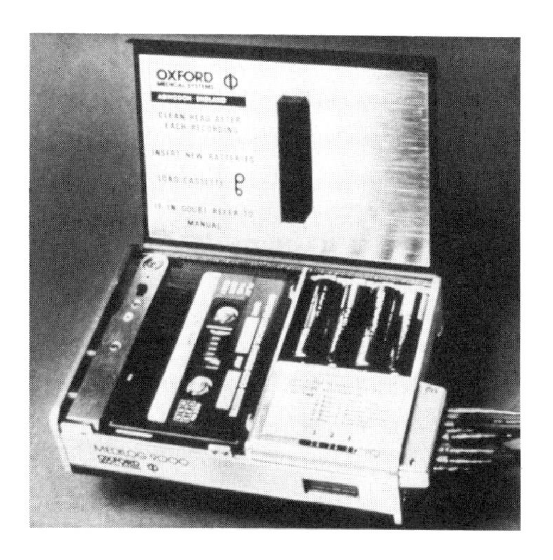

FIG. 4. The Oxford Medilog 9000 was the first commercial 8-channel ambulatory cassette EEG recorder.

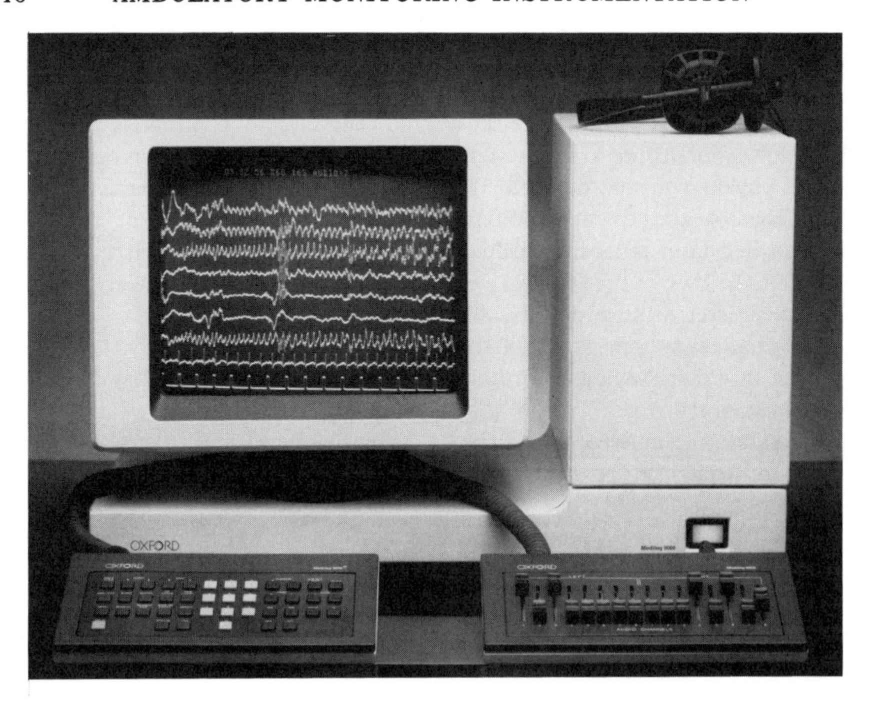

FIG. 5. The Oxford Medilog 9000 8-channel video-audio replay unit was the first of its kind.

possible 2 μV/ pp. The preamplifiers have a frequency band of 0.5 to 35.0 Hz (8).

Apple and Burgess' (11) approach to the preamplifier problem was to create electrodes with built-in 100:1 differential amplifiers. While it is apparent that these "active electrodes" perform superbly, the electrode/preamplifier unit is bulky, and it is impossible to hide underneath the hair. Turbans or stockings are usually put on the head to cover the assemblies. Patients, therefore, are not apt to go about their usual day-to-day activities.

In 1978, Quy (12) introduced a preamplifier that reduced artifacts significantly and was small enough to be hidden underneath most patients' hair. The preamplifier unit is constructed of a microchip encased in a small (13 × 13 × 6 mm) plastic case.[1] Each unit represents a single channel with its own two electrode inputs. After affixing the electrodes to the scalp, montages are created by connecting each pair of electrodes to the appropriate preamplifiers. Electrodes with bifurcated leads are necessary if bipolar montages of linked channel configuration are desired.

Quy reported that electrode and 60-cycle artifact are reduced with his system as compared with previously available EEG preamplifiers. He related the reduction in artifacts to the signal being amplified close to the electrodes. Quy's

[1]Oxford Medilog marketed the preamplifier under the trade name HDX-82.

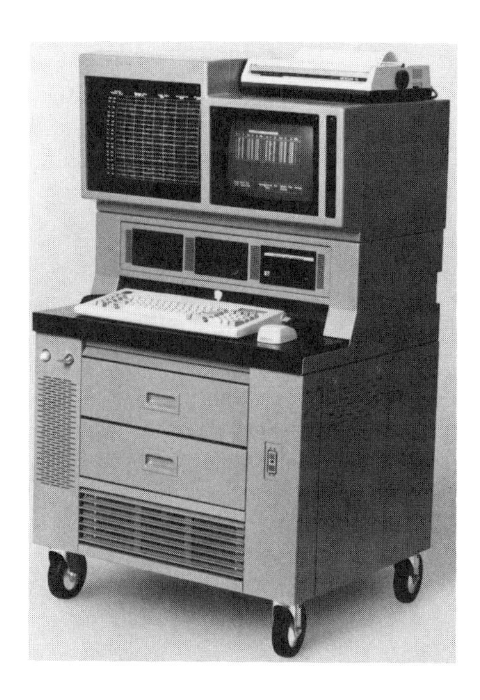

FIG. 6. The Spectrum 32 of Cadwell Laboratories can be modified to replay cassette EEG tapes that have been recorded in blocked-analog format.

preamplifiers used shorter electrode lead wires than the previous systems, on the order of 50 to 120 mm. Subsequent clinical evaluations revealed, however, that, for the desired reduction of artifact to be achieved, the Quy preamplifiers must be securely affixed to the scalp with collodion. Otherwise, patient movement will cause the preamplifier to move and produce its own artifact. If this happens, the recording will likely be rendered uninterpretable.

In 1983, Sams and Wasson introduced a preamplifier system[2] that combined the advantages of the off-head preamplification developed by Ives and Woods with the quality of recording available with the Quy and Burgess/Apple technique. The heart of this system is an anchor point on the cable about 1 in. from the electrode disk. As the electrodes are applied to the scalp, both the anchor point and the electrode disk are affixed to the skin with adhesive. The net effect is identical to having the electrode very close to the preamplifier, that is, electrode wire movement cannot rock or otherwise move the electrode disk. Artifact is dramatically reduced because the electrode-scalp interface is not disturbed, or only slightly so, when the patient moves.

With the Sams and Wasson Q.P. Preamplifier System,[3] a body harness with one pouch for 4 channels, or two pouches for 8 channels, is used (Fig. 7). After the electrodes are affixed to the scalp, the connectors are attached to the

---

[2] U.S. Patent No. 4,503,860.

[3] Available from Bio-Scan, Inc., Dallas, TX.

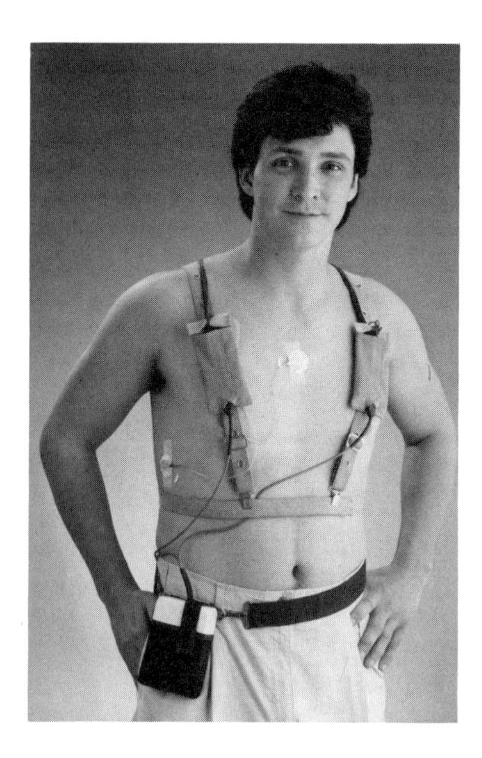

FIG. 7. The Q.P. Preamplifier System is worn from a body harness, as pictured here.

appropriate inputs on the preamplifier(s) (see Fig. 20 in Chapter 3). Once this is accomplished, the preamplifier units are placed in the pouches.

In 1986, Oxford Medical eliminated the HDX-82 on-head preamplifiers by releasing a recorder with built-in preamplifiers. The electrode input connectors are terminated into small plastic boxes, which are inserted into a neck collar; nine cables (eight for the recording electrodes, one for the ground electrode) then extend from the neck collar to the recorder (see Fig. 19 in Chapter 3).

Calibrator Unit

To keep recorders as small as possible, an external calibration system is used. A separate calibrator unit, which generates a 50- or 100- μV square wave pulse, is temporarily connected to the recorder. The calibration signal is recorded onto tape so that it can subsequently be played back to provide a standard of amplification. As on a clinical EEG instrument, the sensitivity of each channel must be checked and adjusted as necessary prior to processing data.

Interface Unit

After the patient is hooked up and the recording begun, the technical quality of the electrode application and recorder operation must be evaluated. To do this, an interface unit is connected between the cassette recorder and an EEG instrument. Ongoing physiologic activity can then be written out onto chart paper. Technical problems with the electrode application or the recorder amplification systems can be identified and corrected before the patient is released. If checking the integrity of the electronic components is desired, it is necessary to review the tape with a playback unit. (See Chapter 3 for details.)

CASSETTE RECORDERS

4-Channel

As previously described, an industrial 4-channel cassette recorder was the first to be used to record ambulatory EEG (7,8). Although available from other commercial sources, it was the Oxford Medical version with HDX-82 preamplifiers that made the recorder popular. The Oxford recorder is small, lightweight, and internally powered with four small Mercury cell batteries.

Cables from the HDX-82 preamplifiers (now discontinued) were attached to the recorder via a small box (CC-4) on its end. In the event of a broken preamplifier or cable, the unit can be detached, opened, and a new preamplifier installed.

8-Channel

When Oxford Medical offered their 9-channel (eight channels of physiologic data and one channel for time/event) system, it was considered a major advance in ambulatory technology. Attempting to record more than four tracks of data on a ⅛-in. cassette tape is difficult due to head-alignment difficulties and channel crosstalk.

Oxford's recording/playback system overcame this problem by using so-called block-analog technology, which permits the recording of up to three channels of data per tape track. In essence, analog data are collected from three channels in short segments, digitized, temporally compressed, combined in set sequence into one new segment, converted back to analog, and recorded on one tape track. With a 4-channel recording head, data channels 1 to 3 are recorded on the first track, channels 4 to 6 on the second, and channels 7 and 8 and time/event signal on the fourth. Channel 3 is reserved for a signal that the playback unit uses to synchronize the data on the other three tracks. A reverse-order transcription is used to replay the data.

The Oxford recorder uses a standard C-120 cassette tape and is powered by four AA alkaline batteries. Measuring 11.2 (W) × 4.05 (H) × 15.4 cm (L), the 8-channel recorder is not much larger than the 4-channel version with the CC-4 side unit attached.

The Bio/Scan Bio-log 8+1 8-channel recorder with Q.P. off-head preamplifiers and separate time/event channel was introduced in 1986 (Fig. 8). The device is powered by a single 9-v alkaline transistor battery. Since the recording technology is similar, its C-120 tapes can be reviewed on the Oxford 9000 8-channel playback unit. It is slightly smaller [8.9 (W) × 8.8 (H) × 13.3 cm (L)] and lighter (19.2 oz with battery) than the Oxford Medical unit.

AUDIO-VIDEO RAPID PLAYBACK SYSTEMS

Reviewing 20-min EEG recordings can be tedious; reviewing a 24-hr EEG on chart paper would be physically exhausting and emotionally draining. If 24 hr of standard EEG recording were printed at 30 mm/sec paper speed, approximately 8650 pages (8.6 boxes) of paper would be required; at 15 mm/sec, 4320 pages (4.3 boxes). Allowing only 3 sec per double page, data review at 30 mm/sec would take over 3½ hr.

Oxford Medical's answer to this problem was the rapid-playback unit. The 4- and 8-channel systems consist of a CRT display and a playback unit for the cassette deck, audio output, and control panel. The data displayed on the screen can be written onto chart paper by connecting a polygraph to the playback unit with a special coupler.

Features common to both 4- and 8- channel playback systems include:

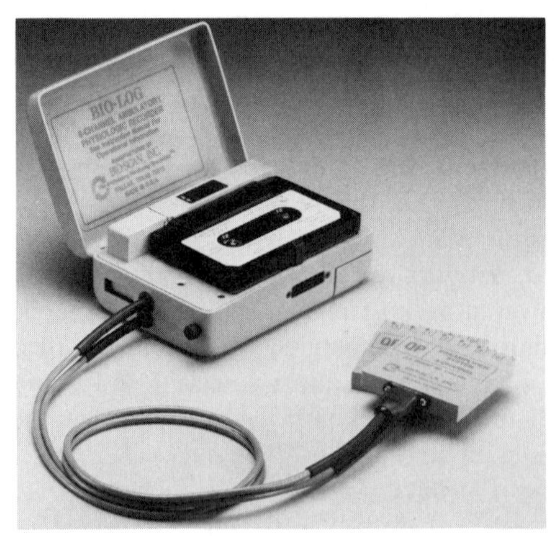

FIG. 8. The Bio-Scan Bio-log 8+1 8-channel ambulatory cassette EEG recorder.

8-Sec or 16-sec "pages"

The multiple channels of recorded data are displayed on the CRT screen in 8- or 16-sec pages. The 8-sec page is equivalent to 30 mm/sec paper speed; the 16-sec page, to 15 mm/sec paper speed. Experience has shown that epileptiform activity (such as spikes, sharp waves, and generalized spike and wave discharges) plus nonepileptiform activity (such as slow-wave activity and discharges) are all very recognizable in the compressed format. Some reviewers, though, prefer an 8-sec page when analyzing certain segments for detail.

Review speeds of ×20, ×40, and ×60

The data can be played back at 20 or 60 times the recorded speed; some units can also scan at ×40. At ×20, it takes 72 min to scan a 24-hr tape; at ×40, 48 min; and at ×60, 24 min. Most reviewers use the ×60 speed routinely for scanning, reserving the ×20 or ×40 speed to focus on interictal abnormalities or singular clinical events, such as electrographic seizures.

Sensitivity and low-frequency filter controls

The sensitivity (gain) of the displayed activity must be adjusted for each tape. On some scanner models, calibration adjustment is automatic, being done electronically. Low-frequency (time constant) controls allow accentuation or attenuation of slow activity. The setting values are similar to those on standard EEG instruments.

Recorded time and "stop on event"

4-Channel replay. If accurate time-and-event or stop on event is desired on a 4-channel recorder, one channel of physiologic data must be sacrificed in order to record a time code onto tape.

8-Channel replay. On the Oxford and Bio-Scan 8-channel recorders, a ninth channel is encoded with the time; it also notes and records any events signaled by the patient or observer pressing the event button. Time is displayed on the CRT screen, while the event signal triggers a tone or automatically stops the playback unit, depending on the reviewer's preference.

Scanner clock display

4-Channel. If the recorder is equipped with a time-code and event channel, the time is accurately portrayed on the control panel's digital clock. If a fourth channel of physiology is preferred, the time is still displayed, but it is an estimate based on the playback unit "counting" the turns of the capstan as the tape is played. Since frequently stopping and starting the playback unit can produce gross errors in the displayed time, the clock should be set at the end of the calibration period and the tape reviewed without stopping. The times of questionably abnormal or abnormal activity can be noted on a work sheet, which will allow the occurrence of certain activity and discharges to be pinpointed with only a few seconds' or minutes' error. If hourly or frequent data samples are being written out, about halfway through the tape rewind to the end of calibration. Reset the clock, fast-forward the tape to the desired time, and continue the printing process.

8-Channel. The time code is retrieved from the tape and continuously displayed on the CRT screen. The time and displayed data are synchronized to 1-sec accuracy.

Audio output

The combined audio and video presentation is essential for the maximum identification of specific waveforms. For this reason, all data, whether they be physiologic or artifact, are converted to an audio signal. Either an external speaker or headphones may be chosen to listen to the data. So that more than one channel can be listened to simultaneously, an audio mixer can be used to combine the sound from two or more channels. Each visual page is presented rapidly (at $\times 60$, a new page appears every 0.27 sec), so the audio is heard one page before the video is seen. In practice, the time difference often allows the reviewer to stop the video display on the page containing the event just heard.

Data output connector

The playback unit can be connected to an EEG instrument or other type polygraph so that the data on tape can be written onto chart paper. Representative samples of the data can be written for subsequent interpretation by the electroencephalographer and for record storage.

8-Channel playback system (Oxford) features

Scrolling display. An internal memory stores up to 64 sec of data, which can then be "scrolled" across the screen. The context and detail of prolonged runs of physiologic data such as seizures can be examined at leisure.

Channel invert control. If any channel's Input 1 and Input 2 are inadvertently reversed, the data can be inverted to correct the signal polarity.

Continuous print function. The control allows long periods of recorded data to be printed onto chart paper in real time. The feature is especially beneficial in writing out seizures or other long trains of activity.

Search feature. The reviewer can enter a specific time on the keyboard. The playback unit will then automatically search and find the desired time. Once found, the data recorded at the time specified will be presented on the CRT screen.

THE FUTURE

A major consideration in ambulatory monitoring is the reviewer's expertise (13,14). Only highly trained, experienced professionals, specifically physician-electroencephalographers and credentialed EEG technologists, are qualified to analyze ambulatory EEG tapes. Because of the extensive analysis and process time required, personnel whose time is valuable (and perhaps critical) to clinical situations, operations, or research are tied up for extensive periods. Computer analysis of the EEG, which would greatly aid in freeing up these professionals, is now available, but existing systems analyze in real time or no faster than 20 times real time. Because of the extensive amount of physiologic information, the time required to process the data makes computer interpretation too impractical. However, advances in computer technology will no doubt lead to the development of a semiautomated scanning/reading system. When the technology is developed, there will be a dramatic reduction in the amount of personnel time required to review and process tapes. Detection of spikes and other significant waveforms may also increase.

It is unlikely that ambulatory systems will continue with cassette-tape technology. Although the format is convenient, there are certain technical limitations. For example, the cassette-recorder size cannot be reduced beyond certain limits, there is always variability in the tape speed, and the number of recording channels is limited. Bubble memory or some other advanced microprocessor-based technology will likely supersede today's cassette systems.

A new recording technology will lead to 16 or more channels of continuously recorded data. While 16 channels may not be essential for the detection of epileptiform features in the EEG, such a system would be ideal for the characterization of ictal and interictal events and for multiparameter work. All-night complete polysomnographic recordings at home become possible, as well as the ability to record simultaneously many different tests on an individual patient.

REFERENCES

1. Holter NJ and Generelli JA. Remote recording of physiological data by radio. *Rocky Mtn Med J* 1949;46:747–750.
2. Ives JR, Thompson JJ, Gloor P, et al. Multichannel EEG telemetry-computer monitoring of epileptic patients. In Neukomn N, ed. *Biotelemetry II.* Basel: Karger, 1974:216–218.
3. Porter RJ, Wolf AA, Jr, Penry JK. Human electroencephalographic telemetry: a review of systems and their applications and new receiving system. *Am J EEG Technol* 1971;11:145–159.
4. Marson GB, McKinnon JB. A miniature recorder for many applications. *Control and Instrumention* 1972;46–47.
5. Cashman PMM, Stott FD. A semi-automatic system for the analysis of 24-hour EEG recordings from ambulatory subjects. *Biomed Eng* 1974;8–54.
6. McKinnon JB. A miniature 4-channel cassette recorder for physiologic and other variables. In: Neukomn N, ed. *Biotelemetry II* (Second international symposium, Davos, May 1974). Basel: Karger, 1974;67.
7. Ives JR, Woods JF. 4-Channel 24-hour cassette recorder for long-term EEG monitoring of

ambulatory patients. *Electroencephalogr Clin Neurophysiol* 1975;39:88–92.
8. Ives JR. Electroencephalogram monitoring of ambulatory epileptic patients. *Postgrad Med J* 1976;52 (suppl 7),86–91.
9. Stokes G. Ambulatory EEG monitoring in neuropsychiatric patients using the Oxford Medilog 4-24 recorder with visual play-back display. In: Stott FD, Raftery EB, Goulding L, eds. *ISAM 1979: Proceedings of the third international symposium on ambulatory monitoring.* London: Academic Press, 1980;399–406.
10. Ives JR. A completely ambulatory 16-channel cassette recording system. In: Stefan H, Burr W, eds. *Mobile long term EEG monitoring: proceedings of the MLE symposium,* Bonn, May 1982. New York: Fischer, 1982;205–217.
11. Apple HP, Burgess RC. An analysis of the use of active electrodes in electroencephalogram ambulatory monitoring. *Postgrad Med J* 1976;52(suppl 7),79–84.
12. Quy RJ. A miniature preamplifier for ambulatory monitoring of the E.E.G. *J Physiol* (Lond.),1978;284:23p–24p.
13. Ebersole JS, Bridgers SL, Silva EG. Differentiation of epileptiform abnormalities from normal transients and artifacts on ambulatory cassette EEG. *Am J EEG Technol* 1983;23:113–125.
14. Ebersole JS, Leroy RF. An evaluation of ambulatory, cassette EEG monitoring. II. Detection of interictal abnormalities. *Neurol (NY)* 1983;33:8–18.

Ambulatory EEG Monitoring,
edited by John S. Ebersole.
Raven Press, Ltd., New York © 1989

3

Techniques of Cassette EEG Recording

Sandra L. Clenney

Oxford Medical, Inc., Clearwater, Florida 34620

A successful ambulatory EEG (AEEG) is dependent on the skill and expertise of the EEG technologist. The application of stable low-impedance electrodes is critical to the success of the study. The information and instructions given to the patient will determine in large part how well he assists in obtaining a satisfactory test. Unlike standard tests done in the laboratory, the AEEG is usually obtained without supervision of allied health personnel. For this reason, every effort should be made during the hookup to assure that minimal problems occur once the patient leaves the laboratory. This chapter will be presented in a manner that assumes that the EEG or polysomnographic technologist has a thorough understanding and experience in basic electrophysiology. Its goal is to expand on those skills and apply them to AEEG.

SCHEDULING THE APPOINTMENT

There are several things the technologist or secretary can do at the time the patient is scheduled.

1. Ask the patients to wash their hair the night before the test. Hair should be dry and free of oils and hairspray.
2. Try to schedule patients for early-morning appointments. The patients will look their very best right after the electrodes have been applied. If they have clean hair, the electrodes can be better concealed and the patients will be more likely to go about their normal day's activities. If the patients are hooked up late in the afternoon and are expected to wear the recorder the next day after sleeping all night and not being able to comb their hair, they will be less willing to go to work or school. The electrodes will be more stable and have the lower impedance in the first few hours after the patient leaves the laboratory. Significantly fewer environmental artifacts are seen when impedances are not only low but balanced. As impedances start to rise, it will be closer to the patient's bedtime and environmental artifacts are less likely to

occur. If the laboratory does many studies, it may not be possible to do all hookups in the early morning. Occasionally, hooking up the patient in the afternoon is desirable, as with patients who are being evaluated for a possible sleep disorder. Since children often have bursts of paroxysmal EEG activity shortly after awakening, it may be beneficial to hook them up later in the day so an extended early-morning recording may be obtained the next day.

3. If the recording is to be obtained on a 4-channel ambulatory recorder, ask the patient to wear a watch. Accurately correlating time with the patient's symptoms and activities can be difficult, as 4-channel recorders do not have a built-in clock. A wristwatch at least ensures that the patient will always use the same timepiece rather than several clocks over the next 24 hr, all of which may be different.
4. Patients should be instructed to continue taking medications, unless their physician has specifically asked them to stop. The majority of AEEGs are obtained on outpatients; anticonvulsants should only be discontinued if the patient is hospitalized and under the observation of trained medical staff.
5. Ask the patient to wear a shirt or blouse that buttons. Not only will it be easier to attach the recorder and ECG electrodes to the patient, but the patient will be less likely to pull off electrodes or disturb the recorder when undressing for bed.

BEFORE THE PATIENT ARRIVES

Just before the patient arrives, lay out everything that is needed to do an AEEG. This will include those items listed in Table 1. Electrodes required for the montage for that particular patient should be laid out in the order they will be applied. They will usually include both single and bifurcated electrodes. The application of Collodion USP may be made easier by placing it in a small plastic bottle that has a hole in the top, a medicine bottle with dropper, or a 5-cc plastic syringe. Collodion may also be obtained in aluminum tubes with a special applicator top. Figure 1 shows supplies commonly used during a collodion hookup.

Inserting Batteries

Fresh batteries are required for each 24-hr study. If the study is to be performed over several days, new batteries must be used every day. Observe the correct polarity when inserting batteries. One or more reversed batteries will allow the recorder to record only a short period of time. Remove the batteries immediately after the test. Do not store the recorder with batteries in the battery bay.

TABLE 1. *Supplies needed for an AEEG hookup*

Tape measure and marking pencil	Two disposable ECG electrodes
Recorder	Collodion USP (nonflexible)
Calibrator	Acetone
Monitor box or interface unit	5-cc syringe with blunted needle
A C-120 cassette tape	Hair clips
Batteries	Low-salt conductive jel or cream
Electrodes needed for the montage	Air source (usually an airpump) with electrode applicator and foot pedal

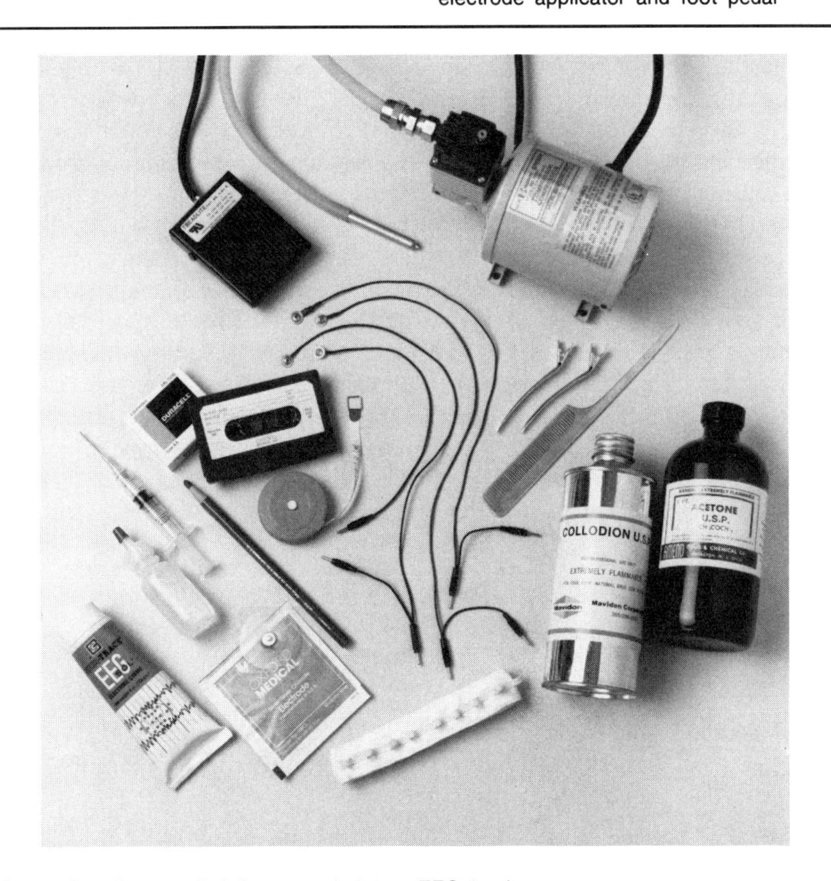

FIG. 1. Supplies needed for an ambulatory EEG hookup.

Preparing a Tape for Recording

A new C-120 cassette tape should be used for each AEEG recording. The manufacturer of the recorder should be consulted as to type and quality of tape that is required. In general, Maxell C-120 UD and Maxell C-120 Communicator Series are tapes that perform well. Since a tape may occasionally not transport properly, the technologist should fast-forward and rewind all new tapes in a conventional tape recorder or the scanner replay before using. All tapes should be labeled with the following information: patient's name, procedure number, date of study, recorder serial number, the montage, and the "start time" if using a 4-channel recorder.

Each cassette has a length of clear plastic at the beginning, which is called the leader. The leader should be advanced until the brown recording tape extends entirely across the cassette before placing the tape in the recorder. In this way, the calibration signal will go onto tape, not the leader. Hold the cassette in your left hand so that you are looking down on the cassette and the arrows on the leader are going toward you. The label, or "A" side, will face away from your hand. With your finger, turn the spool that is closest to you counterclockwise until the clear plastic is no longer seen and the tape is over the small brown pad in the center of the cassette. This is illustrated in Fig. 2. The tape is now ready to be inserted into the recorder.

Since both 4- and 8-channel recorders use all four tape tracks to record physiology, the tape is placed into the recorder with the A side up. Some tapes only have a label on the A side. After putting the tape in the recorder, take a moment to verify that the tape is in front of the capstan, and not behind it, or caught on top of it. Figure 3 shows correct placement of the tape. It is extremely important to do this before closing the arm that contains the recording head. Once the head arm is closed, it is impossible to tell if the tape is correctly inserted. The single most common cause for lost recordings is a tape correctly inserted. When this is done, the recorder may run sporadically for several hours before stopping. After verifying correct placement, close the head arm and turn on the recorder.

The Clock

If the correct time of day does not appear when the recorder is turned on, insert new clock batteries and follow the manufacturer's instructions for setting the clock.

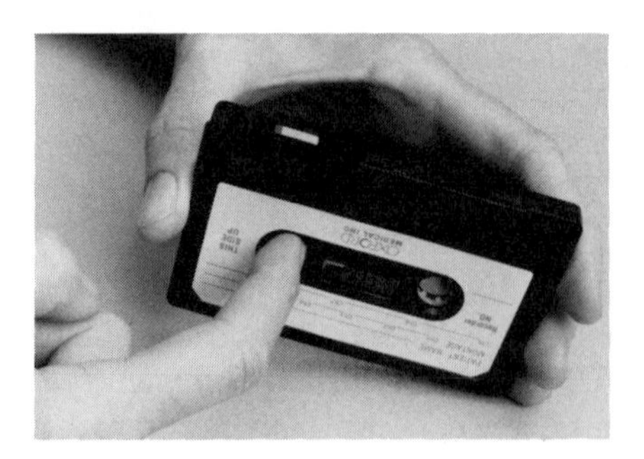

FIG. 2. Advancing the leader counterclockwise prior to placing the cassette in the recorder.

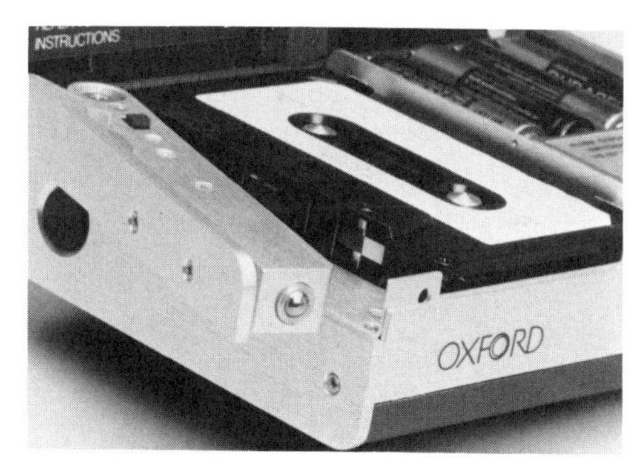

FIG. 3. The tape must be in front of the metal capstan before closing the recorder head arm.

Calibration

Calibration should be done just before or after the patient's scheduled arrival. As with standard EEG, it is important to calibrate immediately before the study to be sure the recorder is working properly at the time of use. The tape must also be calibrated in the recorder that will be used for the test. The recorder should be attached to the calibrator via the preamplifiers or channel connectors. Each preamp or channel connector has a mark that identifies Input 1. Match it with the dot by each channel of the calibrator that also identifies Input 1. Figures 4 and 5 illustrate methods of attachment. Calibrators provide several known voltages and morphologies. A 50- or 100- μV signal is commonly used, and a square wave provides a signal shape familiar to technologists and physicians. If a channel of ECG is to be recorded, attach the ECG snap leads to the posts on the calibrator that are labeled with a 1-mV voltage input. Correct polarity will be achieved if the red snap lead is attached to the "+" post and the black or white lead to the "−" post, as illustrated in Fig. 6. The red and black snap leads may be wired directly to the amplifier in the recorder or may be part of a special adaptor that allows the technologist to use a channel for either EEG or ECG.

Calibrate all channels for approximately 20 min. This ensures that the person scanning the tape will have adequate time to evaluate the recorded calibration signal.

Interfacing with an EEG Instrument or Polygraph

After the calibrator and recorder are connected and both have been turned on, they should be connected in turn to an EEG instrument or polygraph so the technologist can verify that all channels have been attached correctly and that each channel is working properly. The manufacturer will provide an interface unit or "monitor box" that allows the technologist to connect each channel of the recorder to a channel of the EEG machine. This interface can also be used when the recorder is attached to a patient instead of a calibrator. Figure 7 illustrates how the components are joined.

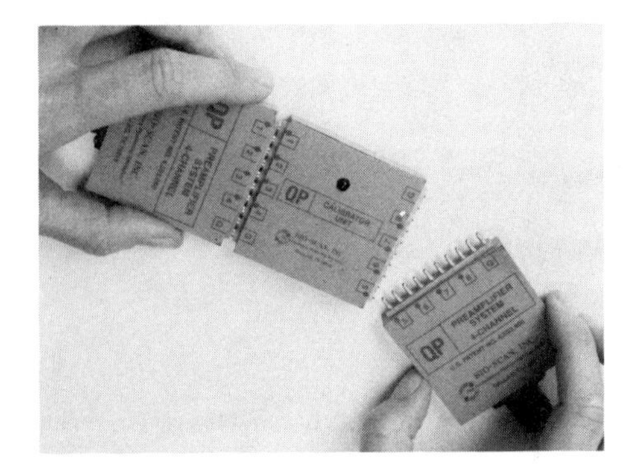

FIG. 4. QP preamplifiers being attached to the calibrator.

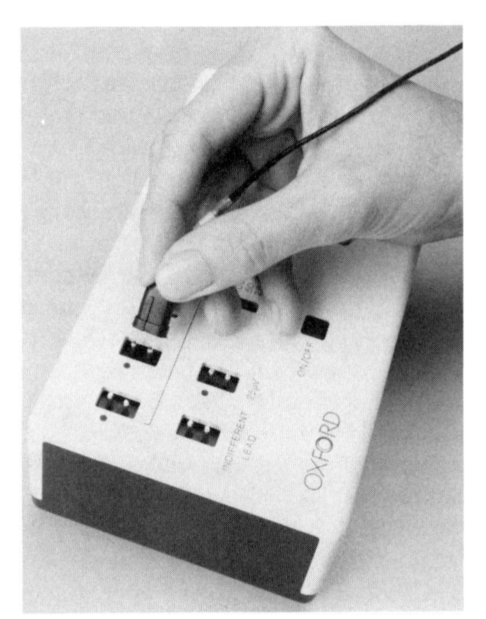

FIG. 5. Oxford Medilog channel connector being attached to the calibrator.

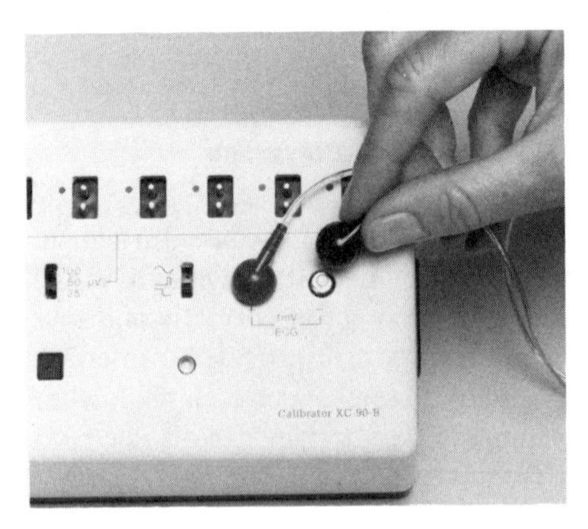

FIG. 6. ECG snap-leads are plugged into special posts in the calibrator.

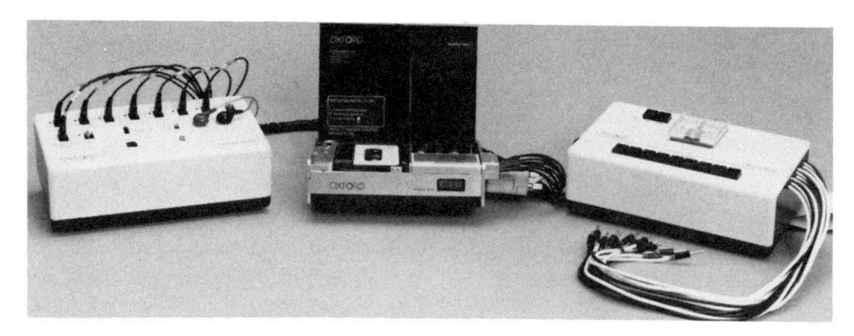

FIG. 7. A monitor box (*far right) is provided to interface the calibrator and recorder with an EEG instrument.*

The cables of the monitor box are numbered according to the AEEG channel each represents; each white cable carries the channel signal and the corresponding black cable is an indifferent to complete the circuit. They are plugged into the electrode terminator or jack box of the EEG in set combinations so that the AEEG channels can be easily derived at the channel selector or "overrides" of the EEG instrument. To avoid confusion, a standard pattern for connecting the black and white cable of each AEEG channel into the electrode jack box is suggested, such as the one illustrated in Table 2. Note in Fig. 8 that the black cables form rows of electrode positions that will be used as Input 1 for the various EEG channels and that the white cables form rows of electrode positions that will be used as Input 2. Different manufacturers may use other cable colors; therefore, check the operator's manual to see which is meant to be Input 1 and which Input 2.

After the cables are plugged into the electrode terminator box, the same combinations of electrode positions must be chosen in the same order on the selector panel of the EEG instrument in order for AEEG channels to be written out properly on the polygraph. This is illustrated in Fig. 9. For example, if black and white cables from AEEG channel #1 were plugged into jack box positions FP1 and FP2, respectively, then these same positions must be selected as Input 1 and Input 2 for the first channel on the EEG, etc. It is essential to understand that the AEEG montage is determined by the input to the recorder and not at the EEG instrument. The electrode positions chosen on the selector panel of the EEG bear no relation to the electrodes on the patient's head, which are used at the recorder to make the AEEG montage. The EEG instrument is being used only as a writer to show what is going on the tape. This will be the calibration signal now and eventually the EEG from the patient. Technologists using 4-channel recorders would only use channels 1 through 4 of the suggested interface combinations.

The preamplifiers in ambulatory recorders markedly increase the size of the EEG activity. Because of this, the signals must be reduced when printing data from the recorder or scanner. Table 3 gives the EEG instrument settings that

TABLE 2. *Suggested pattern to interface the ambulatory recorder with the EEG instrument*

Channel	Black (Input 1)	White (Input 2)
1	FP1	FP2
2	F3	F4
3	C3	C4
4	P3	P4
5	01	02
6	F7	F8
7	T3	T4
8	T5	T6

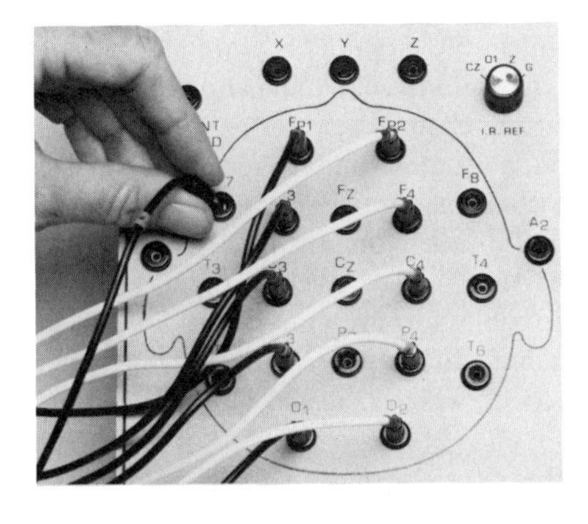

FIG. 8. Black and white cables are plugged into the EEG input box in set combinations.

will approximate certain sensitivities in the resultant AEEG write-out. The technologist should print out the calibration signal from the recorder and label the resultant hard copy as to sensitivity according to the pen deflection caused by the AEEG calibrator voltage. The sensitivity setting of the EEG instrument is not the same and should not be used.

The calibration signal seen on printout is taken from the recorder before it reaches the tape head. Interfacing with an EEG instrument verifies that all amplifiers are working but not that the tape has been correctly inserted. The technologist needs only to observe several pages of calibration. After trouble-shooting and correcting any problems, the technologist may turn off the EEG instrument and begin working with the patient while the tape finishes calibrating.

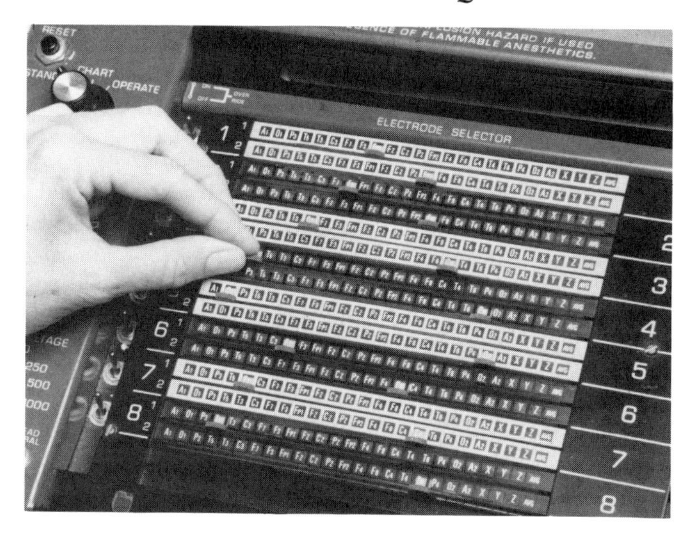

FIG. 9. The same combinations of electrode positions are chosen in the same order on the selector panel of the EEG.

TABLE 3. *EEG instrument settings for hard-copy printouts*

EEG Instrument individual sensitivity must be set on	To get a printout equivalent of
For 4-channel recorders and replays	
70 μV/mm	5 μV/mm
100 μV/mm	7 μV/mm
150 μV/mm	10 μV/mm
200 μV/mm	15 μV/mm
For 8-channel recorders and replays	
20 μV/mm	5 μV/mm
30 μV/mm	7 μV/mm
50 μV/mm	10 μV/mm
70 μV/mm	15 μV/mm
100 μV/mm	20 μV/mm

PREPARING THE PATIENT

Measuring the Head

Have the patient sit in a chair or lie on a bed. Measure his head according to the International 10-20 System of Electrode Placement. Not all of the standard electrode positions will be used, but the head should be measured to assure anatomically correct placement of the electrodes. Positioning the patient so his head can rest against the back of a chair or on a bed gives the technologist more control when applying the electrodes.

Applying the Electrodes

These instructions for electrode application assume that the technologist is right handed. Position the foot pedal of the airpump next to your right foot. Hold the airpump applicator in your right hand. Try to work without putting it down. Although awkward at first, putting on electrodes goes faster and more smoothly if the applicator is held continuously in the right hand. With fingers or a hair clip, part the patient's hair so that the mark for the first electrode position is exposed. Clip the hair up and away from the area where the electrode will be applied. This will keep the working area clear and the hair free of collodion.

Pick up the first electrode with the left hand and put it directly over the electrode position mark. With the right hand, insert the pointed end of the applicator into the hole of the electrode and apply enough pressure so that, when you remove your left hand from the electrode, it is held in the correct position. From this point on, the electrode is maintained in place by this means.

Pick up the collodion bottle or tube in your left hand. Position the opening of the collodion source very close to and directly over the electrode. Gently squeeze the bottle or tube until a generous amount of collodion is totally covering the electrode disk and shaft. These steps are illustrated in Fig. 10. When first learning collodion application, technologists are usually afraid to use "too much." You will quickly learn how much is enough and more problems arise from applying too little than too much collodion. When the collodion has been applied, set the bottle down and step on the air compressor foot pedal. Allow a steady and continuous flow of air to dry the collodion. Continue to apply steady pressure with the applicator, as this is the only way the electrode will remain tightly against the scalp until the collodion has dried. With your left hand, smooth the hair away from the area of the collodion. When the area around the electrode has dried, twist the applicator slightly to break the collodion seal that may have formed between the applicator and electrode. This will prevent the applicator from pulling the electrode away from the scalp.

To anchor the electrode further and apply strain relief, take several strands of hair and glue them down over the disk-wire junction. Place the applicator back in the hole of the electrode. This will prevent the additional liquid collodion that will be applied to the hair from loosening the electrode from the scalp. The applicator will be used to keep the electrode tight against the scalp while collodion that spreads to the electrode dries again. Pull the hair down over the junction and then hold it in place with the fourth finger of your right hand. Apply collodion over the hair from above, then set the bottle down. Apply a continuous stream of air while pressing the hair against the scalp and disk-wire junction with the fingers of your left hand to assure that the hair dries to the electrode wire as well as to the scalp above and below the wire. Figure 11 illustrates how a collodion-applied electrode may be stress-relieved with hair. Electrodes may be further stress-relieved by covering the wire with a small amount of hair at one or more additional points and gluing both to the scalp. This not only anchors the electrode wires more securely but also serves to camouflage them. You are now ready to apply the next electrode.

It is not necessary to cover the electrodes with gauze for most AEEG applications. If the patient is bald, however, or if a sleep study requires electrodes to be placed on the face or legs where there may be minimal hair to anchor the electrode, covering the electrodes with small gauze squares soaked in collodion is recommended. From 1-in. gauze rolls, squares are cut to a size that allows the electrode and shaft to be covered completely. These are then soaked in a small amount of Collodion USP poured into a shallow dish.

Place the electrode on the scalp with the left hand. Pick up the gauze square with the right hand, which is holding the electrode applicator, and place the soaked gauze square over the electrode and shaft. Hold the gauze square in place over the electrode with the left hand, and insert the electrode applicator through the gauze and into the hole of the electrode. Apply a steady stream of air using the left hand to press the gauze onto the scalp, smoothing it flat as it dries. When the gauze has dried to the scalp, stop the air flow and gently twist the applicator

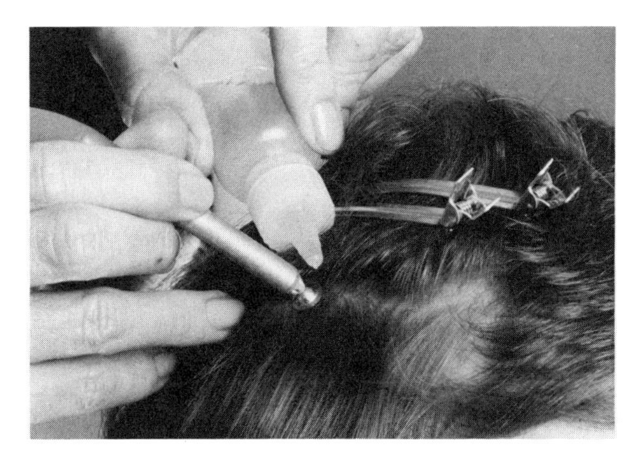

FIG. 10. An electrode is applied to the scalp using Collodion USP.

to break the seal between the electrode and the applicator. Figure 12 shows an electrode that has been applied with gauze.

Technologists who do hospitalized children or patients with severe behavioral problems find wrapping the head with Kling gauze an effective way of keeping the electrodes and wires out of the reach of the patients.

Single-ended electrodes are used when input to only one channel is needed. Bifurcated electrodes are used when the position is common to two channels. For example, in the montage starting Channel 1: T5-T3, Channel 2: T3-F7, the T5 and F7 electrodes would each use a disk with a single wire. One bifurcated electrode would be used for T3 and would plug into both Channels 1 and 2. Although commonly used with the 8-channel recorders, bifurcated electrodes are not recommended with 3- and 4-channel recordings. If one bifurcated electrode becomes unstable or falls off during the recording period, two (or one-half) of the available channels are no longer of value. Two single electrodes should be used for the patient ground. These electrodes may be placed anywhere

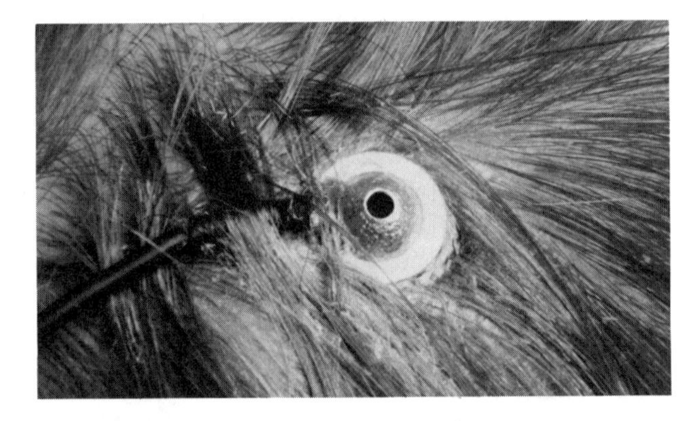

FIG. 11. A collodion-applied electrode is further anchored by gluing hair down to the electrode disk-wire junction.

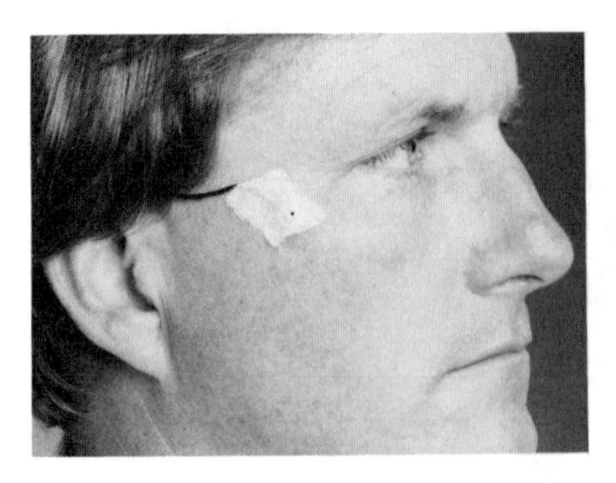

FIG. 12. Collodion-soaked gauze squares securely anchor electrodes to skin areas with no hair.

on the patient's head. Since the majority of AEEG montages do not use electrodes in the parietal regions, the area around P3, Pz, and P4 provides a site that is inconspicuous and protected from head movement during sleep.

When all electrodes have been applied, fill a 5-cc syringe with a low-salt conducting gel or cream. Attach a blunted needle to the syringe, and insert gel through the hole of each electrode, as shown in Fig. 13. The electrode is filled when a little gel comes out the hole. If any gel appears around the outer edges of the electrode, the disk has not been firmly applied and it must be reapplied with collodion. As each disk is filled, apply slight downward pressure to the syringe, and rock it back and forth, so that the blunted needle abraids the top layer of skin. This will reduce impedance under each electrode. Hold the index finger of your left hand against the electrode's disk-wire junction to stabilize it during the procedure. Scratching the very top layer of skin removes the surface coating of natural body oils, hairsprays, or creams. The skin itself should not be broken. The impedance of the applied electrodes should then be measured. Any impedance meter and most of those that are part of the electrode input box of new EEG instruments may be used to check the electrodes. Impedances must be verified prior to attaching the patient to the recorder, as it is not possible to do so afterward. Under no circumstances should a DC ohmmeter be used to check the applied electrodes. This will polarize the electrodes, which will attenuate the signal and produce artifacts during the recording. An ohmmeter may also deliver a small but painful current to the patient (1). Do not attach the patient to the recorder until all impedances are below 5000 ohms. With experience, technologists will find that impedances of 3000 ohms can be achieved routinely.

Many technologists use a skin preparation cream that is mildly abrasive prior to standard EEGs. Caution should be exercised in using such creams in AEEG, particularly when coupled with a conducting gel high in salt. Leeming et al. (2) report electrochemical burns with devices with voltages as low as 3 V DC, when they are applied over long periods of time. Over-vigorous use of a skin prep cream or the blunted needle will lower the impedance too much and can allow excessive current to form. Conducting creams rich in saline will break down by electrolysis as a result of this increased current flow and produce skin irritation or burns. This is seen most commonly under electrodes applied to the face and

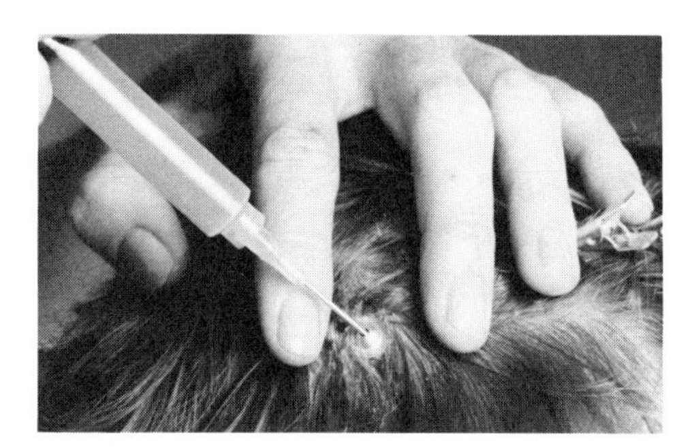

FIG. 13. A conductive cream is inserted with a blunted needle into each applied electrode.

in any patient with very sensitive skin. Use of conducting creams low in salt and conservative use of skin preparation creams will prevent skin irritations that have been reported with long-term cassette monitoring (3).

Hookup Techniques for 1-Channel ECG

ECG monitoring is a useful addition to AEEG. ECG may be recorded by dedicating one channel of the recorder with ECG leads that are hard-wired to the amplifier or by using special adaptor leads that plug into the input of any channel. This allows ECG to be recorded whenever needed on an EEG channel. Abnormalities of rate and rhythm are easily detected using the modified V5 electrode placement shown in Fig. 14.

Preparation of ECG Electrode Sites

Dry-shave the electrode sites. Prepare the skin with Omniprep or a similar skin abrasive. Wipe off the excess and allow the skin to dry. Attach disposable ECG electrodes to the patient lead wires. Applying a thin layer of Betadine solution or tincture of benzoin to the skin surface around the electrode site will help hold the electrode securely. This substance has a sticky quality and works well during hot, humid weather or on people who perspire heavily.

Placement of ECG Electrodes

The electrode attached to the positive, red snap-lead is placed on the fifth rib space on the left anterior axillary line. The electrode attached to the negative, black snap-lead is placed on the right first or second rib space at the

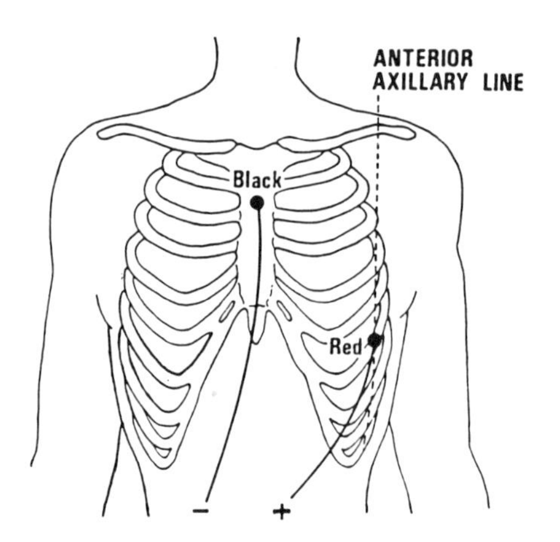

FIG. 14. A modified V5 electrode placement is recommended for 1-channel ECG monitoring.

midclavicular line. It may also be placed directly on the sternum at the level of the second rib. Since the color coding on some ECG cables may differ, always verify the positive and negative lead wires for each channel before attaching them to the patient.

Check the electrode impedance. Impedances must be 5000 ohms or lower. If they are higher, prepare the skin more aggressively and apply a new electrode. About 1 in. back from the electrode form a loop in the lead wire and attach that loop to the skin with nonallergenic tape, as shown in Fig. 15. This stress loop will prevent body movement from reaching the ECG electrode and producing artifact. Electrodes should not be placed over scar tissue, bone, large muscle areas, or directly under the breast.

ATTACHING THE PATIENT TO THE RECORDER

After the electrodes are applied, unplug the calibrator from the recorder. Leave the recorder on, and allow the patient to hold it in his lap. If he is not able to cooperate, place the recorder in a safe position close to his head or in a book bag that has been strapped to his back.

HDX-82 On-Head Preamplifiers

If the recorder uses on-head preamplifiers, plug the electrodes into the correct pins of the appropriate preamplifiers to make the desired montage. A dot on

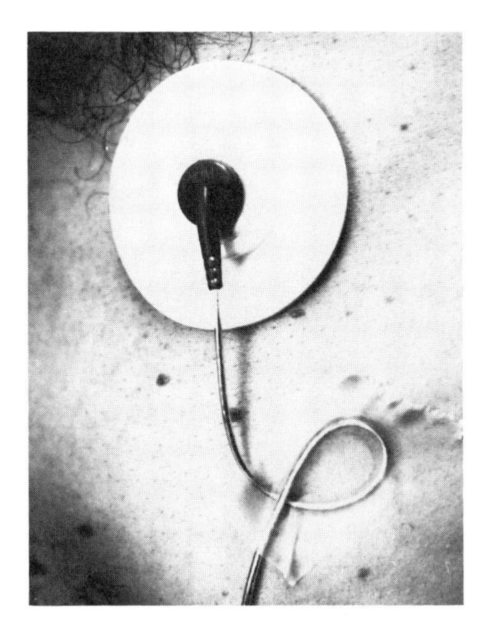

FIG. 15. ECG electrodes may be stress-relieved by looping the wire 5 cm back from the electrode and taping it to the skin.

each HDX indicates the Input 1 pin. After verifying the quality of the signal through an EEG instrument, the HDX should be anchored to the scalp with collodion. A small piece of hair should be glued down over the HDX or the electrode-pin junction to anchor the preamplifier further. Figures 16 and 17 illustrate these two steps.

QP Preamplifier Packs

If the recorder uses QP preamplifiers, they should be harnessed to the patient's chest as shown in Fig. 18. Since each pack contains four preamplifiers, one pack in used for a 4-channel recording and two packs for an 8-channel recording. Once the packs are securely anchored, the electrodes must be

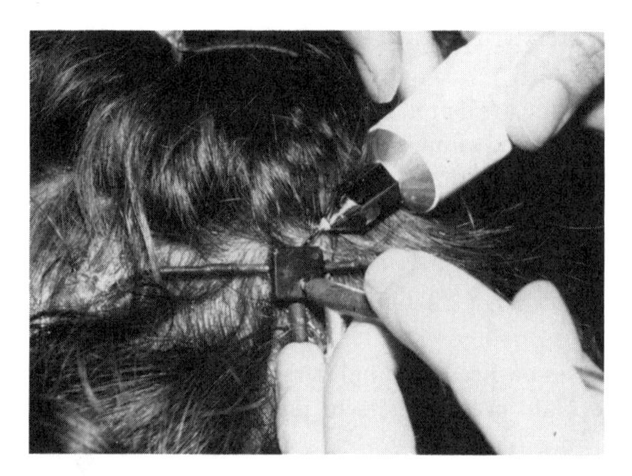

FIG. 16. The HDX-82 should be glued to the scalp after the patient pretest.

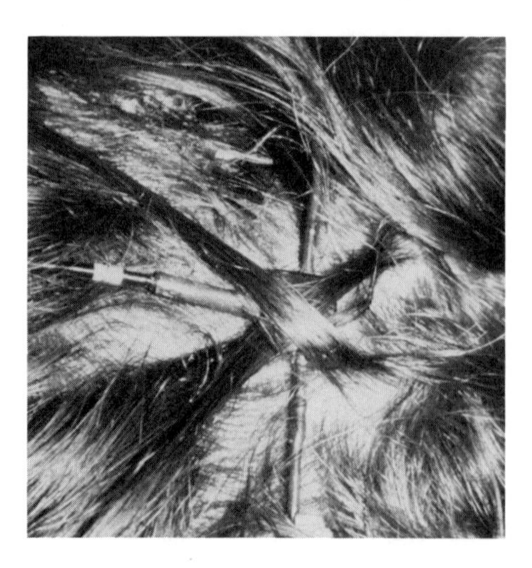

FIG. 17. Gluing hair down over the HDX-82 further anchors it to the scalp.

attached to the QP preamplifier connectors that conform to the desired montage. A dot indicates the Input 1 connector for each channel.

Amplifiers in the Recorder

If all four or eight amplifiers are housed inside the recorder, the channel input connectors should be inserted into the elastic loops of the Velcro collar. The electrodes may then by plugged into the appropriate connectors, as illustrated in Fig. 19. A raised line on each channel connector indicates the Input 1 position. Figure 20 summarizes the three methods of connecting electrodes to ambulatory EEG recorders.

ECG Monitoring

If ECG is to be recorded, the cable for that channel should be separated from the others, which are held together by a plastic spiral. Attach the red and black snap-leads to the disposable ECG electrodes and apply to the patient's chest.

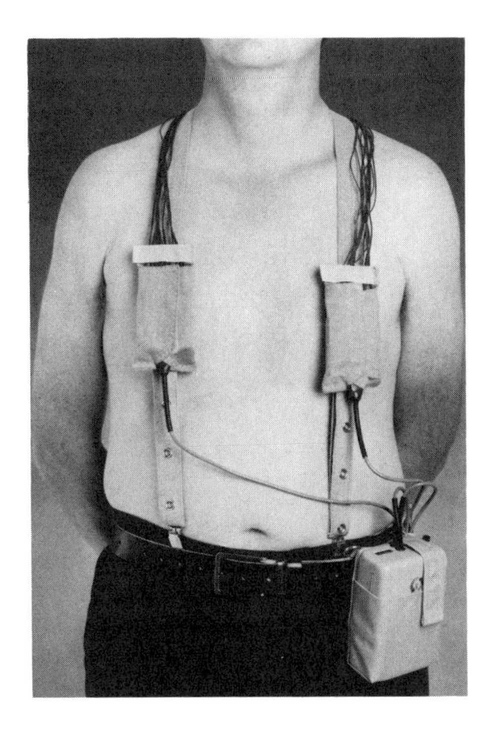

FIG. 18. QP preamplifiers are harnessed to the chest to provide stability.

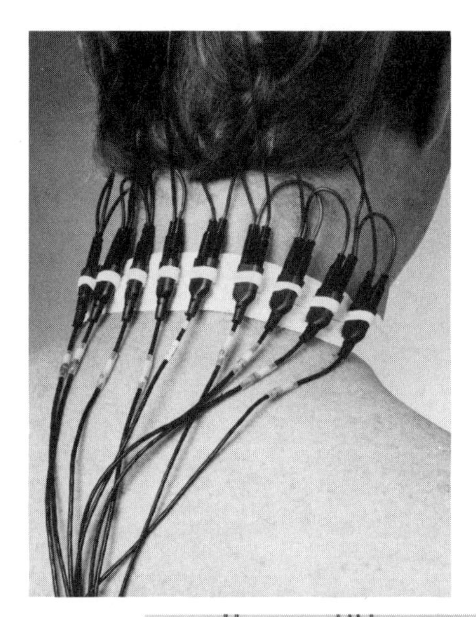

FIG. 19. Electrodes are plugged into each channel connector, which has been inserted through the loops of the Velcro collar.

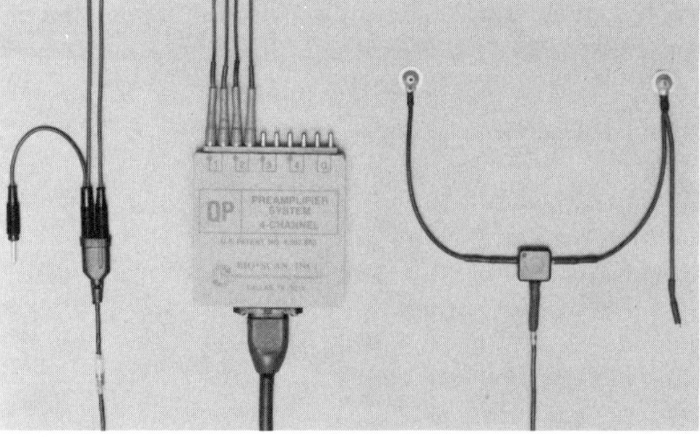

FIG. 20. Three methods of connecting electrodes to ambulatory EEG recorders are shown.

EMG Monitoring

If a sleep study requires one or more channels of leg EMG, cables for those channels should also be taken out of the plastic spiral before attaching to the electrodes.

THE PATIENT PRETEST

After the hookup is completed, the patient and recorder should be connected to an EEG instrument or polygraph to verify electrode stability and correct montage hookup. Use the interface unit in the same manner as when looking at the calibration signal. During a standard EEG, the EEG technologist goes to great lengths to relax the patient and to minimize both physiologic and external artifacts. During this pretest, however, the technologist must give the patient and electrodes every opportunity to display any problems so they may be corrected before the patient leaves the laboratory. Printing some of the many artifacts that will be seen over the next 24 hr, particularly during active wakefulness, will be helpful to the person analyzing the tape. During the pretest, the patient should be asked to open and close his eyes, look left and right, and swallow and chew, as illustrated in Fig. 21. The patient should also be asked to nod his head up and down and to vigorously shake it from left to right. Although movement artifacts will be generated with these various activities, the technologist should be watching for electrode artifacts that may also occur. These electrode "pops" indicate unstable electrodes that need to be changed, reapplied, or re-gelled. Each applied electrode should also be tapped in sequence during the pretest to make sure that it has been attached to the correct channel. The calibration printout and pretest should be given to the individual or scanning service who scans the tape. It is usually discarded after being scanned.

All problems must be corrected before the patient leaves the laboratory. Conditions that are marginal at the time of hookup and pretest will quickly deteriorate during the recording. When all problems have been identified and corrected, place a small drop of collodion over the hole of each electrode. Let it air-dry. This will help prevent the gel from drying out. Sending a syringe full of gel home with a spouse or parent and asking them to add more gel at bedtime is an alternative way of preventing the gel from drying out.

INSTRUCTIONS TO THE PATIENT

The majority of patients will have had a standard EEG prior to the ambulatory recording. Some will have also had a Holter ECG recording. The similarities with these two common tests should be drawn upon in helping the

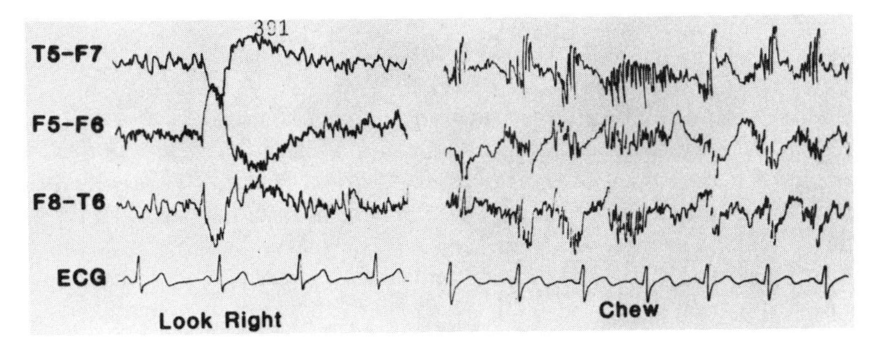

FIG. 21. The patient should be asked to perform various activities during the pretest.

patient understand the AEEG. Begin explaining to the patient early in the hookup procedure what the test involves and what is expected of him. In order to obtain the most positive results, he should be encouraged to go about his normal daily activities. There are very few limitations during the 24-hr recording and patients should be encouraged to go to work or school or to participate in most athletic activities. While patients should not engage in heavy contact sports like football during an AEEG, other activities such as jogging, bike riding, fishing, and bowling should be encouraged. Patients should be told not to chew gum or eat hard candy during the testing period, as this produces a continual artifact on tape that makes identifying true paroxysmal events difficult.

The patient must understand that under no circumstances should the recorder or recording electrodes get wet. The patient should be instructed not to wash his hair, take a shower, or go swimming. A bath should also be discouraged, as the recorder may fall off the closed toilet lid or off the edge of the bath tub. When recording infants, place the recorder in the crib above their head so it will not be damaged when they urinate.

The patient may wear the recorder on a belt or hanging from a shoulder strap. Many technologists prefer the belt, as it holds the recorder close to the body and does not interfere with movement of the patient's arms. The belt should not be in the pant loops but should be worn tightly around the waist like a holster, so that the patient may remove his pants without having to also hang onto the recorder. This will help ensure that the recorder does not fall into the toilet when the patient goes to the bathroom and also makes it easier to undress for bed. Inquisitive children and confused or demented patients should wear the recorder in book bags strapped like knapsacks to their backs. At night, patients may sleep with the recorder under the pillow.

There are very few patients who, because of their age or emotional status, should not have an AEEG. The EEG or sleep lab should always have the right to refuse a test if it is the judgment of the medical director or supervising technologist that the patient is an inappropriate candidate.

The Diary

The importance of keeping an accurate diary should also be stressed. The individual reviewing the recording would prefer to have too much information that can be easily edited rather than have important activities left out that the patient was unsure about entering. The technologist must be able to access the patient's willingness and ability to keep a useful diary. At the very least, the patient must use the event button and make a diary entry when he is symptomatic, as well as note in the diary when he eats and goes to bed. He should be encouraged to write as much as he wishes about his activities, as entries such as "riding in the car," "reading on my waterbed," and "scouring bathtub" will assist the interpreter in differentiating artifacts from cerebral activity. Patients being evaluated for a possible sleep disorder should clearly indicate their "lights out" and "lights on" times with both the event button and a diary entry.

Give the patient a pencil along with the diary, and help him make his first several entries (i.e., "11:05 looking at brain waves on EEG," "11:12 leaving lab"). Tell him to make an entry when he gets in the car or on the bus. If the patient does not have a pencil and makes no diary entries before leaving the lab, it is less likely that he will make use of the diary during the rest of the recording period.

WHEN THE PATIENT RETURNS

Ask the patient if he had any "spells" during the test. See if the spell is noted in the diary, and ask the patient the time of the spell if it is not noted. Then open the recorder and verify that the tape has transported to the take-up spool. Turn the recorder off; take the tape out and place it in the replay unit. Rewind the tape a short distance and play it to verify that all eight channels were recording. If one or more channels are flat, rewind the tape several more hours and check again. Keep rewinding the tape until it can be determined when the problem(s) began. At this time, a decision needs to be made whether there is enough information on tape to answer the clinical question or whether the study needs to be repeated.

Laboratories without a scanner should connect the patient and recorder to an EEG instrument or polygraph and print out a short sample to verify that all channels are working. If they are not, the technologist should troubleshoot the problem before doing another patient. In general, it is best not to repeat the study until the scanning service returns a technical report.

If the patient needs another study because he did not have a clinical spell, or because of technical problems that have been identified and corrected, insert fresh batteries and cassette, re-gel the electrodes, and check the impedances. Interface the patient and recorder with the EEG instrument and do another pretest before sending the patient home. If the test does not have to be repeated, unplug the electrodes from the recorder or preamplifiers. Remove the electrodes from the patient's head and body with cotton balls or gauze soaked in acetone. Using a comb and more acetone-soaked cotton balls, clean the patient's head. Acetone makes the collodion transparent when wet, but it dries quickly. Running a comb through the hair will soon identify areas needing more attention.

Once removed, the electrodes should be soaked in hot water and then gently brushed with a soft tooth brush to dislodge any residual gel or cream. After they are cleaned and dried, check the continuity of the electrode disk, wire, and plug ends with a DC ohmmeter or AC impedance meter as illustrated in Fig. 22.

Electrodes with erratic readings or readings of infinity should be discarded. Because electrodes cannot usually be changed during the study, it is imperative that you use only electrodes known to be good.

The tape recording head, capstan, and pinch roller should be cleaned with a Q-tip dipped in denatured alcohol. Oxide from the tape and dirt from the environment will build up on these parts of the recorder, which may prevent the tape from transporting correctly. Commercial head cleaners should not be used, since they can leave an oily residue on surfaces or may scratch the recording head.

QUICK GUIDE TO OBTAINING A 24-HR CASSETTE EEG RECORDING

Insert batteries in the battery bay of the recorder. Observe the correct polarity.

Prepare a new C-120 cassette tape for insertion by advancing the leader until tape is in front of the brown pad. Place tape in the recorder label side (A side) up. Make sure tape is in front of capstan before closing the head arm.

Turn on the recorder.

Verify that the clock updates to the correct time. If the time is incorrect, insert two fresh internal clock batteries and reset the time.

Attach the recorder to the calibrator. Observe the correct polarity. Turn the calibrator on.

Interface the calibrator and recorder with a polygraph or EEG instrument and verify that all recorder amplifiers are working. Troubleshoot and correct any problems.

Turn off EEG instrument and allow tape to calibrate for 20 min.

Measure the patient's head.

Use Collodion USP to apply all electrodes needed for the montage.

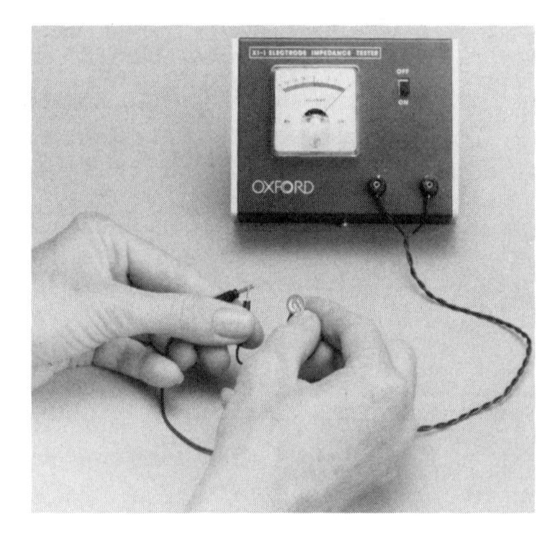

FIG. 22. An impedance meter or ohmmeter is used to verify electrode continuity.

Insert a low-salt conducting gel or cream through the hole of each electrode.
Abraid the skin gently with a blunted needle to lower skin impedance.
Check impedances of electrodes with an impedance meter. Re-abraid the skin under any electrodes with an impedance over 5000 ohms. Impedances of all applied scalp electrodes *must* be under 5000 ohms.
Use alcohol or a skin prep cream to prepare the chest for application of two ECG electrodes. Apply the ECG electrodes in a modified V5 electrode placement. Check the impedance of the applied ECG electrodes. Reprepare the skin if the impedance is above 5000 ohms.
Disconnect the calibrator from the recorder. Leave the recorder on.
Attach the electrodes on the patient's head and body to the recorder channel by channel, making the desired montage. Observe correct polarity.
Interface the patient and recorder with the EEG instrument. Write out at least 5 min of the patient's brain-wave activity. Ask him to blink, chew, and shake his head to help identify unstable electrodes. Tap each electrode to verify correct channel assignment. Troubleshoot and correct any problems.
Disconnect patient and recorder from EEG instrument. Put recorder in case and secure to patient's body. Fix patient's hair.
Give final instructions to the patient. Stress the use of the event button when patient is symptomatic and the importance of regular diary entries.

When the patient returns the next day

Verify that the majority of tape did transport during the test.
Take the tape out and replay selected portions in the scanner (or interface patient and recorder with the EEG instrument) to verify that all channels are working.
Turn recorder off. Unplug electrodes from recorder.
Remove electrodes from patient and clean his head.
Clean electrodes. Clean tape recorder head, capstan, and pinch roller with alcohol.
Check the electrodes with an impedance meter. Discard any that are unstable or read infinity.

If patient is to have a second 24-hr recording

Add more electrode gel and check impedances.
Reapply any unstable electrodes.
Insert a new cassette and four more fresh AA batteries.
Interface patient and recorder with the EEG instrument and record at least 5 min of physiology.

REFERENCES

1. Seaba P, Reilly EL, Peters F. Patient discomfort related to measurement of electrode resistance. *Am J EEG Technol* 1973;13:7–12.

2. Leeming MN, Ray C, Jr. Howland, WS. Low-voltage, direct current burns. *JAMA* 1970;214:1681–1684.
3. Sewitch DE, Kupfer DJ. A comparison of the Telediagnostic and Medilog systems for recording normal sleep in the home environment. *Psychophysiol* 1985;22:718–726.

Ambulatory EEG Monitoring,
edited by John S. Ebersole.
Raven Press, Ltd., New York © 1989

4

Montage Design for Cassette EEG

John S. Ebersole and Samuel L. Bridgers

Department of Neurology, Yale University School of Medicine, New Haven, Connecticut 06510; and Neurology Service, Veterans Administration Medical Center, West Haven, Connecticut 06516

Over the past 20 years, the evolution of laboratory EEG has been reflected principally by a progressive increase in the number of recording channels. Spatial resolution has thereby been enhanced, and fewer montages are needed to cover the head adequately. In the diagnosis of paroxysmal disorders, however, temporal sampling is as important or may in fact be more so. Ambulatory cassette EEG (AEEG) has evolved as a diagnostic test the greatest utility of which is in the evaluation of these disorders, epilepsy in particular. The question most often asked by physicians requesting AEEG is whether there are objective electrographic findings to support or refute a clinical diagnosis. Usually, this means the presence or absence of epileptiform features. For this task, AEEG is well suited, and, as will be discussed below, the limited number of EEG recording channels (three to eight) do not hamper its ability in diagnosis. Characterization of epileptiform abnormalities once identified is more a spatial function; hence, AEEG can be expected to do less well. Reliable differentiation between generalized and focal features and the ability to lateralize the latter are the most important data clinically. This AEEG can also do with proven accuracy. The success that has been met by AEEG in epilepsy evaluation has been dependent on recognizing where modifications in routine EEG protocol were necessary. Montage design has been a critical aspect of the development of cassette EEG as a practical clinical tool, at least for those systems with restricted numbers of channels, continuous recording, and rapid video/audio review capability.

For the cassette system that uses epoch recording, 16- or 24-channel reformattable montages, and examination of transcribed paper EEG, this is not the case. That approach allows presentation of EEG in conventional montages with full spatial representation, in accord with the recommendations of the American Electroencephalographic Society (1). The rationales behind those guidelines and the development of the 10-20 system of electrode placement are thoroughly discussed in several well-known reference works on clinical neurophysiology, and no unique problems arise in their application to ambulatory recording of this type. Consequently, this chapter will be devoted entirely to montage issues regarding continuous recording with rapid video/audio review, exemplified by the Oxford Medilog systems.

Since the spatial limitations of this approach to ambulatory EEG were in large part responsible for the initial resistance to acceptance within the community of electroencephalographers, it is important to understand the factual basis on which both the capabilities and the true limitations of cassette EEG montages have been defined. It is clear that our success in the application of cassette EEG has resulted from the attention we have devoted to montage development and testing. In this effort, we have attempted to remain mindful that we are working within limits, but with an optimistic eye toward what can be accomplished despite those limits.

From the outset, we have studied cassette EEG montages within a context of comparison to something better. This approach of comparison to a "gold standard" has been commonly employed in the evaluation of new medical technology. For EEG, at least where epilepsy evaluation is concerned, the gold standard is a well-established one—continuous long-term EEG monitoring in concert with video recording of behavior, under the supervision of trained personnel, in an inpatient epilepsy center (2). Our resource for comparative studies has been a unique one—the inpatient unit of the Epilepsy Center at the Veterans Administration Medical Center, West Haven, Connecticut. Under the direction of R. H. Mattson, M.D., the Epilepsy Center was one of the first to provide continuous EEG/video monitoring on a routine basis and had been doing so for more than a decade when the first comparative studies of cassette EEG montages were undertaken.

SPATIAL DISTRIBUTION OF EPILEPTIFORM ABNORMALITIES

Underlying the initial comparative studies was a presumption, based on clinical experience and logic, that epileptiform activity is not randomly distributed across the scalp. Corollary to this was an expectation that a limited number of channels, even three, could result in detection of a substantial percentage of abnormalities associated with epilepsy. In order to determine the extent to which a few electrode positions could serve, and to determine which positions would be most likely to be productive, a review of results of continuous EEG monitoring of epileptic patients in the Epilepsy Center over a 10-month period was undertaken (3).

It is standard practice in the Epilepsy Center to retain representative examples of epileptiform abnormalities on all patients monitored. These were reviewed on those patients monitored between January and October 1980. Analysis was performed of each epileptiform abnormality retained on each patient. Some patients had more than one spatially distinct abnormality, and thus contributed multiply to the analysis. The epileptiform abnormalities detected in these retained samples were characterized as to spatial distribution by region (anterior temporal, posterior temporal, frontal, and "posterior," encompassing central, parietal, and occipital) and laterality. Generalized epileptiform abnormalities were included as a separate category, together with bilaterally synchronous frontal or temporal discharges.

During the study period, monitoring was performed on 198 patients. Distinct epileptiform abnormalities totaled 139 and were found in the recordings of 115 patients. The proportional distribution of these abnormalities according to region is illustrated in Fig 1. It can be seen that one-third of abnormalities were generalized, more than a third were anterior temporal, and another quarter were in the frontal or posterior temporal regions. In all, 94% of the abnormalities might confidently be expected to appear clearly on a montage covering the frontotemporal areas, even if only three or four channels were used.

MONTAGE DESIGN PRINCIPLES

Montages for ambulatory cassette must fulfill two goals to be entirely successful. First and foremost, they must provide a spatial coverage that will maximize the likelihood of recording epileptiform features. Unlike laboratory EEGs, which use multiple montages to ensure complete coverage of brain activity from multiple perspectives, a single fixed montage is used throughout an ambulatory record. Electrodes must be placed where the yield will be greatest, realizing that certain head regions will necessarily go uncovered. Given the above results, frontotemporal electrode placements take priority over all others in general screening montages. Second, abnormalities once recorded need to be perceived by the reviewer in order to be of diagnostic help. Rapid playback of EEG on a video screen adds a new dimension of complexity to the interpretive process that is very different from traditional manual review of paper records. Montage design features that enhance the perception of epileptiform features presented in this fashion will greatly assist in the recognition of these abnormalities.

Generalized or bilateral EEG discharges, either ictal or interictal, pose little problem even for montages of limited coverage. Focal seizures usually evoke EEG changes over a large portion of one hemisphere, if not both hemispheres, even if the onset is localized. Furthermore, as will be reviewed in Chapter 5, detection of seizures, whether generalized or partial, is achieved for the most part by recognizing the unique sounds of the ictal patterns on audio review. As long as there is coverage of both hemispheres, most seizures can be identified in this manner. Seizure detection per se does not place great demands on a montage. Characterization of the seizure, on the other hand, is a function of visual inspection, which clearly benefits from a well-designed montage. It is,

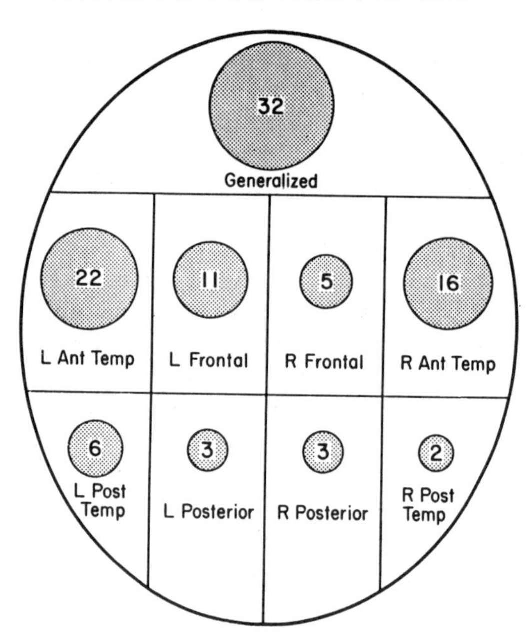

FIG. 1. Scalp distribution of epileptiform abnormalities. Numbers indicate percentages of the total of 139 morphologically distinct epileptiform abnormalities identified in each area on review of EEG records of 115 Epilepsy Unit patients with epileptiform abnormalities. Note frontal and temporal preponderance.

however, the identification of focal abnormalities, in particular focal interictal transients, that will be the most difficult. The field of these discharges may be limited to one region. Statistically, in adults and adolescents, this area will most likely be frontotemporal. It would thus seem worthwhile to direct special attention to montage designs that would routinely provide detection and allow perception of the common frontotemporal abnormalities of the partial epilepsies.

Many of the basic rules for formulating laboratory EEG montages are applicable to cassette EEG with modifications that take into account special requirements associated with rapid video replay, need for one or more channels for audio monitoring, artifacts during most of the waking record, and multiple changes in level of consciousness. Since artifacts are a pervasive problem with AEEGs recorded during active wakefulness and since focal epileptiform features present the greatest challenge to identification, bipolar channel derivations that reduce the former and emphasize the latter would seem a logical choice. Similarly, as in traditional montage designs, it would seem unwise to end a chain of bipolar channels in a location that is likely to be the field maxima for many of the abnormalities sought. Doing so will sacrifice the appearance of phase-reversals, which make transients easier to recognize on a static page and most certainly with rapid video pagination.

THREE-CHANNEL MONTAGE TESTING

A number of 3-channel montages were designed and tested by comparison to simultaneous standard recording (4), based on the results of the above investigation. Although the Oxford 4-24 cassette recorder featured four recording channels, it was presumed that one channel would be needed for non-EEG data, such as electrocardiographic monitoring. We felt that a limitation to two EEG channels would be impractical, since this would allow only a single channel per hemisphere. Such an approach would eliminate any possibility for focal discharges to produce phase-reversing waveforms, as discussed above. Others who did attempt 2-channel EEG monitoring encountered a high percentage of uninterpretable recordings (5).

Montage testing was performed on a group of patients in the Epilepsy Center, chosen because of the abnormalities present on their standard monitoring records. Each test recording was continued for at least 4 hr, and included one or two test montages and an 8-channel reference montage. Appearance of epileptiform abnormalities on the test montages was graded as equal to the reference montage appearance, less clear but still identifiable, or unidentifiable. The total number of identifiable epileptiform abnormalities was tabulated for each montage in each scalp region.

Twenty-three patients with more than a thousand examples of 33 distinct epileptiform abnormalities were studied with five 3-channel montages. The distribution of abnormalities was similar to that found in the study described above. A circumferential frontotemporal montage (1. T5-F7, 2. F7-F8, 3. F8-T6) provided the best overall detection rate, with 92% of generalized and 80% of frontotemporal abnormalities detected. A montage that substituted parasagittal longitudinal channels for the temporal longitudinal channels improved detection of generalized abnormalities to 100%, but at the cost of missing an additional 12% of the more common temporal abnormalities. This investigation was concerned with side-by-side comparison of individual complexes. As such, it underestimated the capability of the 3-channel montages when actually applied to cassette EEG recording, where the crucial issue would be recognition of the epileptiform nature of the recording as a whole, rather than sure identification of every single complex.

Once the 3-channel montages for recording had been proven on paper, they were tested on tape, first by a similar approach of comparison of individual complexes (4) and then by blinded review of entire tapes (6,7). Throughout, the 3-channel montage with frontotemporal coverage held up well. In the transition from experimental inpatient to clinical outpatient cassette recording, the transverse channel of the montage was modified from F7-F8 to F5-F6 in order to separate the longitudinal channels from the transverse channel for clearer identification of electrode artifacts and to provide a greater safety margin against channel loss. This montage is illustrated in Fig. 2. In the 3-channel montage with true linkage, the F7 or F8 electrode serviced two channels. Loss of or artifact in either would obscure two-thirds of the data.

Subsequently, 3-channel recording served us well through several years of clinical use, although we have now all but abandoned it in favor of 8-channel recording, with between five and all eight channels devoted to EEG. Nevertheless, we have learned of occasional failures of the montage, which was never expected to be perfect. We had anticipated that a particularly troublesome area would be in the detection of Rolandic discharges in children, with no central coverage and a risk of cancellation of midtemporal discharges on the longitudinal channels. However, we have accumulated a number of examples of such patterns, documented by standard EEG, that were readily detected on the 3-channel montage.

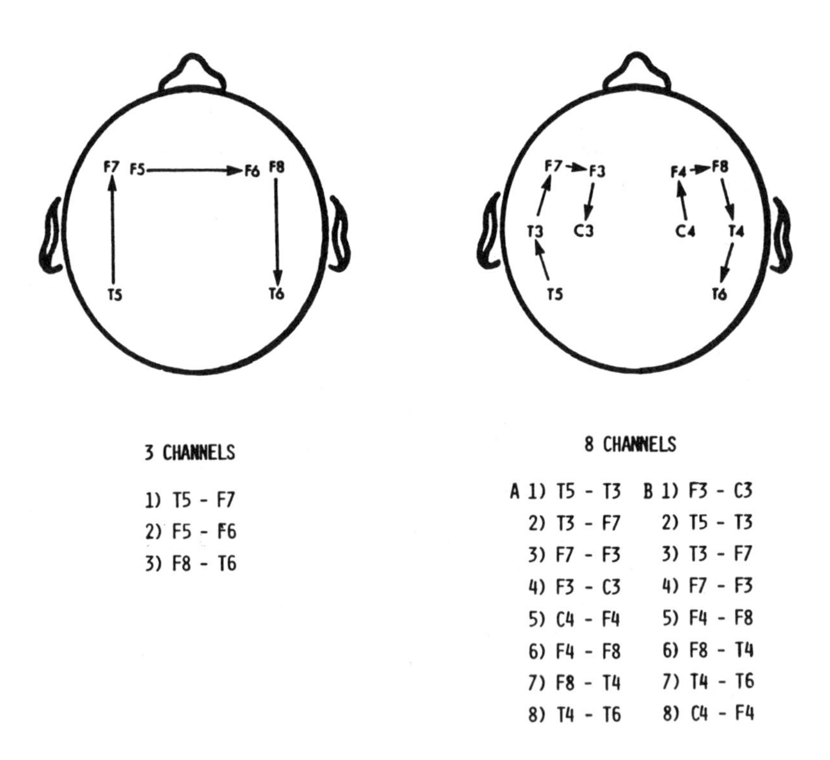

FIG. 2. Three- and 8-channel montages. Our standard 3-channel, circumferential, "unlinked chain" montage is illustrated at *left,* and our standard electrode placement for 8-channel recording is shown at *right.* For the latter, there are two reasonable options for channel ordering. We favor option **B,** which puts the less-productive frontocentral channels at the periphery.

MONTAGE DESIGN CONSIDERATIONS—EIGHT CHANNELS

Even as we were establishing the reliability of recording with the 4-channel Oxford system, it was viewed as an intermediate technology. By 1983, a cassette recording system with eight data channels had been developed. The task to design ambulatory EEG montages using this new capability ensued. From our prior experience in cataloging epileptiform abnormalities and from the impressive results of 3-channel montage testing, it was apparent that the statistical improvement in detection rates with the transition to eight channels would not be numerically impressive no matter where the additional electrodes were placed. With exposure to the interpretive difficulties of others, who did not have the opportunity to build their cassette EEG analytical skills on simultaneous monitoring studies, we had seen that misinterpretation of artifacts as either epileptiform abnormalities or seizures was common. Therefore, it seemed that better frontotemporal resolution might improve the overall accuracy of cassette EEG interpretation more than the extension of electrodes into other areas simply for the sake of broadening coverage regardless of likely yield from those new regions. To accomplish this, midtemporal (T3, T4) and frontal (F3, F4) electrodes were added. This still allowed an opportunity to provide two additional channels. These could have involved occipital, parietal, and/or central electrodes. Because parasagittal frontocentral channels would have the additional advantage of improving recognition of focal frontal or generalized abnormalities, as demonstrated in the first montage study (4), we elected to complete an 8-channel montage with central electrode sites as illustrated in Fig. 2.

Since the 3-channel montage was arranged in a continuously linked or nearly linked bipolar fashion, it was logical to display the derivations in a circumferential sequence, in this instance left posterior temporal to right posterior temporal. As a result, many frontal artifacts, such as eye blinks, and most sleep transients, such as vertex sharp waves or K-complexes, appeared as waveform patterns that, on the video display, had mirror-image symmetry around the middle, transverse frontal channel. We soon realized that this pattern of symmetry was disrupted by lateralized epileptiform discharges and that recognition of this asymmetry was a key to distinguishing these focal transients on video review of AEEG. A typical example is illustrated in Fig. 3. It is true that generalized or bifrontal spike-wave discharges also produced visual patterns that were symmetrical and thus could be confused with normal sleep complexes on rapid visual review. The spike component of the abnormal transient, however, results in a characteristic snap or click in the audio output, which can be used to differentiate the two even before inspecting a static page.

The 8-channel recorder afforded the opportunity to design montages with four channels symmetrically covering each hemisphere. Rather than run the four channels from each side front to back, as in traditional montages, our experience with the perceptual advantage granted by a circumferential arrange-

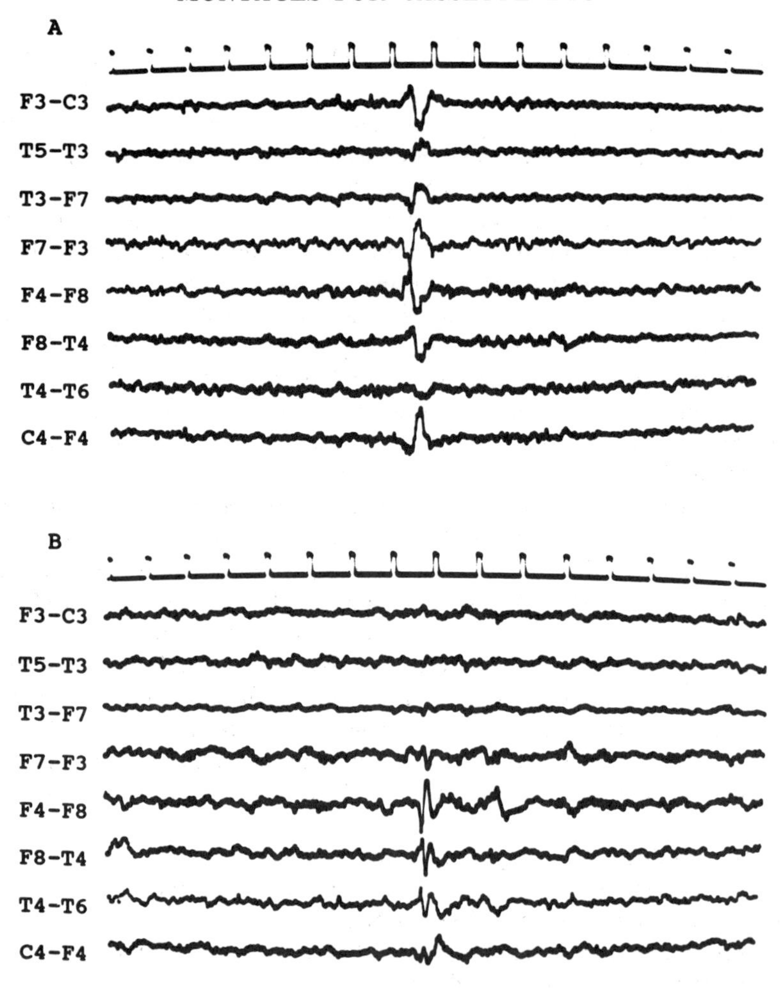

FIG. 3. Asymmetry on the circumferential montage. Note in **A** the typical symmetrical distribution of a normal sleep complex when using a circumferential montage, whereas the frontotemporal focal epileptiform abnormality in **B** is readily distinguished by its asymmetry.

ment led us to maintain this overall design. The added complexity of searching eight rather than three channels for focal transients was in this manner partially compensated by a montage that helped the reviewer distinguish between normal and epileptiform sharp waves. We soon learned that an additional advantage could be gained by a slight rearrangement in the way the channels were displayed on the video screen. It was our common experience that four channels could be seen in clear central vision. It would seem worthwhile to place in four adjacent traces those channels most likely to contain focal interictal features so that it would not be necessary to scan the eyes up and down continually. This was accomplished by relegating the two frontocentral channels to positions 1 and 8 while maintaining their same derivation. These channels participate mainly in generalized discharges that are easily recognized and thus would require the least attention during rapid review. The frontotemporal channels would now occupy the four center traces of the screen and could be the focus of the majority of visual attention.

Some, however, were tempted to revert to miniaturized traditional montages, such as temporal and parasagittal longitudinal bipolar chains of two channels each that run from frontal to posterior temporal and parietal regions. It is very likely that one or more of the electrodes of such a montage would record the majority of focal frontotemporal transients; however, the four longitudinal chains in this configuration all end in this same region of likely field maxima. Phase reversals would not be evident on the video display, and this would make recognition of the interictal abnormality more difficult. It is a well-established practice to run bipolar chains through areas of likely epileptiform abnormality so that the resultant phase reversals can localize the field of the spike or sharp wave. If frontopolar electrode positions are avoided in cassette EEG montages because of the high-amplitude eye movement artifacts recorded there, an alternative that we have found very useful is the circumferential design, as discussed above, where F7 is connected to F3 and F4 to F8. In practice, for the common sharp waves or sharp-slow wave complexes of complex partial epilepsy, the voltage gradient between the frontal and frontotemporal electrodes is often larger than any other electrode combination so that the amplitude of the discharge is greatest in this channel, which obviously also makes the abnormality easier to perceive. The differences in straight-chain and circumferential representation are illustrated in Fig. 4.

EIGHT-CHANNEL MONTAGE TESTING

When given the opportunity to evaluate the 8-channel Oxford 9000 system before its commercial introduction, our immediate response was to undertake another comparative study involving not only conventional 16-channel continuous monitoring, but 3-channel cassette EEG as well (8). To do this, trifurcation of electrode lead cables from monitoring rooms in the Epilepsy Center was used, allowing simultaneous recording in all three modalities. With careful attention to timing, we were able to transcribe corresponding segments from both cassette systems for comparison to the Epilepsy Center's polygraph paper records for correlation of individual complexes. Additionally, the interpretation of the entire tape was compared to the results of interpretation of the standard monitoring records by the Epilepsy Center staff.

In the comparative study, 30 patients underwent simultaneous cassette EEG recording, using both 4- and 8-channel devices, and standard monitoring. In identifying records as epileptiform, the scores of 3- and 8-channel recording were identical, with 93% agreement with the standard, although the actual

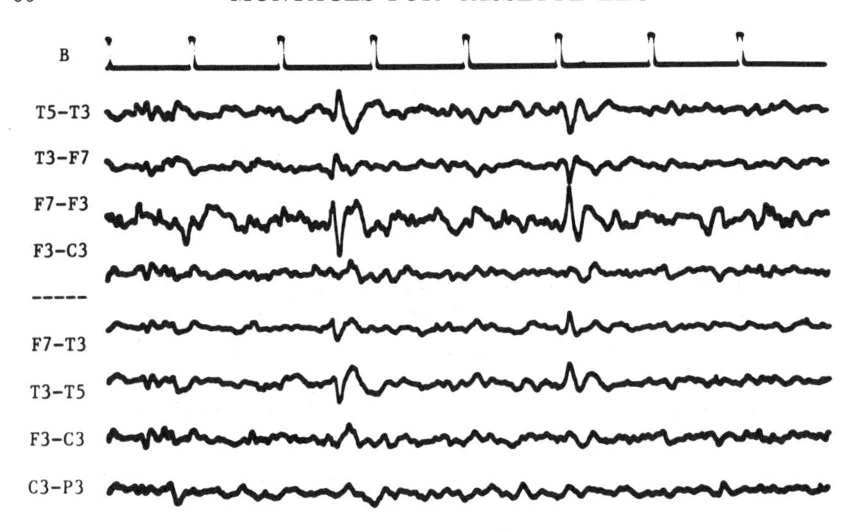

FIG. 4. Influence of linkage on the appearance of epileptiform abnormalities. Illustrated are frontotemporal sharp waves recorded with a "split" montage in which the top four channels are the left side of a circumferential chain, while the bottom four channels are short longitudinal bipolar chains from the same side. The epileptiform abnormalities are clearly enhanced by the circumferential display.

subjects for whom errors occurred were not the same for both systems. Three-channel and 8-channel interpretations were in agreement for 87%. The major failing of 3-channel cassette EEG in this study was misinterpretation of rhythmic artifacts as seizures, which occurred in two patients. This did not occur with 8-channel cassette EEG. Also, 8-channel recording provided the better spatial definition of abnormalities that would have been expected. In retrospect, it seems likely that the 8-channel montage suffered in this comparative study because of our limited experience with 8-channel rapid review at the time. We think it unlikely that either of the epileptiform records called normal at the time would have the same interpretation if presented to us now.

The 8-channel montage that we employed from the first included the same scalp coverage, though not the same order of channels, that had been used routinely for monitoring in the Epilepsy Center for its first decade of operation, when 16-channel recording was reserved for depth-electrode recordings. Since it had performed adequately in the comparative study, we saw no need for further testing of this sort and proceeded to routine use of the montage. It was altered slightly to create a 7-channel montage that would allow simultaneous ECG monitoring. Because we have found that rapid review is facilitated by a reasonable consistency of analytic strategy, we have departed from these two montages only infrequently, when circumstances demanded occipital or parietal coverage, until embarking on a novel approach for recording in emergency situations (see below).

ALTERNATIVE APPROACHES

With the initial use of Oxford 4-channel recorders, the playback devices allowing rapid video/audio review were not yet available. Ives and Woods, who reviewed their EEG data on paper after rapid transcription, used conventional longitudinal bipolar derivations (9). A number of other investigators used similar arrangements in 4-channel recording. Having been called on by others to provide interpretation of 4-channel tapes using either bilateral 2-channel chains or four single-channel longitudinal bites, we can only observe that rendering confident interpretation was difficult for us. This may have been related to the problems with the perception of focal transients with open-ended channels or chains that end in the frontal regions, as discussed above, or this may have simply reflected the concentration of our practical experience on circumferential montages.

Little published information exists on 7- or 8-channel montages other than those we have employed, which have been adopted by others (10). Aminoff and associates have used bilateral longitudinal parasagittal chains with temporal and midline bites (11). Powell et al. used longitudinal bipolar chains that were positioned between the standard temporal and parasagittal locations in combination with a transverse midtemporal-central chain (12). There is no reason to expect that either approach could not be effective, in light of our own Epilepsy Center's previous experience in the use of similar montages for 8-channel cable telemetry, but we would expect that isolated epileptiform abnormalities would be less reliably identified on rapid review for the reasons discussed previously.

If one concurs with Aminoff's skeptical opinion on the value of detecting interictal epileptiform abnormalities on AEEG (11,13), the visual aspects of channel arrangement become less crucial. Under such circumstances, reliable identification of EEG seizures becomes the only purpose of cassette recording, and the ear serves quite well for this purpose on rapid review. Suspicious ictal-like events identified aurally can then be examined visually on a static page with less need for perceptual help. We would point out, however, that seizures are recorded far less frequently in clinical practice than are interictal abnormalities (see Chapter 7). It would seem wasteful to discard this information simply because it is not ideal and/or is somewhat more difficult to extract from the record.

SPECIAL DESIGNS

The most frequent modification necessary in the 4- or 8-channel general screening montage is one that incorporates a channel of ECG. This is commonly used in patients with sudden loss of consciousness, syncopal-like episodes, dizzy spells, and the older patient in general (see Chapters 7 and 11). When using 4-

channel recorders, the fourth channel is most often used for ECG. This allows three channels for EEG so that the suggested screening montage can be maintained. However, in the Oxford 4-24 system, this means that time and event markers will not be encoded on tape. Further reduction in EEG to two channels is not recommended by us, nor does it meet American EEG Society guidelines for ambulatory monitoring (1). With 8-channel recorders, the EEG channel that is sacrificed should be one of statistically lesser diagnostic value. In the suggested 8-channel screening montage, the frontocentral channels usually only emphasize generalized abnormalities that are evident on the other frontal channels. In practice, we have used three approaches to accommodate the ECG channel. The simplest is to omit one of the frontocentral channels. Although the resulting presentation is imbalanced peripherally, the symmetry of the middle channels on the video screen is maintained. To maintain symmetry of the seven EEG channels, a single bihemispheric transverse channel may be created. Trading the two transverse frontal channels for a single F7-F8 derivation allows preservation of the parasagittal channels, but the long interelectrode distance results in a noisy, disproportionate channel that is difficult to examine. Omission of the frontocentral channels in favor of an F3-F4 derivation yields a more readily interpreted presentation, although all central coverage is lost. In adults, that is not a costly sacrifice, but it may not be desirable in children. Since most of our patients undergoing simultaneous EEG/ECG monitoring are adults, we usually chose to sacrifice central coverage. Both montages are illustrated in Fig. 5.

If two channels are needed for physiologic measures other than EEG, both

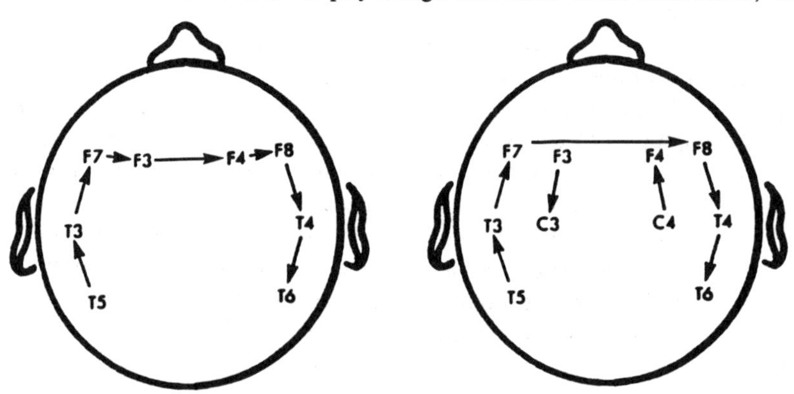

FIG. 5. Seven-channel montages. Two alternative 7-channel montages are illustrated. A free channel for simultaneous ECG monitoring is available with each. **A** provides enhanced frontal resolution by means of the F3-F4 transverse channel but sacrifices central coverage. **B** provides a single bihemispheric channel for audio monitoring, F7-F8, and preserves frontocentral coverage but renders the display more difficult to interpret due to the disproportionate amplitude of the single transverse channel. Seven EEG channels: **(A)** 1. T5–T3; 2. T3–F7; 3. F7–F3; 4. F3–F4; 5. F4–F8; 6. F8–T4; 7. T4–T6; 8. ECG. **(B)** 1. F3–C3; 2. T5–T3; 3. T3–F7; 4. F7–F8; 5. F8–T4; 6. T4–T6; 7. C4–F4; 8. ECG.

frontocentral channels could be replaced. This leaves the essential circumferential montage skeleton of six channels intact. In this instance, rather than having the non-EEG data on channels 1 and 8, the six channels of EEG may be shifted to positions 1 to 6. Mirror-image symmetry is maintained among the EEG channels. When the number of EEG channels is reduced to five, the advantages gained over the older recorders in terms of characterization, ease of differentiation from artifact, and safety margin for linked channels begin to erode. Use of separate electrodes for individual channels again becomes a consideration, since loss of one site could result in a 40% reduction of data if common to two channels. A single transverse frontal channel can be combined with temporal chains of two channels each, when three channels of non-EEG physiology are required.

When the Oxford 9000 system was first introduced, audio monitoring was limited to one channel. Our experience with the 4-channel system, where there was a similar limitation, pointed to the importance of bihemispheric representation in this audio output. Lateralized seizures or spikes that could have been detected by sound were sometimes overlooked when listening to the EEG from the other hemisphere. Accordingly, it became common practice to audio-monitor the wide transverse frontal channel when using a 3-channel montage. The 8-channel recording systems lent themselves to montages with four channels from each hemisphere with necessarily no bihemispheric derivation. This deficiency quickly became apparent in our comparison study of the two systems (8). Initially, one solution was to create an 8-channel montage with one channel designed specifically for bihemispheric audio monitoring. A better answer to the problem came with the introduction of stereo sound output derived from any number of channels (see Chapter 5).

The general screening montages discussed above were based on data from adults and adolescents. They are equally good with generalized epileptiform features of children, as well as adults. The increased incidence of posterior epileptiform abnormalities in children may, in certain instances, warrant additional coverage in these regions. A useful approach with eight EEG channels is to substitute occipitotemporal channels (O1-T5, T6-O2) for the two frontocentral channels in positions 1 and 8, respectively. Alternate montages are also worthwhile when recording from neonates, particularly the premature. Four-channel recorders and associated montages are commonly used (see Chapter 9). With 8-channel devices, a reduced number of EEG channels is reasonable, given the small size of a neonate's head. In addition, the remaining channels can be used to monitor other physiologic parameters that may be useful in characterizing sleep state.

The attempt to use common reference recording in AEEG has met with little practical success. In theory, by doing so one could create any number of bipolar derivations when printing out selected epochs onto paper, by putting separate AEEG channels into grid 1 and grid 2 of each polygraph channel. Commercial scanning services sometimes claim 16-channel capability from 8-channel recorders by this method. In fact, this technique is fraught with difficulty and compromise when applied to clinical situations. First, only eight electrode sites can be recorded, not 10 or more, as is routine with bipolar chains. Second, the epochs to be printed using this capability must first be identified by reviewing data recorded in common reference fashion. Artifacts are enhanced, and localization of focal abnormalities is more difficult. There has been no documentation that this technique offers any advantage in routine diagnostic recordings.

SUBHAIRLINE MONTAGES

The setup for AEEG is somewhat time-consuming. It requires all the skills of standard EEG technology and more. However, the cassette recorder itself is quite simple to operate. This simplicity, plus the small size of the recorder, would make it a natural means of obtaining EEG, and even EEG monitoring, quickly and unobtrusively in emergency situations, were it not for the stringent technical demands of electrode placement and skin preparation.

In attempting the novel approach of cassette EEG recording with disposable, adhesive electrodes placed outside the hairline, we were inspired by the report of Dyson and co-workers on a similar approach to overnight recording for the purpose of sleep-stage quantification (14). They placed disposable, adhesive-backed, pre-gelled electrodes just beneath the hairline frontally, approximately 1.5 cm above standard Fp1 and Fp2 positions, with referential recording to ipsilateral ear electrodes (A1 and A2). Using standard polygraph write-out, sleep-stage scoring based on 2-channel recording with these novel electrode positions was compared to scoring based on simultaneous overnight monitoring with 2-channel EEG using C3-A1 and C4-A2 derivations in six individuals undergoing overnight recording. Good interobserver agreement for the novel positionings and within-observer agreement for the novel positions versus standard placement were demonstrated. In fact, within-observer agreement for the two montages was higher than interobserver agreement for the standard recording for scoring of most sleep stages. As in all sleep-stage recording, however, judgment was based not on EEG alone, but also on information provided from other physiologic recordings such as the electro-oculogram.

It is a long step from adequacy for sleep staging to adequacy for detection of epileptiform abnormalities and seizures. Characterization of sleep by EEG depends on identification of straightforward and fairly widely distributed transients that can be seen relatively easily on a single channel, provided one electrode is close to the midline and the other is more laterally placed. Vertex waves and sleep spindles occur repeatedly in Stage II of sleep and disappear with both lighter and deeper stages. There is little from which they must be differentiated. Defining epileptiform abnormalities is a trickier undertaking, for these must be clearly and accurately differentiated from other activity, including sleep transients. Nevertheless, our own experience had shown that this could be accomplished with only three channels of EEG. Since anterior temporal electrodes, usually located at the margin of the hairline, serve quite well in defining epileptiform abnormalities, it did not seem farfetched to expect that an entire array of electrodes outside the hairline might prove sufficient to justify clinical use.

To test this proposition, we performed simultaneous EEG recordings using a 7-channel subhairline montage and a standard longitudinal bitemporal 8-channel montage in 25 Epilepsy Unit inpatients, all of whom had definite epileptiform abnormalities (15). The novel montage consisted of mastoid, preauricular, suprazygomatic, and frontal electrode positions as illustrated in Fig. 6. We chose these positions because they corresponded somewhat to a typical temporal chain, and could be easily and consistently identified without head measurements, or even knowledge of the 10-20 system. We used disposable, adhesive-backed electrodes with inset polymer gel electrolyte pellets (Meditrace Pellet Electrodes, Graphic Controls Corp.). These electrodes have snap-on lead attachments, having been originally used for pediatric ECG monitoring.

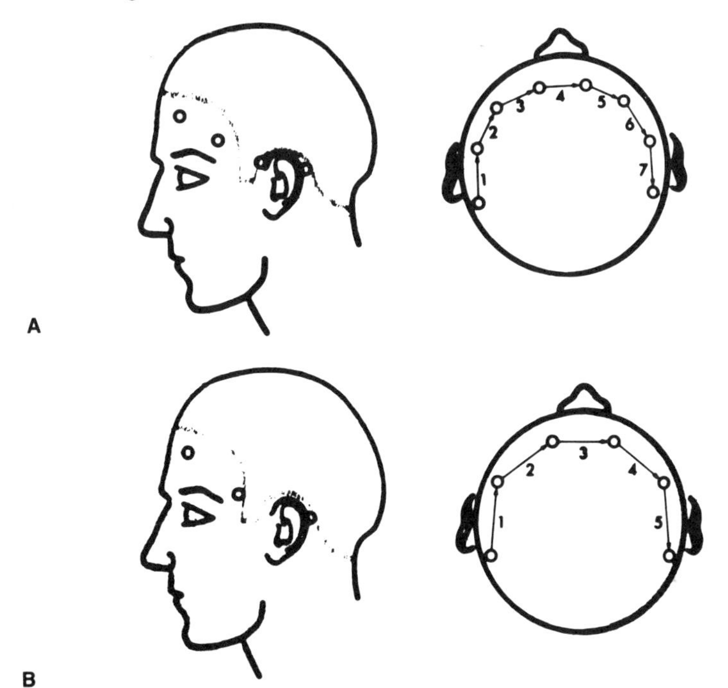

FIG. 6. Subhairline montages. A 7-channel circumferential montage with subhairline electrode positions is illustrated *above* **(A)** and a 5-channel version *below* **(B).** These montages compare favorably in yield to those of standard EEG monitoring. Elimination of the preauricular electrodes in the 5-channel montage enhances the appearance of both normal and abnormal posterior temporal activity. It is our routine montage for emergency cassette EEGs.

Open examination of the EEG recordings revealed that at least some epileptiform abnormalities could be identified in all records with the subhairline montage. To provide a more rigorous test, four 10-sec segments were selected from each record. After coding and separation of the two portions with simultaneous subhairline and standard montage tracings, the segments were presented randomly for blinded analysis.

Complete correspondence in blinded identification of all epileptiform abnormalities with the two montages was achieved in only 11 patients (44%), but correspondence for a majority of complexes was achieved in 24 patients (96%). Considering the 100 individual 10-sec segments presented for each montage, there were partial agreement for 96%, majority agreement for 92%, and only agreement for 79%. Of 30 segments without epileptiform activity on the reference montage, 28 (93%) were similarly labeled with the test montage. Of a total of 160 epileptiform abnormalities identified by either montage, 82% were seen on both, 10% were false positives, and 8% were false negatives on the subhairline montage, assuming reference montage identifications were all correct. Open reexamination showed that the false negatives were just that. Posterior temporal abnormalities presented the greatest problem. Most of the false positives, however, were epileptiform abnormalities that just could not be clearly identified on the reference montage.

Subsequently, we found that a 5-channel montage, eliminating the preauricular electrodes, appeared to work somewhat better. Both posterior temporal epileptiform discharges and the posterior dominant rhythms of relaxed wakefulness were enhanced by the greater interelectrode distance of the zygomatic-mastoid electrode derivation. The montage is illustrated in Fig. 6.

With the reliability of these subhairline montages demonstrated, we felt confident in proceeding to actual recording in emergency situations. Our subsequent experience with this technique is discussed in Chapter 14.

CONCLUSIONS

In considering montage design for cassette EEG, we have been forced to concentrate on our own efforts. In the absence of competing opinions, we have to assume that others have been satisfied to accept what we have done or have not considered this a crucial aspect of cassette EEG development. To the extent the latter may be true, we think this is unfortunate. A willingness to continue thinking about and testing montages has allowed us to move into the fruitful new area of emergency cassette EEG recording. No doubt there are other areas where specific montages could be designed and tested with specific purposes in mind. To those who might be so tempted, we can only repeat the principal lessons of our own experience with montage design—that trade-offs will always be necessary, that something short of perfection may still prove quite useful, and that nothing is quite so convincing as a careful comparison with the conventional.

REFERENCES

1. American Electroencephalographic Society. Guidelines in EEG and evoked potentials. Guideline 1: Minimal technical standards for performing electroencephalography. *J Clin Neurophysiol* 1986;3:1–6.
2. Mattson RH. Value of intensive monitoring. In: Wada JA, Penry JK, eds. *Advances in epileptology. The Xth Epilepsy International Symposium.* New York: Raven Press, 1980;43–51.
3. Leroy RF, Ebersole JS. An evaluation of ambulatory, cassette EEG monitoring. I. Montage design. *Neurology* (*Cleve*) 1983;33:1–7.
4. Ebersole JS, Leroy RF. An evaluation of ambulatory, cassette EEG monitoring. II. Detection of interictal abnormalities. *Neurology (Cleve)* 1983;33:8–18.
5. Blumhardt LD, Oozeer R. Simultaneous ambulatory monitoring of the EEG and ECG in patients with unexplained transient disturbances of consciousness. In: Stott FD, Wright SL, Raftery EB, et al., eds. *ISAM 1981. Proceedings of the Fourth International Symposium on Ambulatory Monitoring.* London: Academic Press, 1982;171–182.
6. Ebersole JS, Leroy RF. Evaluation of ambulatory cassette EEG monitoring. III. Diagnostic accuracy compared to intensive inpatient EEG monitoring. *Neurology (Cleve)* 1983;33:853–860.
7. Bridgers SL, Ebersole JS. The clinical utility of ambulatory cassette EEG. *Neurology (Cleve)* 1985;35:166–173.
8. Ebersole JS, Bridgers SL. Direct comparison of 3 and 8-channel ambulatory cassette EEG with intensive inpatient monitoring. *Neurology (Cleve)* 1985;35:846–854.
9. Ives JR, Woods JF. A study of 100 patients with focal epilepsy using a 4-channel ambulatory cassette recorder. In: Stott FD, Raftery EB, Goulding L, eds. *ISAM 1979: Proceedings of the Third International Symposium of Ambulatory Monitoring.* London: Academic Press, 1980;383–392.
10. Keilson MJ, Hauser WA, Magrill JP, et al. ECG abnormalities in patients with epilepsy. *Neurology (Cleve)* 1987;37:1624–1626.
11. Aminoff MJ, Goodin DS, Berg BO, et al. Ambulatory EEG recordings in epileptic and nonepileptic children. *Neurology (Cleve)* 1988;38:558–562.
12. Powell TE, Harding GFA. Twenty-four hour ambulatory EEG monitoring: development and applications. *J Med Eng Tech* 1986;10:229–238.
13. Goodin DS, Aminoff MJ. Does the interictal EEG have a role in the diagnosis of epilepsy? *Lancet* 1984;1:837–839.
14. Dyson RJ, Thorton C, Dore CJ. EEG electrode positions outside the hairline to monitor sleep in man. *Sleep* 1984;7:180–188.
15. Bridgers SL, Ebersole JS. EEG outside the hairline: detection of epileptiform abnormalities. *Neurology (Cleve)* 1988;38:146–149.

Ambulatory EEG Monitoring,
edited by John S. Ebersole.
Raven Press, Ltd., New York © 1989

5

Audio-Video Analysis of Cassette EEG

John S. Ebersole

Department of Neurology, Yale University School of Medicine, New Haven, Connecticut 06510

When ambulatory EEG (AEEG) recorders were first developed, analysis of the recorded data necessitated transcription onto paper. Real-time playback would have been terribly inefficient, taking as long to print out as to record, and would have, in itself, created technical obstacles to the recovery of low-frequency analog signals, such as EEG. A more rapid transcription was required to improve both. Ink-jet writers, with high paper transport speeds and an upper frequency response of nearly 600 Hz, were the original solution. Even with these, playback of data could only be done at 20 times real time; thus, 72 min were required to make a copy of one day's record even before analysis could begin. Trying to operate an ink-jet writer at a paper speed of 600 mm/sec, so that the EEG would have the standard appearance of 30 mm/sec, was a formidable task for only the daring. Consequently, cassette EEG analysis was usually limited to writing out seizures that could be appreciated despite the temporal compression accompanying a more manageable paper speed.

This type of analysis suffered from the same drawbacks as did intensive inpatient monitoring of the day, namely, that there was no easy way to review all the data that were recorded and extract what was pertinent. Tape review was effectively limited to writing out clinical events, such as seizures of which the patient was aware or that were witnessed, and to sampling the EEG at random during other times. Infrequent interictal features or subclinical seizures were easily missed.

What made cassette EEG a viable and unique clinical tool was the development of the audio-video replay unit. With this device, EEG and other biologic signals were displayed as video pages, advanced at rates up to 60 times real time, and transformed into audio outputs, which could be heard concurrently. Efficient analysis of the entire record became feasible for the first time.

It quickly became apparent to early users that rapid audio-video analysis of cassette-recorded EEG from ambulatory patients was unlike any other type of

EEG interpretation. Totally new skills had to be developed if analysis was to proceed at anything faster than traditional hand-turning speed. The freedom that was gained for the patient by this technique assured that the recording would be made in conditions unheard of in the EEG laboratory and experienced only to a limited extent in intensive monitoring facilities. Artifacts, which are the subject of an intense effort at elimination during routine recordings, were pervasive during much of each AEEG, including those never before seen in EEG recordings. Reliance on new features of the EEG had to be learned. Protocols were needed that would provide a schema for an orderly analysis of taped data and in which time and effort were spent on segments of the recording in proportion to what was likely to be gained.

It is the purpose of this chapter to review techniques for the analysis of ambulatory cassette EEG. Since this is a personal account, I will provide as much rationale for my opinions as possible. I hope these will serve as guides for those who wish to extrapolate on their own. The methodology that I will discuss is based on tape reviews using the Oxford Medilog PMD-12 and 9000 replay units. Although certain details may be applicable only to these devices, basic principles will apply to rapid analysis with any audio-video playback unit. I will concern myself mainly with techniques used in the identification of epileptiform EEG abnormalities, both ictal and interictal. These methods conform to the guidelines for long-term neurodiagnostic monitoring that were established for ambulatory monitoring by the American EEG Society (1). Rapid analysis of ECG and polysomnographic data will be reviewed in Chapters 11 and 16, respectively.

PLAYBACK SETTINGS

When a cassette tape is inserted into the replay unit, certain adjustments in playback settings may have to be made before review can properly begin. This depends on whether the default parameters of the machine meet the requirements of a particular review. Gain, high-frequency filtering, and time constant for each channel, replay speed, page length, which channel is to be heard over the speaker, and which channel combination is to be heard via headphones may be selected.

Sensitivity

Display gains are continuously adjustable over an arbitrary 0 to 2.0 scale, with 1.0 being the default value. The vertical deflection of a signal at gain settings 2.0 and 0.5 will be twice and one-half the size, respectively, of the signal display at gain 1.0. Display gains are usually adjusted so that 50- or 100-μv calibration pulses at the beginning of each tape produce a video deflection equal to the amplitude of the 1-cm cursor scale. When this adjustment is made, EEG amplitude can be read from the video screen.

This standardized sensitivity setting is a good place to begin a review and to determine the overall amplitude of the EEG rhythms. The reviewer can return to this setting whenever an amplitude reading is needed. However, it need not be used, and in most instances should not be used, for the entire analysis. One definite advantage of tape-recorded EEG is that the reviewer can adjust the settings at will to produce a display that is most easily interpreted. In general, gains are reduced during active wakefulness when the EEG is full of high-amplitude artifact, increased during quiet wakefulness and light sleep, and again turned down in slow-wave sleep, when the amplitude of delta activity becomes large. Sensitivities should always be reduced when the signals from individual channels begin to overlap frequently and the screen is so cluttered that distinguishing individual channels becomes difficult (Fig. 1).

Filters

The recording technology used in continuous cassette EEG recorders tends to limit the high-frequency response of the device. The upper-frequency limit for the Oxford Medilog recorder, for example, is 40 Hz. In most situations, additional high-frequency filtering (30 or 15 Hz) is not needed. Muscle activity present during much of active wakefulness is of such amplitude that it is seldom eliminated by this filtration, and it is more important not to reduce the amplitude of epileptiform spikes. As will be discussed later, these are mostly identified during periods of quiet or sleep, when muscle artifact is not a problem and thus when high-frequency filtration would not only be unnecessary, but would also be detrimental. Occasionally, slower frequencies in the alpha, theta, or delta range, which comprise a seizure discharge, may be discerned more clearly when accompanying muscle artifact is reduced by high-frequency filtering. As in standard EEG, one should be cautious about beta frequencies revealed by such filtration, since muscle artifact may take on this appearance under these conditions.

Time constant (TC) adjustments are also infrequently necessary in cassette EEG analysis. Most reviews should be performed at a TC of 0.1 sec. This is similar to standard practice in many labs. This setting results in a flatter baseline and thus makes isolated sharp transients easier to discern (Fig. 1). Interictal abnormalities are more difficult to appreciate on a wildly undulating background, even when they are of the same amplitude. Delta activity is quite apparent at a 0.1-sec TC, and the diagnosis of lateralized or generalized slowing or the analysis of sleep rhythms is usually not impaired. If it is crucial to measure the amplitude of slow waves, which is seldom the case in epilepsy evaluations, longer time constants can be used.

The 0.1-sec TC may give high-amplitude slow waves, such as those of spike-

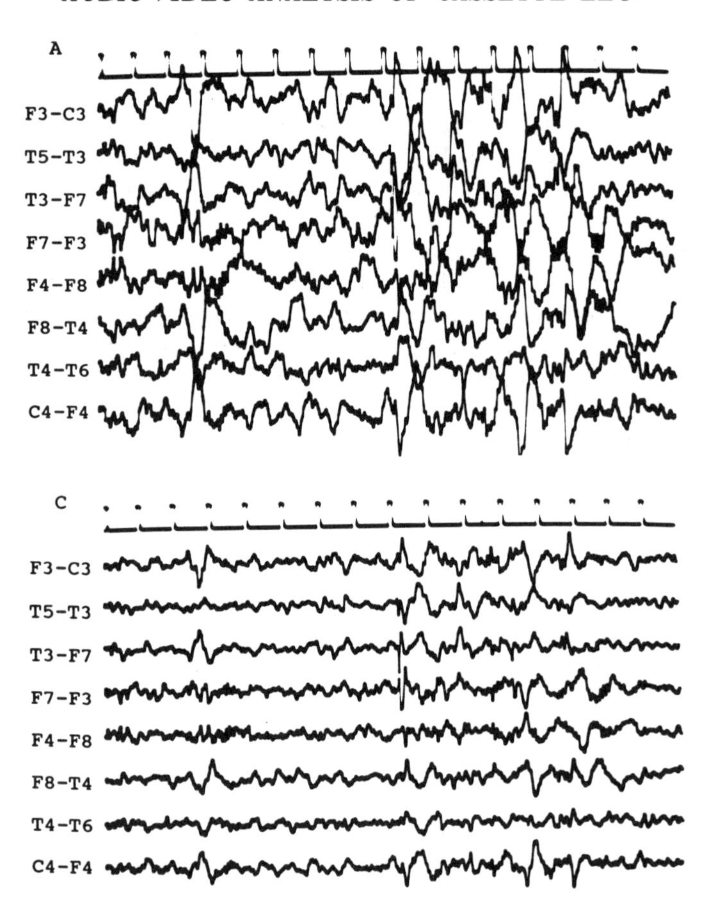

FIG. 1. Perception of epileptiform features in the EEG is enhanced by appropriate filter and gain settings as noted in these examples of the same left frontotemporal spike during Stage 3 sleep. **A:** Sixteen-sec page; DC time constant; gain that was appropriate during wakefulness, but results in trace overlap during sleep. **B:** Original settings, except a 0.1-sec time constant. (TC). **C:** Original settings, except 0.1-sec TC and reduced gain. **D:** Eight-sec page; 0.1-sec TC; reduced gain. Unless otherwise noted, all EEG examples in the figures of this chapter are displayed with a 0.1-sec TC.

wave discharge, an unusual appearance, if the amplitude of the waveforms results in amplifier blocking. The truncated top of each wave has a decaying slope typical of a square-wave calibration signal under similar conditions (see Figs. 2 and 3). When slow-wave morphology is crucial, the longer TCs of 0.3 sec or DC should be used for visual analysis of static pages. Obviously, signals with a slow time course, such as respiration and thermistry measures, must be viewed with a DC time constant for the video display to be accurate.

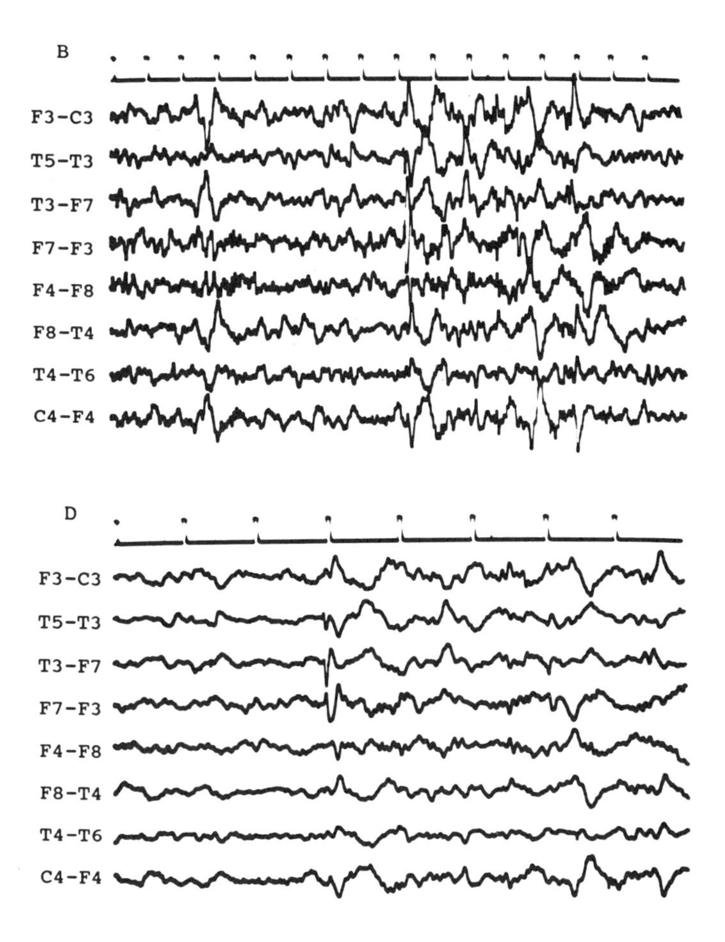

FIG. 1. *(continued).*

Page Lengths

Two page lengths are available on the Oxford replay units, 16 sec or 8 sec, each equivalent to paper speeds of 15 and 30 mm/sec, respectively. Page length and replay speed interact to determine how long each page appears on the video screen during dynamic review. Persistence of a 16-sec page at 20, 40, and 60 times real time is 0.80, 0.40, and 0.27 sec, respectively. These times are halved for an 8-sec page. Transient features such as interictal events, particularly if focal, are obviously easier to identify with a longer visual analysis time per page. In most instances, rapid review is performed with a 16-sec page. The temporal compression resulting from this page length also improves the recognition of spatial patterns of activity in much the same way that slow paper speeds will enhance them on routine EEG.

Although new AEEG reviewers often approach 16-sec pages with some

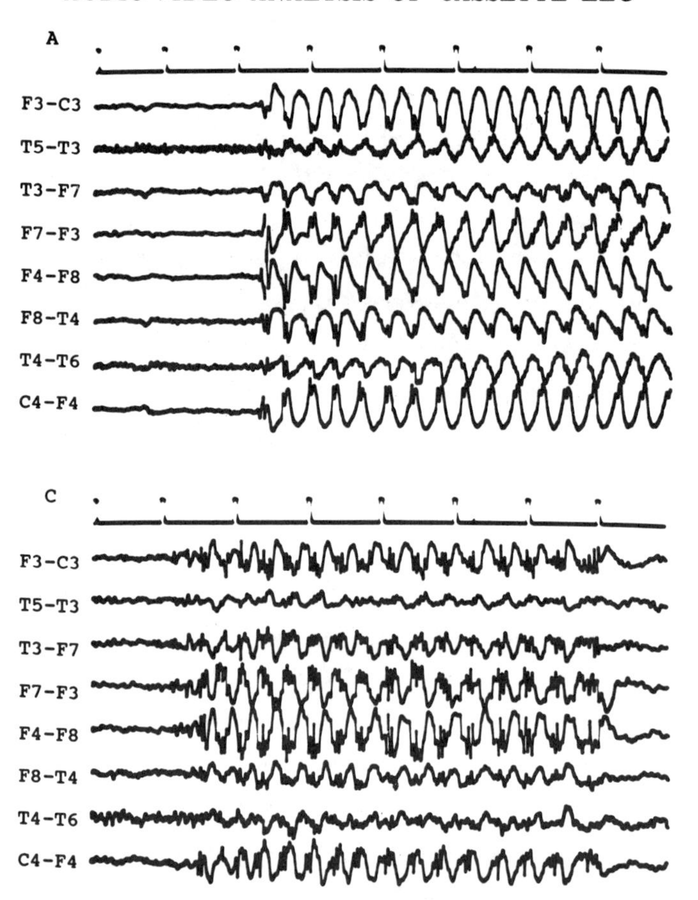

FIG. 2. Generalized spike-wave discharges illustrated in 8-sec pages. **A:** Three-Hz spike-wave run from a patient with absence seizures. **B:** Fragmentation of spike-wave activity during sleep from the same patient as in **A. C:** Polyspike-wave discharge from a patient with atypical absence seizures. **D:** Irregular spike-wave, polyspike-wave discharge from a patient with myoclonic seizures.

hesitancy, most quickly appreciate the advantages of this format in dynamic review and quickly become accustomed to it, just as do neonatal electroencephalographers and polysomnographers. Events do appear sharper at this setting, but this only assists initial detection. The close visual scrutiny necessary for a final analysis and interpretation is usually done on static data. In this instance, an 8-sec page and a 30 mm/sec presentation represent a diagnostic advantage rather than the opposite.

Some replay units offer further temporal compression such that a minute or more of EEG can be seen on one screen. These levels of compression are useful for seeing slowly evolving patterns, such as sleep or even seizures; however, individual interictal transients become nearly unrecognizable. The compromise

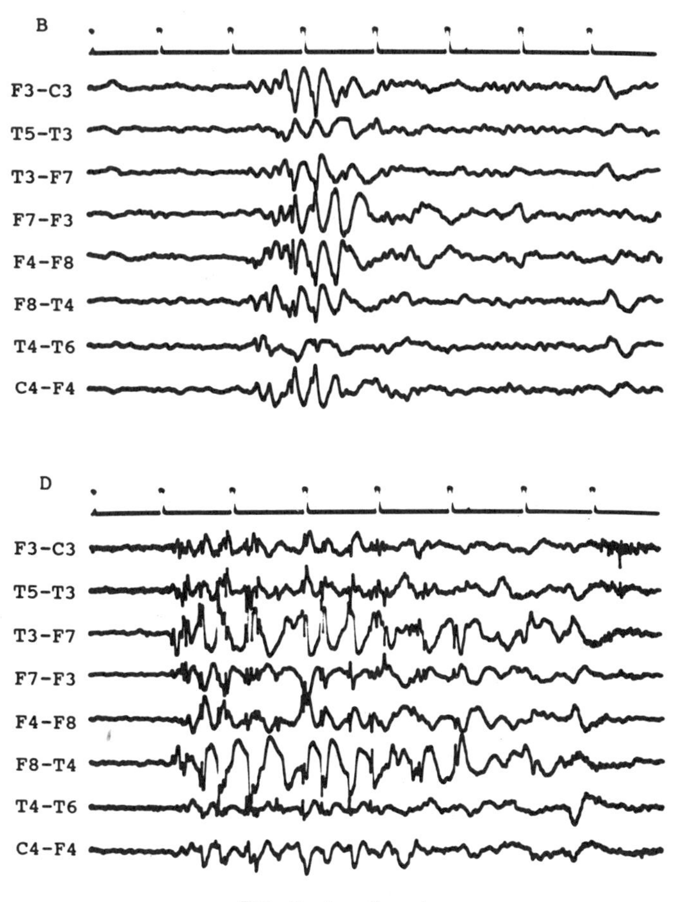

FIG. 2. *(continued).*

of a 16-sec page length seems to fit best the need for identifying both seizures and interictal features confidently. Later detailed analysis, rather than the initial detection, can use the entire extent of temporal expansion or compression abilities of the replay device without penalty.

Replay Speeds

Cassette replay units provide a range of scanning speeds, usually from 20 to 60 times real time. Data that took minutes or hours can be played back in seconds or minutes. At the fastest replay speed, 24 hr of EEG can be reviewed in 24 min. This ability offers tremendous advantages when dealing with long-term EEG data. Video "page turning" is done in discrete updates with variable persistence, depending on page length, as noted above. Pagination allows visual

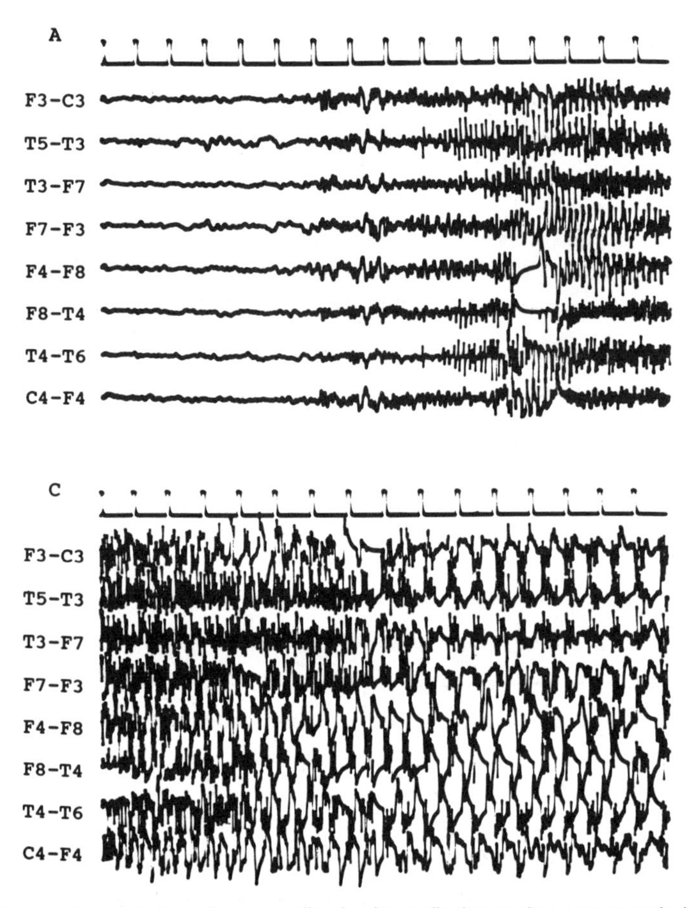

FIG. 3. Progressive evolution of a generalized seizure discharge that accompanied a clinical tonic-clonic seizure. Note in **A** the low-voltage, high-frequency onset, which is followed in **B** by widespread high-amplitude tonic EMG activity. Lower frequency, high-amplitude EEG waveforms accompanied by EMG bursts mark the clonic phase of the seizure seen in **C.** Less rhythmic, intermittent discharges, a sudden termination, and postictal depression characterize the latter portion of the seizure, as depicted in **D.**

analysis to proceed at rapid rates. A scrolling, continuous display is available at a real-time or slightly faster rate. It would be unintelligible at the higher scanning speeds of 20 to 60 times real time. Auditory analysis of the EEG frequencies resulting from rapid replay is, on the other hand, a continuous process, so long as the tape is in motion.

Adjustments in replay speed during analysis are meant to assist one or the other perceptual process. Audio review is more sensitive at 60 times real time, since higher frequencies in the normal hearing range are produced. Serendipitously, this also results in a shorter review time. Visual analysis benefits from a slower review rate and, consequently, longer persistence of each page of data.

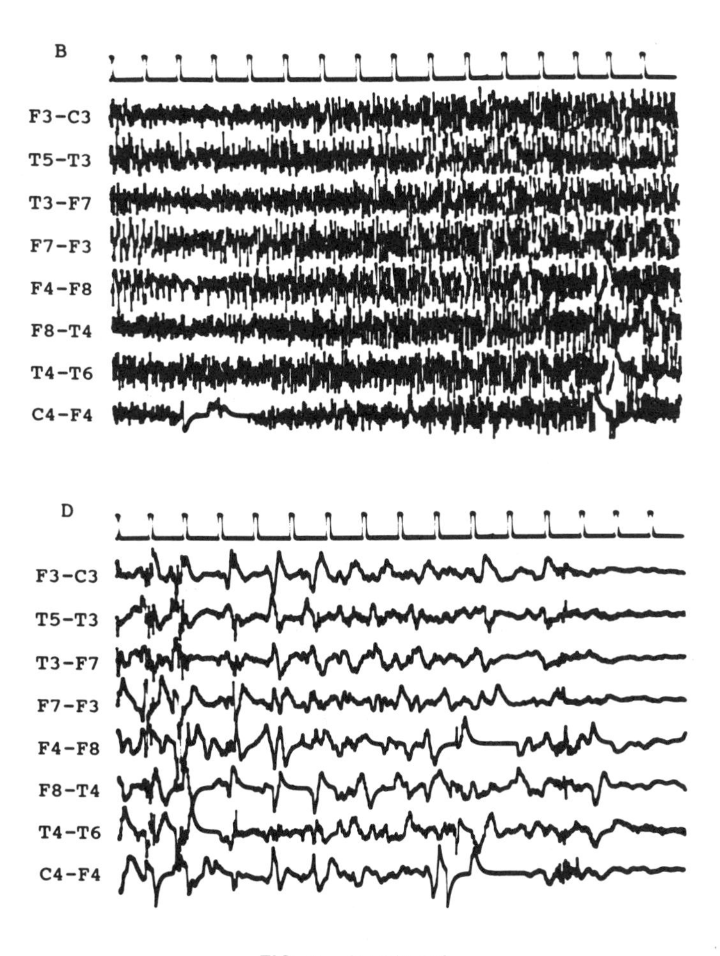

FIG. 3. *(continued).*

Unfortunately, this means that the analysis is protracted. These two factors must be balanced to provide an ideal review protocol. There is no one replay speed that is best for all circumstances. Just as with display gain, scanning speeds should be adjusted throughout the recording as necessary to maximize the accuracy and efficiency of review. In general, when dependent on auditory cues, replay at 60× is best. When using visual cues, replay at 20× is best; 40× is a compromise.

Audio Channel Selection

The original Oxford PMD-12 replay units provided a speaker output of the signals from one data channel, which one could select. Similarly, a single channel can be heard via a speaker when using the Oxford Medilog 9000 playback unit. With the latter, however, multichannel combinations can be aurally perceived by means of an audio mixer unit and headphones. This was a significant improvement over single-channel sound.

At the beginning of a tape review, it is necessary to select which channel(s) will be heard. As a general rule, unless the location of the patient's EEG abnormality is known ahead of time or it is known that the patient has only generalized epileptiform features, it is wise to listen to EEG activity from both hemispheres. With early systems, this could be accomplished by using montages that derived at least one channel in a bihemispheric fashion, usually across the frontal region. The same is necessary for 8-channel AEEG analysis, if only the speaker is used. Several errors in the interpretation of 8-channel tapes, noted in early controlled trials of cassette EEG versus telemetry (2), occurred when the patient's EEG abnormality was on the side opposite the one chosen for audio monitoring. The ability to listen via headphones to several channels from both hemispheres has obviated this problem.

Audio cancellation of a focal discharge can occur if two adjacent and linked channels are monitored together. Signals of equal amplitude, but opposite polarity, when applied to the same speaker or earphone result in no sound. This can be avoided by choosing channels for audio monitoring that do not have the same electrode used as both Grid 1 and Grid 2 input. A practical solution, when using linked bipolar montages such as those suggested in Chapter 4, is to listen only to every other channel in the circumferential sequence.

I usually listen to two channels from each hemisphere, one temporal and one frontal, and play those into one ear. The corresponding contralateral channels are played into the other ear. This resultant stereo effect enables the reviewer to be very sensitive to lateralized events. Dichotic properties of auditory perception can be used to great advantage in the recognition of minor events masked in noise or background rhythms. How audio analysis is used specifically to identify interictal and ictal events and distinguish them from artifacts will be discussed in detail in the following sections.

CASSETTE TAPE REVIEW

As indicated earlier, a number of factors interact to determine the best review protocol for AEEG cassette tapes. These include modes of replay most conducive to auditory and visual perception of epileptiform events and seizures, the sleep-waking cycle and the resultant distribution of periods of maximal artifact or epileptiform activity, and the clinical question being asked, e.g., initial diagnosis, seizure detection only, quantification, etc. An optimal protocol is obviously one that maximizes both information gain and efficiency. As in all endeavors, compromises are usually necessary, however. Page-by-page analysis is, of course, possible and may be very accurate, but it is highly impractical.

Rather, the question is how best to use the rapid review capability of cassette EEG replay devices (see also refs. 3 and 4).

On average, two-thirds of a 24-hr cassette recording will contain the signals of active wakefulness. In terms of EEG, these are mainly low-voltage mixed frequencies, a relatively minor contribution compared to the overwhelming abundance and variety of artifacts that dominate this portion of the recording. This is the price paid for ambulatory freedom during a cassette EEG. Most of this artifact is of physiologic origin—EMG of head muscles and eye or tongue movements. Other artifacts are related to movement of the electrode or cabling, which disturbs the electrode-scalp interface. Either type, particularly the former, is unavoidable. It becomes quickly apparent to anyone who reviews the EEG of an active patient that confident identification of isolated epileptiform discharges is very difficult, unless they are very prominent and confirmed during intermittent quiet periods that are relatively free of artifact (5,6).

Almost always a 24-hr recording will contain sleep. Usually it comprises about one-third to one-fourth of the data. During these periods, obfuscating muscle and movement artifacts cease and EEG rhythms are seen clearly for the first time. Not only can interictal discharges now be identified with confidence, but they are naturally more prominent during these periods, particularly Stages 1 through 3 of sleep. These two opposing relationships make sleep the best time to identify interictal features.

Seizures may occur at any time of day, although proportionally more occur during wakefulness. Seizures of nearly all types are notable for the rhythmic nature of their electrographic discharge. Typically, seizure activity also involves a rhythm of changing frequency and amplitude, usually from low-voltage faster frequencies to higher amplitude lower frequencies as the end of the seizure approaches. This regular progression of waveforms stands in marked contrast to the white-noise background engendered by artifact of active wakefulness. It can be appreciated by auditory analysis even when intermixed with artifact.

Logic would have us conclude that seizures should best be identified by frequency analysis and that this is the domain of auditory perception. Furthermore, active wakefulness is a good place to look, i.e., listen. Visual identification of interictal features is unadvised during this same time period, however, because of artifacts. All factors point to the same conclusion, namely, that the 16 or so hours of active wakefulness in a cassette EEG would be spent most productively in search of seizures using principally auditory cues, which are best heard at the fastest replay speed. This, in turn, means that the majority of the record can be reviewed in the least amount of time, without undue concern for what might be lost by doing so.

Epileptiform spikes are of sufficiently short duration that a snapping or popping sound is heard as a sonic representation at all scanning speeds, even a slow 20×. This, however, is not true of isolated sharp waves, which may not be identifiable by sound because of their longer duration and thus lower frequency. Therefore, interictal features are best identified visually. Furthermore, the spatial pattern of these events is important, i.e., whether they are focal, lateralized, or generalized. As will be made clear later, visual clues are also very useful in the differentiation of epileptiform complexes from other normal sharp transients. Thus, we can conclude that auditory cues may help in the detection of interictal features, but visual identification is the mainstay.

The interplay of the above factors results in the second recommendation, namely, that interictal transients are best sought during the sleep portion of the record using visual identification, which is aided by a slow scanning speed. In practice, at least the first part of the normal sleep period should be reviewed at 20× or 40×. After several sleep cycles are scrutinized without yield, the likelihood of seeing interictal features during later sleep diminishes. High-yielding slow-wave sleep becomes proportionately less, and REM sleep, which is often devoid of interictal abnormalities, increases. Commonly, therefore, replay speeds are increased progressively during the latter portions of the sleep period in continued search for seizures.

SEIZURE IDENTIFICATION

In the evaluation of epilepsy, the most useful information is undeniably obtained by recording seizures or at least clinical attacks that are thought to be seizures. Generalized seizures are easily identified by either visual or auditory means. Given the ease with which auditory, as opposed to visual, concentration can be maintained over a long period of time, it is far simpler to detect these seizures by sound and later inspect them visually on static pages once found.

The 3-Hz spike and wave discharge of absence seizures produces a very characteristic and easily identifiable sound, as well as a striking visual pattern (Fig. 2). The "Bronx cheer" or "raspberry" sound, likened by some to flatulence, is so characteristic that identification on review hardly needs visual confirmation on the screen. In fact, simple quantification of the number of spike-wave discharges can be performed at the fastest replay speeds by sound alone, if need be.

Runs of polyspike-wave are equally distinctive on auditory review, although the resultant sound is less musical and has a more "scratchy" sound due to the high-frequency polyspike components of the discharge (Fig. 2). The irregular, spike-wave and polyspike-wave discharges commonly seen in myoclonic epilepsy are the least distinctive of the generalized seizure discharges (Fig. 2). The mixed frequencies contained in these discharges result in a sound that is often similar to that of muscle and movement artifact, which makes it difficult at times to identify them during active wakefulness. Often they are first appreciated during quiet periods or drowsiness when artifact is diminished.

Generalized tonic-clonic seizures on dynamic replay are quite impressive both visually and aurally. Thus, detection is no problem. EEG seizure activity is usually seen only at the beginning and end of such seizures, since the muscle activity associated with the tonic and, to a lesser extent, clonic phase all but obscures the record (Fig. 3). The main source of difficulty comes in differentiating these from periods of intense muscle activity sometimes seen during pseudoseizures or other nonepileptic attacks. In these cases, auditory analysis is often more helpful than visual inspection. The underlying rhythmic activity of the electrical seizure discharge can often be heard despite the intermixed myogenic potentials. Listening to a supposed seizure can often provide the differentiation that looking at it cannot.

Convulsive seizures, both generalized and partial, and nonconvulsive partial seizures have a similar electrographic evolution in terms of frequency and amplitude. In contrast to spike-wave discharges, which have a sudden onset that is without buildup and only a slight change in frequency during the course of the ictus, these seizures show a characteristic progression of frequency and amplitude change (Fig. 3). Although varying tremendously, these seizures in general show a gradual buildup, in which low-voltage higher frequencies are replaced with higher amplitude lower frequencies. Intermittent or "stuttering" discharges near the end and a sudden termination also mark the typical seizure. A tone burst of changing frequency and loudness thus is the hallmark of a seizure discharge. These translate into a characteristic seizure sound that is similar to a lion's roar or to a speeding car going by. Variations on the theme are legion, but once the basic pattern is learned, reviewers can achieve remarkable accuracy in seizure identification. As will be discussed later, artifacts seldom mimic this evolving pattern and, thus, can be distinguished.

Partial seizures have the same basic pattern, only a localized distribution, in which the amplitude of discharges is less and the frequencies may be lower (Fig. 4). Proper spatial sampling by auditory monitoring is crucial in the detection of partial seizures. Bihemispheric, temporal and frontal, representation is absolutely necessary. Fortunately, most partial seizures induce electrographic alterations over a reasonably wide area of the involved hemisphere and even some change in the opposite side. This is a feature that helps to distinguish true seizure from rhythmic artifacts that may involve only one or two nearby electrodes.

In partial seizures, there is usually less obscuration of the EEG by muscle and movement artifact. Automatisms, particularly chewing, do interfere with identification at times, but, as in the above case, auditory analysis will usually identify the underlying rhythmic seizure discharge, even if it is visually unrecognizable. Lateralization of partial seizures can, however, be difficult. In addition to the customary close visual inspection of the seizure once it is detected, repeated auditory analysis of each EEG channel in succession may provide clues to the site of onset and/or maximal buildup.

Some feel that recording seizures is the only epilepsy-related use for cassette EEG (7). This is a narrow view, in my opinion, which would result in discarding or not attempting to find useful interictal data. This is particularly true, since seizures are far less likely to be recorded without prolonged monitoring, even among a population of known epileptics (2,8,9). Regardless, if the sole purpose

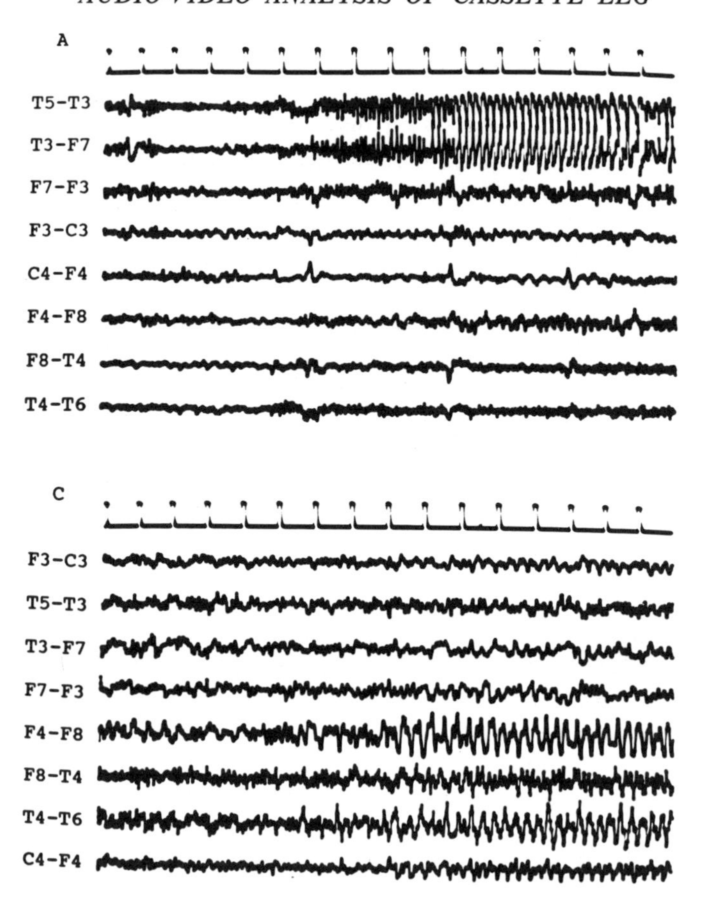

FIG. 4. Electrographic patterns of two lateralized seizure discharges, which accompanied clinical complex partial seizures, are illustrated in **A, B** and **C, D,** respectively. Note the progressive evolution in the frequency and amplitude of the seizure rhythm.

of a recording is to identify seizures, the review protocol can be simplified. Analysis can proceed from beginning to end at the fastest replay speed through wakefulness and sleep without interruption.

RHYTHMIC ARTIFACTS THAT MIMIC SEIZURES

Artifacts must be rhythmic to be confused with seizures. These are predominantly generated by any of a variety of repetitive movements. As such, they occur and confound interpretation only during active wakefulness. The movements either create their own electrical signals, such as physiologic artifacts, or they cause a disturbance of the electrode-scalp interface. In some

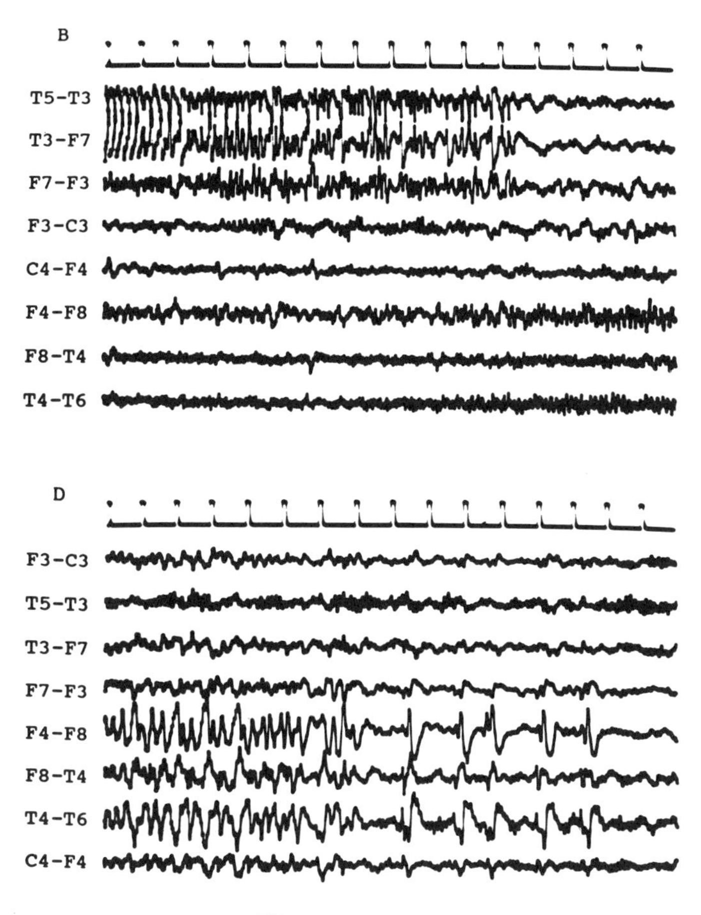

FIG. 4. *(continued).*

instances, seizure-like artifacts can actually be broadcasted to the electrodes from the source of an electromagnetic field.

A common example of physiologic artifacts is eye movements. Eye flutter, in particular, can mimic the rhythmic discharge of a seizure (Fig. 5). Other artifacts in this category include chewing or other activity associated with repeated contraction of facial or cranial muscles. Nonphysiologic artifacts are typified by rubbing, scratching, or shaking the head, thus rhythmically disturbing the electrode disk or leads. Depending on the vigor of the rub, such artifact may involve one or several electrode sites and, thus, channels. Some rhythmic artifacts are created in unlikely circumstances, such as toothbrushing. Not only is there rhythmic arm and head movement, but often there is rhythmic eye movement compensating for head bobbing while maintaining a fixed stare into a mirror.

Some artifacts, such as chewing and toothbrushing, are so common that they

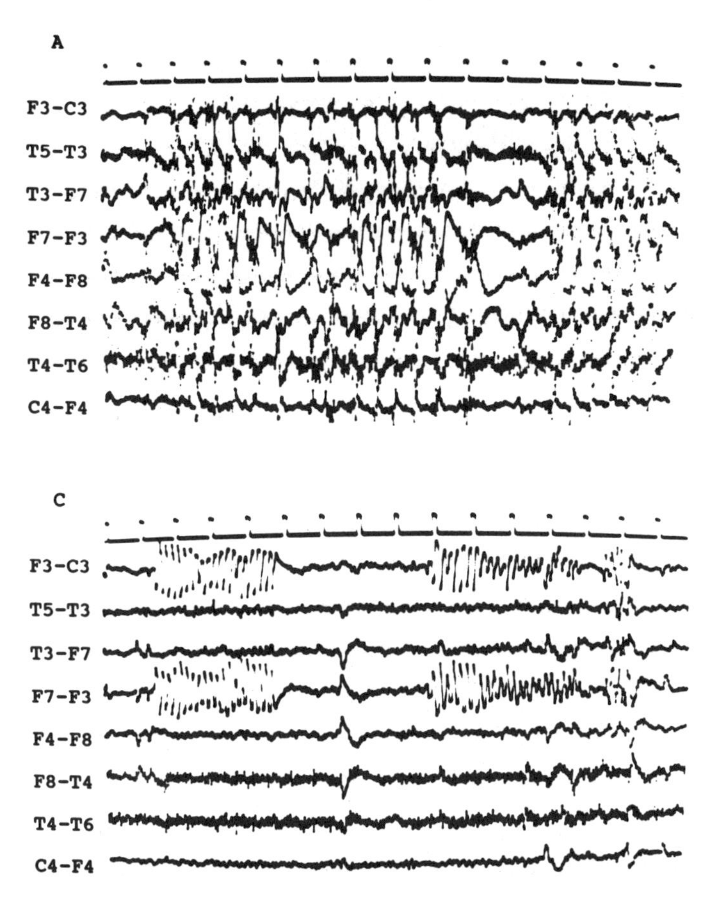

FIG. 5. Rhythmic artifacts that may mimic seizure discharges. **A:** Chewing. **B:** Eye flutter. **C:** Focal rubbing. **D:** External artifact of unknown source. Note in each example one or more typical artifact characteristics (monotonic, no progressive evolution, interrupted, nonphysiologic distribution).

soon become readily identifiable. Other forms of rhythmic movement may be encountered rarely, and a specific cause cannot be ascertained. For example, it took several months and repeated occurrences with accurate diaries to conclude that the unknown rhythmic activity seen in ICU recordings was from postural drainage percussions of the patient's chest. It is, however, not necessary to know what caused every artifact, as long as it is recognized as such. Rhythmic discharges that fail to meet the criteria for true ictal events and occur during active wakefulness, even though seizure-like, should be considered artifact until proved otherwise.

Signals broadcast from electrical appliances used by patients can cause bizarre artifacts. Electric shavers and toothbrushes, hair dryers, even water beds with faulty electric heaters have been documented as the offending agent. These types

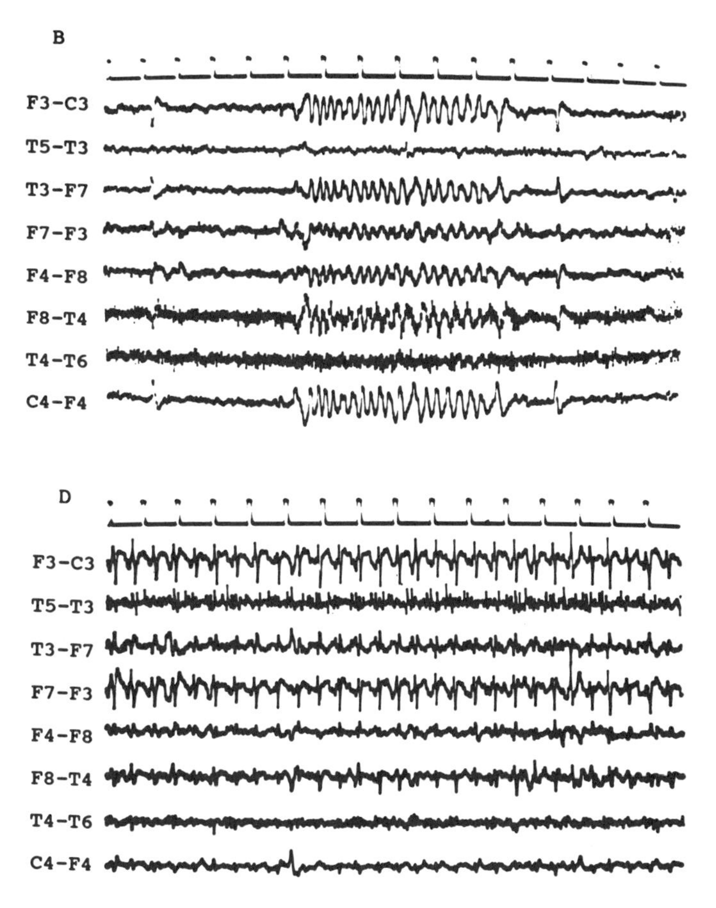

FIG. 5. (*continued*).

of artifact are particularly prominent toward the end of a recording, when electrode impedances grow higher and mismatched.

It is the job of the ambulatory EEG reader to use a variety of information, as well as context, to differentiate artifact from true seizures. Although the experienced observer cannot always distinguish between the two with certainty, certain guidelines are, however, useful in this effort. Both seizures and rhythmic artifacts produce tones as an audio output. It is this feature that sets them apart from the otherwise random white noise of active wakefulness. Seizures, other than spike-wave absences, usually evolve in an orderly progression, as noted above. The usual sequence from low-voltage faster to high-voltage slower activity is not invariable, but there is almost always a progression.

Fortunately, this is not true for many rhythmic artifacts. Typically, they begin abruptly and have a rather monotonic frequency, which yields a single pitched sound. Commonly, a buzzing quality, like a flying insect, is perceived aurally.

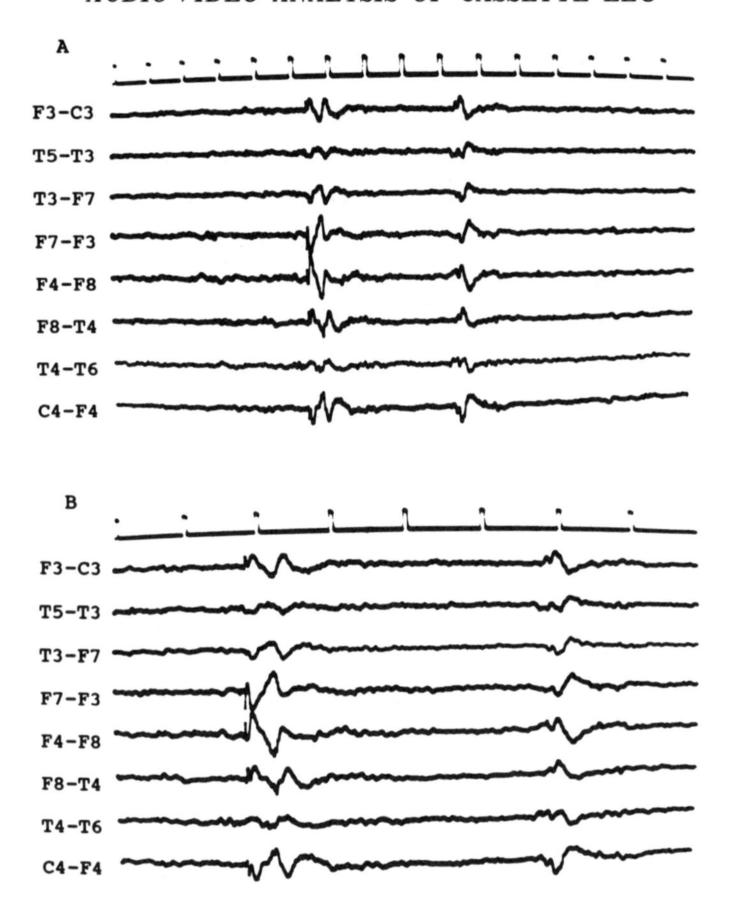

FIG. 6. An isolated, bilateral spike-wave is shown followed by a vertex sharp wave in a 16- and 8-sec page in **A** and **B,** respectively. Isolated spike-wave discharges and vertex sharp waves of sleep may look nearly identical, except for the early spike component, which is visually easier to identify on an 8-sec page.

Often, the artifactual discharge, and, thus, its sound, is interrupted with brief cessations. Seizures seldom, if ever, do this. Multiple seizures can occur in a row, but each typically has an entire frequency-amplitude progression.

In addition to auditory analysis, visual analysis can be of help. Many, but not all, artifacts have a nonphysiologic field and affect only one or two electrodes on a hemisphere. This is highly uncharacteristic of all but the most focal seizures. Eye flutter, for example, produces a frontal pattern that may look like a generalized seizure, except that little of this activity is evident in the more posterior channels, which would not be the case in a genuine generalized ictus.

Sometimes, both auditory and visual analysis fail to clarify the nature of an event. In such instances, context may be the last resort, although often a very useful one. Artifacts can mimic anything once or twice, but usually telltale signs are present before or after the event. Intermittent electrode artifacts, which gradually worsen prior to the discharge in question, can lead the reviewer to the correct conclusion, even though the event itself looks and sounds just like a seizure. This is one of the drawbacks to interpreting AEEG solely from printouts of events. Unless the primary reviewer was skilled enough to notice the preceding or following artifacts, the event out of context may be indistinguishable from a seizure. I have personally reviewed AEEG records as a second opinion in which the printout provided me looked exactly like ictal discharge, yet an analysis of the tape clearly showed artifact development in the same channels that would eventually be involved in the supposed seizure.

Other signs that are associated with a seizure or epilepsy should be sought to help verify the ictal nature of a suspicious discharge. Is there appropriate postictal slowing following the event? This is almost always present following generalized convulsive seizures and many, but not all, partial seizures. Are there interictal abnormalities in other portions of the record that are consistent with the supposed seizure? A left temporal spike focus during sleep would substantially strengthen a provisional diagnosis of seizure for a suspicious left hemisphere discharge. Is there slowing of background rhythms from the region of a supposed seizure, as is often the case with underlying structural lesions? Finally, and very importantly, does the patient, family, or an observer report that the patient had a seizure at this time? Activities producing artifacts are commonly not reported, whereas most seizures, other than absence, are noted. A suspicious discharge during active wakefulness unaccompanied by a report of a seizure must be considered artifact until proved otherwise, particularly if there is no additional supportive evidence.

Seizures out of sleep or subclinical seizures during sleep may not be noted by the patient or observed by others. However, the rhythmic artifacts that mimic seizures do not occur at these times. A seizure-like discharge arising from an EEG background of sleep is most likely of physiologic and probably of cerebral origin. The reviewer's task here is to differentiate seizures from normal paroxysmal cerebral rhythms, such as those generated with arousal. Particularly in children, where it can be quite prominent, the arousal pattern can be confused with ictal discharge, since it, too, is comprised of a progression of frequencies. Context is usually the major discriminant factor, since there are no supportive reports of a clinical seizure and seldom unrelated interictal findings. Awakening or a return to normal sleep patterns is the usual outcome of these events rather than an EEG depression with postictal slowing.

INTERICTAL EPILEPTIFORM TRANSIENTS

As noted earlier in this chapter, the profusion of sharp transient artifacts during active wakefulness makes it difficult to identify interictal features during this time unless they are prominent and occur frequently enough to be seen

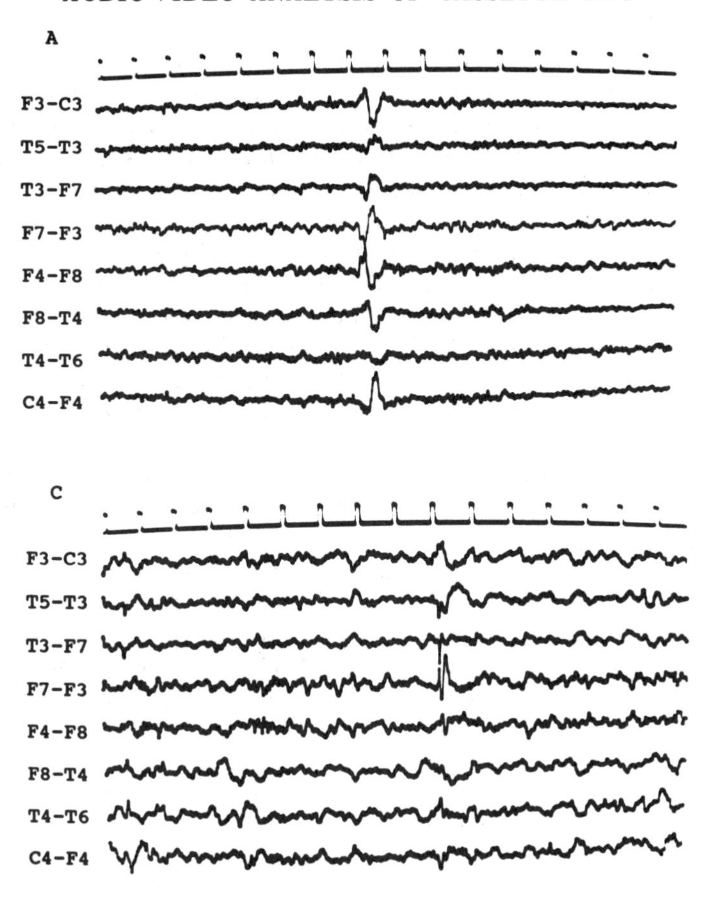

FIG. 7. The left frontotemporal spike embedded in a vertex sharp wave **(B)** is difficult to distinguish from a normal vertex sharp wave **(A).** When seen in isolation **(C),** the spike and the asymmetry between the top and bottom channels produced by it are more apparent. A less-common, posterior temporal spike burst is depicted in **D.**

during occasional periods of quiet during the day. In general, interictal features should be sought during drowsiness, daytime naps, and particularly overnight sleep. At these times, muscle and movement artifacts are minimal, and the problem of differentiation becomes one of distinguishing epileptiform spikes or sharp waves from the normal sharp transients of sleep or the occasional electrode "pop" artifact.

Sleep transients, such as vertex sharp waves or K-complexes, are principally symmetrical in their distribution over the two hemispheres and predominantly frontocentral in location (Figs. 6 and 7). They may be somewhat asymmetrical from time to time, but they are seldom persistently lateralized, unless they reflect an underlying pathologic process or a breech rhythm. Generalized epileptiform discharges of the spike-wave or polyspike-wave type also have

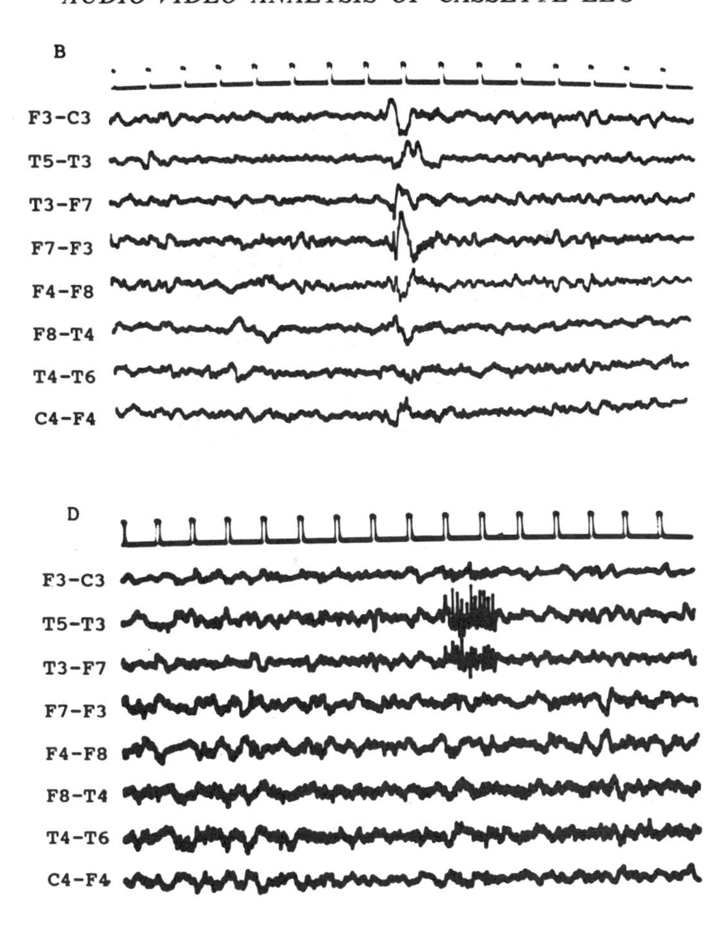

FIG. 7. *(continued)*.

symmetrical fields across the scalp. In fact, the slow waves associated with the spikes are virtually indistinguishable from vertex sharp waves in cassette EEG montages. Differentiation between the two comes not from distribution or symmetry, but from the presence of frank spikes or polyspikes preceding the slow waves (Fig. 6). These can be seen on visual inspection, but they also can be heard on dynamic review as a distinct "snap" or "pop" associated with the usual "thud" of the slow wave. With experience, isolated spike-wave discharges can be distinguished by sound alone from vertex sharp waves, the morphology of which is nearly identical except for the spike.

Spikes, i.e., transients of less than 80-msec duration, can almost always be heard on rapid review, if their amplitude is at least equal to that of background activity. Some sharp waves can also be heard, although as expected from their duration, the sound is duller and less distinctive, unless several occur in succession. Sharp waves of relatively long duration are usually not audible,

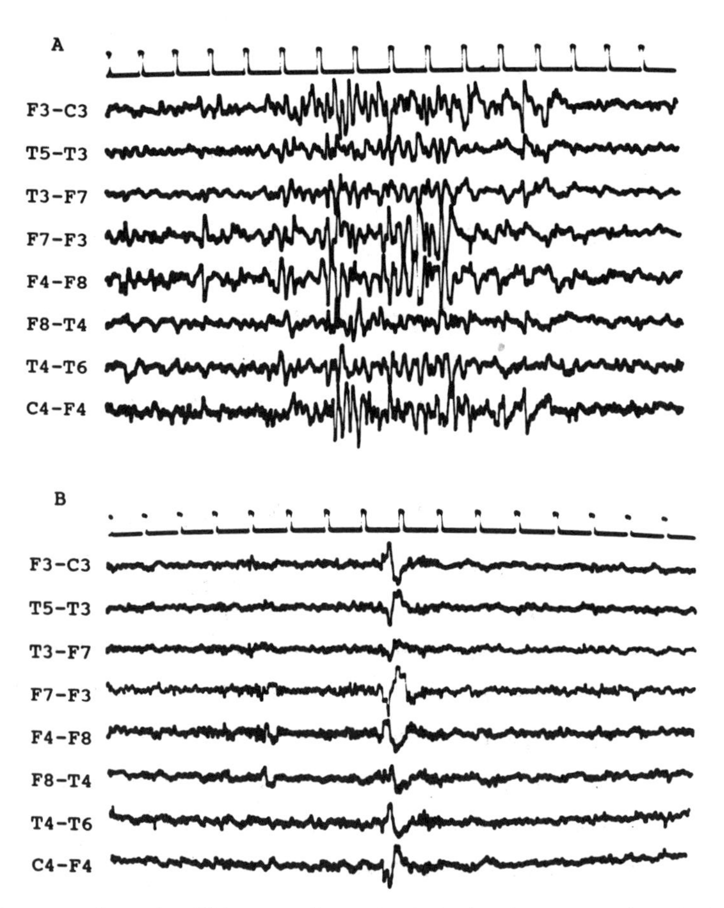

FIG. 8. Sleep complexes in children can be protracted, sharply contoured, and of high amplitude **(A)**, compared with those of the adult **(B)**. Their symmetrical nature and lack of definite spikes distinguish them from epileptiform discharges of partial or generalized epilepsy, respectively.

particularly at the slower scanning speed of 20× that is most useful when visually searching for interictal transients. Therefore, it is unwise to depend solely on auditory cues for the recognition of epileptiform transients. Some will be heard, but others will not. Reliance on visual identification is the more prudent and productive approach.

Interictal features of the partial epilepsies are usually lateralized, whether they are unilateral or bilateral, dependent or independent. Most often, they arise from the frontotemporal areas of the head. A retrospective review of epileptiform abnormalities among patients evaluated in our epilepsy center noted that this latter location was the most common site for all but the generalized discharges (10). The montages discussed in Chapter 4 exploit to advantage the normal distribution of sleep and focal epileptiform features by displaying the EEG in a way that accentuates any asymmetrical event. Most sleep complexes produce a pattern with mirror-image symmetry, whereas lateralized features stand out in contrast. Linked channels that pass through the frontotemporal region, rather than ending there, give these focal events a phase reversal on video display, which helps them stand out even more from the background (Fig. 7). To be considered as a possible epileptiform abnormality, lateralized sharp complexes should have a physiologic field distribution over several electrodes and should be seen in isolation and repetitively during sleep.

Certain normal transients of drowsiness or light sleep may also be lateralized, even though they seldom persist. Small sharp spikes or benign epileptiform transients of sleep are monophasic or simple biphasic events of short duration that are mostly seen during drowsiness. Typically, they wander in location and disappear with deeper sleep. Certain benign rhythmic variants may also be lateralized, such as psychomotor variant, 6-Hz phantom spike and wave, wicket spikes, 14- and 6-Hz positive spikes. These can usually be differentiated from epileptiform transients by their morphology, frequency, and lack of stability in deeper sleep states. Most of these appear in rhythmic runs, have a frequency greater than 5 Hz, and also disappear in Stages 2 through 4 of sleep. Lateralized interictal discharges, on the other hand, seldom have a frequency greater than 5 Hz, and they usually persist or are more evident in Stages 2 and 3 of sleep.

An exception to the 5-Hz frequency rule is bursts of interictal spikes from the posterior temporal region. We have observed several cases of rapid spike complexes in the EEG of patients with complex partial epilepsy. In each instance, the field maxima of these discharges was posterior temporal (Fig. 7), although most of the patients also had more typical anterior temporal transients.

Electrode pops or related artifacts also occur during sleep. They are usually distinguished by their distribution to one electrode and also by their polarity, which is commonly positive or alternatively positive and negative. Increased background noise and high-frequency interference are usually also seen in the same channels. Electrode artifacts of all types and an increased susceptibility to extraneous signals are more typical of the latter half of the recording, when the electrode impedances increase or become mismatched.

The sleep complexes of children must be interpreted with caution. To the reviewer unaccustomed to pediatric EEGs, the vertex sharp waves and K-complexes of children can look particularly sharp and epileptiform (Fig. 8). They are often of long duration and contain high-frequency, spike-like activity. In these cases it is advisable to identify any supposed abnormal spikes in isolation or in sleep stages that do not normally contain abundant vertex activity, such as Stage 1 or REM, or in quiet wakefulness, before considering them frankly epileptiform.

This is not to say that epileptiform transients do not normally associate with sleep complexes. Quite the contrary, interictal transients of partial, as well as generalized, epilepsy commonly lead into a vertex sharp wave or K-complex. This produces an asymmetrical sleep complex, which is the clue to its abnormality (Fig. 7). This association is variable and intermittent, however. Sharp waves or spikes should be seen unaccompanied by sleep complexes before concluding that they are abnormal.

REVIEW OF CASSETTE EEG WRITEOUTS

Writeout of the cassette EEG onto paper can enhance or clarify features of interest. Adjustments in the filter or gain settings of the transcribing EEG machine can produce changes in the EEG signals that are additional to those of the replay unit. A small waveform may be made even larger or more filtering may be employed to extract the EEG from artifact, for example. Seizures can be played out at a slow paper speed to gain additional temporal compression that makes slowly evolving features more evident. With some manipulations of the output of the replay unit, different montages can be created by directing various cassette EEG channels into separate grids of each polygraph channel. The potential advantages and disadvantages of this latter maneuver are discussed in Chapter 4.

Writeout of cassette EEG onto paper can also confuse the practitioner or provide him with insufficient information to make an accurate interpretation. Many neurology or psychiatry practices do not have the patient volume or physician manpower to support cassette EEG analysis locally. Recordings are sent to a scanning service for analysis. In other practices or medical centers, the tape is reviewed by the technologist, who then transcribes pertinent sections onto paper. In either case, the final interpretation is based on hard-copy epochs of EEG, which supposedly contain all or at least a representative sample of the abnormalities present in the recording. Obviously EEG interpretation performed in this fashion can be no better than the data provided.

Interpretation of cassette EEGs solely from paper writeouts has inherent disadvantages, as alluded to previously. Abnormalities that are overlooked by the primary reviewer are an obvious problem. In practice, this is usually not a major factor, since the natural tendency for those who do not have the final responsibility of interpretation is to overread the record and provide samples of even very questionable findings. Regardless, without access to the entire record, interpretation can be difficult. Since artifact can mimic nearly any abnormality for a short time, erroneous conclusions can be reached when the events preceding or following the supposed abnormality are not known to the second reviewer. Whenever possible, it is advisable that the physician making the final interpretation have the capability of reviewing the original data himself or of quickly getting more data if need be.

Since such ideal situations do not always exist and many physicians by necessity or by choice interpret cassette EEGs from printout alone, guidelines may be helpful. Included in the printouts should be an example of every feature that requires comment, including segments of background rhythms and sleep. In particular, any supposed seizure should be written out in its entirety with adequate segments before and after the event to enable the interpreter to assess possible artifactual origins and postictal slowing or epileptiform transients. Multiple examples of interictal spikes or sharp waves should be provided, and some, if not most, of them should be taken from quiet wakefulness or sleep. If the only sharp transients provided for interpretation are intermixed with muscle and movement artifact of active wakefulness, they must be interpreted with caution. Calibration signals, gain and filter settings, and the time of each epoch should be included. A segment of EEG from the end of the recording will show the interpreter which, if any, electrodes or channels were eventually lost or developed artifacts. This may help in understanding an earlier event.

When in doubt about a cassette EEG review performed by an outside concern, seek a second opinion. Send the record to another scanning service or center that routinely analyzes tapes. The second opinion should be based on actual review of the tape and not just the hard copy. Another person can seldom do better from the same confusing segments of printout, particularly when the question is seizure versus artifact.

ROLE OF THE AEEG TECHNOLOGIST

The role of the technologist in the analysis of cassette EEGs varies considerably. In some university centers, there are enough clinical neurophysiology staff, including fellows, that all review and interpretation is done by electroencephalographers. There are other centers or practices in which this is not practical, and most, if not all, of the initial reviewing is performed by the technologist.

It is my opinion that training and experience in cassette EEG review are more important than academic degrees or position in this regard. The person best suited for the job may not even be the one with the most experience in reading traditional EEGs. The role of the primary reviewer is critical, since further analysis and interpretation rely on the data that were provided. The EEG technologist who circles transients of interest or who flags pages that contain possible abnormalities is serving this function in the traditional laboratory EEG setting. Data reduction of this type is worthwhile, so long as that person is competent and the final reviewer does not become complacent and relinquish de facto the responsibility of interpretation.

The primary reviewer must have adequate training in EEG analysis and particularly in cassette EEG analysis. It is perfectly reasonable that this person be the technologist, if he does not object to the additional responsibility. It is unwise and unfair to force this responsibility on a technologist who has not been trained for it or who does not wish it. In such situations, the physician is only deluding himself that quality information is being obtained.

In practice, it is advisable for a registered or senior technologist to undertake cassette EEG review, since this person would have more training and experience. Most commercial scanning services employ only registered EEG technicians for their staff. Although this assures a certain level of competency in routine EEG, this alone is not enough to ensure the quality of cassette EEG analysis. Proper training and sufficient experience are essential. New or unproved scanning services should be critically assessed in regard to personnel and supervision.

SPECIAL ANALYSES

Audio-video scanning techniques are applicable to quantitative, as well as qualitative, analysis of cassette EEG. In terms of epilepsy evaluation, this usually means counting the number or measuring the frequency or duration of epileptiform discharges. Convulsive seizures rarely recur often enough to demand innumeration by EEG, rather than by observation, and quantification of isolated spikes or sharp waves has not proved to be worthwhile prognostically in terms of seizure control.

Absence seizures, other primary generalized nonconvulsive seizures, and associated spike-wave or polyspike-wave bursts can occur multiple times per day or per hour and are difficult to quantitate clinically. As noted in earlier discussion, these discharges are easily discerned even on rapid review of the tape. Not only is it technically feasible to count spike-wave paroxysms; there is also a good correlation between number and duration of discharges and seizure control. Antiepileptic medications, therefore, can be titrated for an individual patient by analysis of his EEG. Cassette EEG can easily obtain the long-term EEG sampling necessary to provide an accurate account of drug efficacy.

The simplest form of discharge quantification consists of identifying bursts of spike wave on rapid review and compiling their number on a note pad. More sophisticated analyses may include the number of bursts within several ranges of durations, the total number of seconds of spike-wave activity per unit time, and/or their temporal distribution over the course of 24 hr. These tasks become increasingly cumbersome for manual record keeping; however, newer versions of the Oxford Medilog replay unit offer an event-logging feature, which compiles such data in computer memory within the replay unit. Once paroxysms are found on standard AV review, their beginning and end are noted by pressing a log button when the screen cursor is at these positions. For each such discharge, the computer retains its length in seconds and time of occurrence. After all bursts are entered, the replay unit can provide all the above-mentioned statistics via a dot-matrix printer. Quite detailed analyses of spike-wave activity can be performed in this manner.

Computer programs that recognize epileptiform transients and ictal discharges have become progressively sophisticated. This methodology, which is reviewed in Chapter 6, can now be used to identify and quantitate certain abnormal patterns in ambulatory EEG recordings. Quantitation of EEG and other physiologic data from cassette tape recordings is also standard practice in the evaluation of sleep and sleep disorders. These analyses are discussed in Chapters 15 and 16.

REFERENCES

1. American Electroencephalographic Society. Guidelines for long-term neurodiagnostic monitoring in epilepsy. *J Clin Neurophysiol* 1986;3:93–126.
2. Ebersole JS, Bridgers SL. Direct comparison of 3 and 8-channel ambulatory cassette EEG with intensive inpatient monitoring. *Neurology (Cleve)* 1985;35:846–854.
3. Ebersole JS. Ambulatory EEG monitoring. In: Aminoff MJ, ed. *Electrodiagnosis in clinical neurology.* New York: Churchill Livingstone, 1986;125–148.
4. Ebersole JS, Bridgers SL. Ambulatory EEG monitoring. In: Pedley TA, Meldrum BS, eds. *Recent advances in epilepsy, vol 3.* Edinburgh: Churchill Livingstone, 1986;111–135.
5. Ebersole JS, Leroy RF. An evaluation of ambulatory, cassette EEG monitoring. II. Detection of interictal abnormalities. *Neurology (Cleve)* 1983;33:8–18.
6. Ebersole JS, Bridgers SL, Silva CG. Differentiation of epileptiform abnormalities from normal transients and artifacts on ambulatory cassette EEG. *Am J EEG Technol* 1983;23:113–125.
7. Goodin DS, Aminoff MJ. Does the interictal EEG have a role in the diagnosis of epilepsy? *Lancet* 1984;1:837–839.
8. Ebersole JS, Leroy RF. Evaluation of ambulatory cassette EEG monitoring. III. Diagnostic accuracy compared to intensive inpatient EEG monitoring. *Neurology (Cleve)* 1983;33:853–860.
9. Bridgers SL, Ebersole JS. The clinical utility of ambulatory cassette EEG. *Neurology (Cleve)* 1985;35:166–173.
10. Leroy RF, Ebersole JS. An evaluation of ambulatory, cassette EEG monitoring. I. Montage design. *Neurology (Cleve)* 1983;33:1–7.

Ambulatory EEG Monitoring,
edited by John S. Ebersole.
Raven Press, Ltd., New York © 1989

6

Automated Analysis of Ambulatory EEG Recordings

Jean Gotman

Montreal Neurological Institute and Department of Neurology and Neurosurgery, McGill University, Montreal, Quebec H3A 2B4 Canada

Ambulatory EEG monitoring allows the recording of EEGs over one or several days. If a 24-hr recording had to be reviewed by traditional means, after replay on paper, it would be an extremely tedious task. This problem has been solved in practice by fast review on a CRT, a convenient and sufficient procedure in most cases. Automated analysis could, however, bring a number of advantages, particularly if used in conjunction with fast visual review. Its advantages are in three areas: automatic detection of infrequent events, quantification of events or background activity, and automatic classification of patterns.

Automatic event detection is particularly valuable, since ambulatory monitoring is mainly used to capture rare and unpredictable events, most often in relation to epilepsy. The automatic detection of events of interest could speed up considerably the review and possibly avoid missing small events, a distinct possibility with fast-review systems. Reliance on an automatic detection system could only take place with an automatic method having a very low rate of false-negative errors (a low probability of missing events).

Quantification of events, such as bursts of spike and wave, or quantification of the background activity is most often not necessary in routine clinical practice. It is necessary in most research applications and helpful in selected clinical situations. It is particularly valuable when measuring the effect of medical treatment. When events are infrequent, quantification can easily be performed visually; when they are frequent and changing in pattern, automated analysis can be helpful.

Finally, automated analysis allows the classification of patterns, a procedure used mostly for sleep staging. Automatic sleep staging can be of great assistance both for clinical practice, since it lightens the burden of visual sleep staging, and for research applications, since it always provides quantified data.

Reviews of automatic EEG analysis methods in epilepsy have been written by Gotman (1–3), Frost (4), Principe and Smith (5), and Ktonas (6). Automatic methods in sleep analysis are reviewed by Smith (7). These are general reviews, not specific to the problems of ambulatory monitoring.

Despite the availability of inexpensive but powerful computers and despite the publication of several methods of automatic analysis showing promising performance, automated analysis has remained absent from the large majority of centers using ambulatory monitoring. In reviewing the different approaches to automated analysis, we shall attempt to identify the factors that have prevented a greater success and those that show a potential for future usefulness. One of the most important difficulties is the problem of artifacts, which are particularly prominent in ambulatory recordings.

DIFFERENT APPROACHES TO AUTOMATED ANALYSIS

There are different practical approaches to automated analysis of ambulatory recordings (Fig. 1); the final purpose of the analysis may be a critical factor in deciding which approach is better, but equally important in this decision is the choice of technology and the cost of equipment. Three broad categories can be distinguished:

1. The automatic analysis equipment, or part of it, may be carried with the portable recording equipment in such a way that the EEG is analyzed on line, before the recording on tape or simultaneously with it (Fig. 1A). This is possible with miniaturized battery-operated electronic components. Computing power is not as great as with a standard computer but is nevertheless significant and will improve rapidly in the future. With this method, results are available during the recording itself.
2. A continuous EEG may be recorded on the cassette and subsequently played back at high speed, as during visual review, into a computer that performs the analysis on line (Fig. 1B). The computer must be powerful or the analysis method simple, since the EEG is played back at high speed and thus little computer time is available for analysis. With this procedure, results of analysis are available immediately at the end of the fast-replay procedure.
3. The above method may be modified so that the cassette is played back at high speed into a computer, but the EEG is simply stored on the computer disk and only subsequently analyzed (off-line analysis, Fig. 1C). This subsequent analysis is freed from the time constraint of on-line analysis and can, therefore, be more complex and sophisticated. This method has the disadvantage that results are only available after the analysis is completed, which can be several hours after the end of replay if a 24-hr recording was analyzed.

It can easily be appreciated that convenience and sophistication of analysis are often in opposition. We will describe below the various methods that have been published for automated analysis of ambulatory recordings, stating for each the

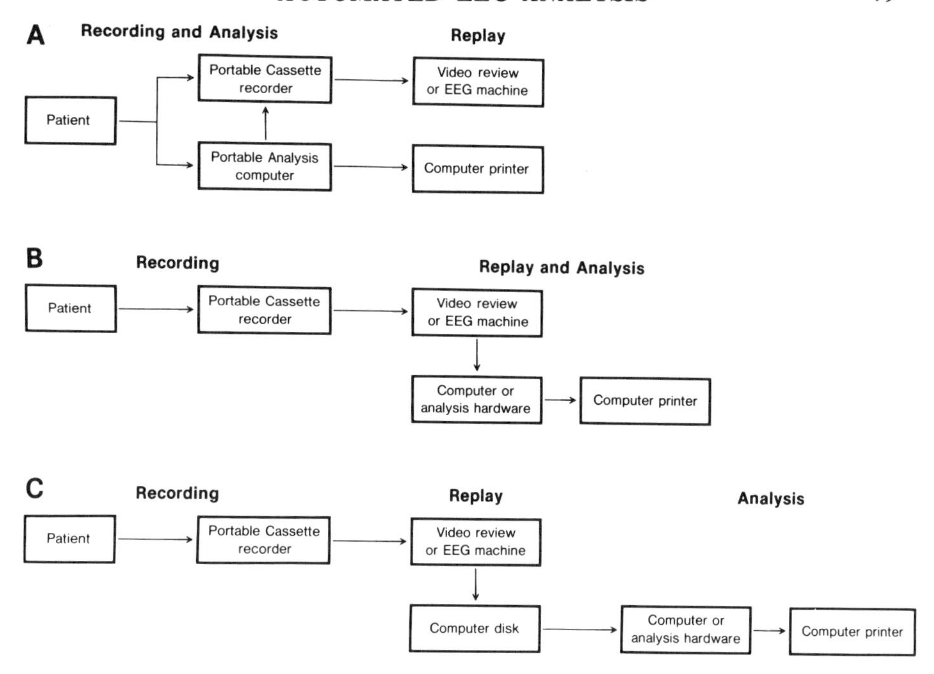

FIG. 1. Schematic representation of the three types of implementation in the automatic analysis of ambulatory recordings. **A:** Analysis equipment is carried by the subject and analysis proceeds on line. **B:** Analysis is performed on replay of the recorded data, replay usually taking place at high speed. **C:** Recorded data are first dumped on a computer disk and subsequently analyzed off line.

type of approach that has been taken. The most common methods relate to the automatic detection of spike-and-wave bursts. Methods for automatic sleep staging have also been implemented. As well as the methods themselves, we will describe the problems related to the validation of automatic methods: How can it be decided whether a method performs adequately?

AUTOMATIC DETECTION OF SPIKE-AND-WAVE BURSTS

The ideal 3/sec spike-and-wave burst found in many patients with absence attacks is a very distinctive pattern: as such, it has long tempted those interested in automatic-detection analysis. This is of particular interest in ambulatory cassette recordings, since the reason for recording is often to determine whether spike-and-wave bursts are present, or to determine the frequency of their occurrence. Most methods rely on the detection of spikes and of slow waves, and on some criterion for alternation of the two patterns at an appropriate repetition rate. Methods must, however, be very flexible, because most bursts of spike and wave seen in clinical practice have patterns that little resemble the classic example: Bursts are often slow and irregular; the spike component is not always clearly present or is present in the form of polyspikes, as during sleep. A system that could only detect ideal 3/sec bursts would be of limited practical utility. Examples of the variety of patterns that are encountered are shown on Figs. 2 and 3.

Methods Not Specifically Designed for Ambulatory Monitoring

Carrie and Frost (8) describe a method that first performs spike detection, relying on the computation of the second derivative, followed by slow-wave detection, relying on the duration between baseline crossings. The second derivative measures sharpness and is frequently used to detect spikes; duration between baseline crossings or between wave extrema is often used to measure wave duration. Carrie and Frost also included a special procedure for the rejection of EMG bursts. Gevins et al. (9) analyzed four channels, detecting spikes, slow waves, and EMG waves; further requirements to declare the occurrence of a generalized burst were a minimum of spatial spread (appearance of the pattern in several channels), a certain degree of synchrony between homologous channels of the two hemispheres, and a minimum total duration. Principe and Smith (10) used a microprocessor to detect spikes and slow waves; they used a technique that has been used by many other investigators: Prior to examination of the time-domain characteristics of spikes and slow waves, they

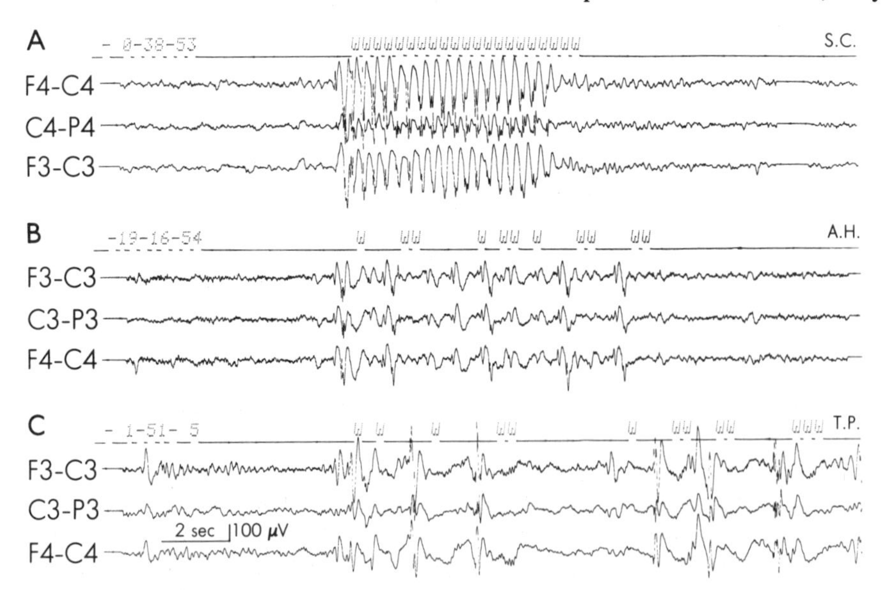

FIG. 2. Examples of variability in the spike-and-wave pattern. **A:** Typical 3/sec pattern; **B:** irregular slow burst; **C:** polyspikes and slow waves during sleep. This illustrates the difficulty in designing systems capable of detecting such a variety of patterns. (From Koffler and Gotman, ref. 16.)

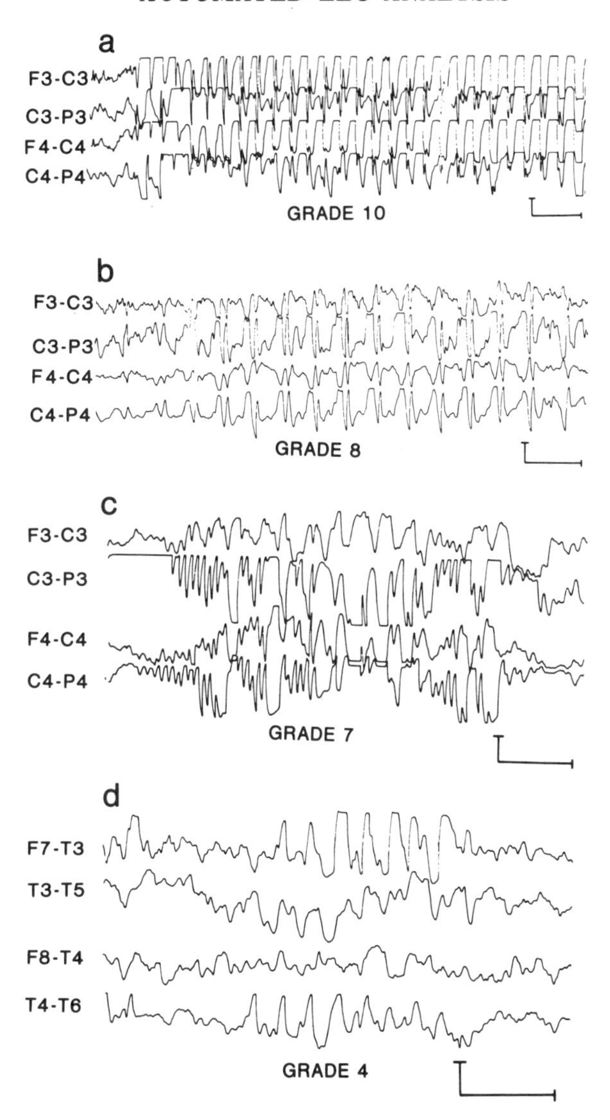

FIG. 3. Examples of different grades of detection of spike-and-wave bursts (from Jayakar, ref. 15). In this method, bursts were not only detected, but also graded with respect to their likelihood of being genuine epileptiform activity.

removed, by filtering, frequencies that are not helpful in the discrimination between these patterns and other EEG activity. In this case, the filtering was digital (done by software in the computer). Others have used analog prefiltering: Quy et al. (11) used a 2- to 4-Hz filter to extract slow waves and a 12- to 18-Hz filter to extract spikes. Analog filtering has the advantage of being able, when properly adjusted, to analyze signals replayed at speeds much higher than real time. Therefore, it is well suited for the analysis of ambulatory recordings at high speed. It can have the disadvantage of distorting the original signal by creating a phase shift at some frequencies.

Methods Specifically Aimed at Ambulatory Monitoring

Whisler et al. (12) presented a device that could be carried by a patient: Using analog filters and a sophisticated detection logic, it performed automatic detection of bursts using two channels for spike recognition and four channels for slow-wave recognition. The system was not actually tested as a portable device but could conceivably be used in conjunction with a portable cassette recorder; in such a situation, results of the analysis would be available immediately at the end of the monitoring session.

Burr and Stefan (13) developed a program allowing replay of a cassette recording into a computer at 20 times the recording speed; automatic analysis was done on line in such a way that sections of EEG in which a detection took place were retained on the computer disk for subsequent visual validation or editing on the computer terminal. Because of the 20-times speed-up factor, only one channel could be analyzed using a PDP-11/73 computer. In this case, results of analysis were available immediately after a replay at 20 times recording speed. Another approach was taken by Mony and Pasquier (14), who used analog equipment and were able to analyze cassette recordings at 60 times the recording speed; although they were mostly interested in analyzing background activity, their system also included a simple detection of epileptiform transients.

Jayakar (15) developed a sophisticated computer program for the automatic detection of bursts of spike and wave in cassette recordings. The system was not fully implemented for the analysis directly from cassette recordings; selected EEG sections from cassettes were digitized and used for developing and testing the algorithms. The method makes use of time-domain descriptors of the EEG, such as duration and sharpness of waves; it takes into account 1 min of context, thus putting more weight on events that are different from the context in which they take place. Rather than providing "yes-no" answers, the system provides results that are graded according to the probability that a detection is truly epileptiform (Fig. 3). Koffler and Gotman (16) developed a software system in which a cassette recording was played back at 20 times the recording speed, stored on a computer disk, and subsequently analyzed off line. The algorithm involved the detection of temporally and spatially correlated groups of spikes or sharp waves; it allowed the detection of very irregular spike-and-wave patterns (Fig. 2). The off-line analysis presents the advantage of being able to use complex detection algorithms and the disadvantage of making results available only some time after replay (it took 6 hr to analyze a 24-hr 3-channel cassette recording). During that time, however, the computer could be unattended (it could, for instance, do the analysis at night). With this system, automatic detection of isolated interictal spikes (17) and seizures not consisting of spike-wave bursts (18) could also be performed.

Performance of Spike-and-Wave Detection Methods

In describing methods of detection, no mention was made of how well, or poorly, they performed. There are two difficulties linked with the evaluation of performance: The first is that, in order to evaluate a method, one should be able to decide with certainty what is to be detected and what is to be ignored, a decision that is not as simple as might be expected. The second is that different authors use different sets of data and different measures of performance; therefore, results are not always comparable.

The problem of deciding what should and what should not be detected appears simple at first sight. In an artifact-free recording, a classic burst of spike and wave is easily classified as an event that must be detected; if, however, there are artifacts of uncertain origin, if the burst pattern is not so clear, or if both take place, then it is not obvious which events should be classified as those that must be detected. Two electroencephalographers may have different opinions in this respect. What should the automatic method detect? This problem has been encountered in every evaluation procedure and has usually been solved by requiring that the automatic method detect at least bursts on which two or more interpreters are in agreement. What about false detections? How can it be decided that an event should *not* be detected? As for events that must be detected, interpreters often disagree. A common method is to consider as false detections those for which all interpreters agree that they are not bursts of spike and wave; in other words, any event that could possibly be considered as a burst, even with great doubts, is not considered a false detection. These approaches for the definition of missed and false detections have been used by Koffler and Gotman (16) and Jayakar (15).

Even if authors use the same procedure for the evaluation of their methods, results are, unfortunately, still not comparable because the methods are evaluated with different sets of data. The same detection method can yield totally different results when applied to different recordings. Authors usually try to include realistic data, such as bursts of varying morphology, artifacts, and periods of wakefulness and sleep, but data sets and performance measures remain so different that comparisons can be meaningless. One example illustrates how the most commonly used performance measure can be misleading with different data sets: Recording A has 100 genuine bursts and recording B has 5 genuine bursts; both recordings last 24 hr. A method detects 95 of the 100 bursts and makes 50 false detections in recording A, for a total of 145 detections; it detects all 5 bursts and also makes 50 false detections in recording B, for a total of 55 detections. In recording A, 66% (95/145) of all detections were valid, and in recording B only 9% (5/55) were valid, whereas the performance is essentially the same in both cases. Rather than the percentage of detections that are valid, a measurement used by most authors, the measurement variables that should be used are the proportion of genuine bursts that were detected (95% in A and 100% in B) and the number of false detections per unit of time (50 per 24 hr in both recordings).

Until there are a standard set of data and a standard evaluation procedure, comparison of methods should be done with extreme caution. Results may be more likely influenced by the selection of data included in the testing set than by the method itself.

Artifacts

The problem of artifacts in ambulatory recordings is a serious one and is discussed elsewhere in this volume. The particular difficulties that automatic methods encounter because of artifacts are of interest here. Most artifacts are large-amplitude transient activity and methods aimed at detecting bursts of spike and wave are extremely vulnerable to such patterns (Fig. 4). In some cases, even the human interpreter has difficulty identifying artifacts with certainty; it should not be expected that an automatic method will make this distinction reliably. Each automatic method may be sensitive to different types of artifact, a reflection of the particular detection algorithm. Most methods have provisions for the handling of one or two particular types of artifact, usually at least transient EMG bursts. The proper handling of artifact is, at present, the major challenge for automatic methods: These methods are most often capable of detecting the large majority of genuine bursts but can make numerous false detections even for artifacts that appear obvious to the human observer. The major reason for this weakness is their inability to use a wide context, i.e., what happened in the EEG in the minutes and hours before and after the section currently analyzed. The human observer may, for instance, see that an electrode contact is becoming slowly worse, giving rise to more and more frequent transients; some may be totally different from spike-and-wave bursts, but some may resemble bursts. The observer will reject all of them, but the automatic analysis device will retain all those having a spike-and-wave morphology; no currently existing system has the ability to follow such a gradual change or to take into account what takes place even in the minutes surrounding the time of analysis. Automatic methods are also relatively poor at determining the spatial distribution of an EEG pattern, a factor often critical in distinguishing artifacts from epileptiform activity.

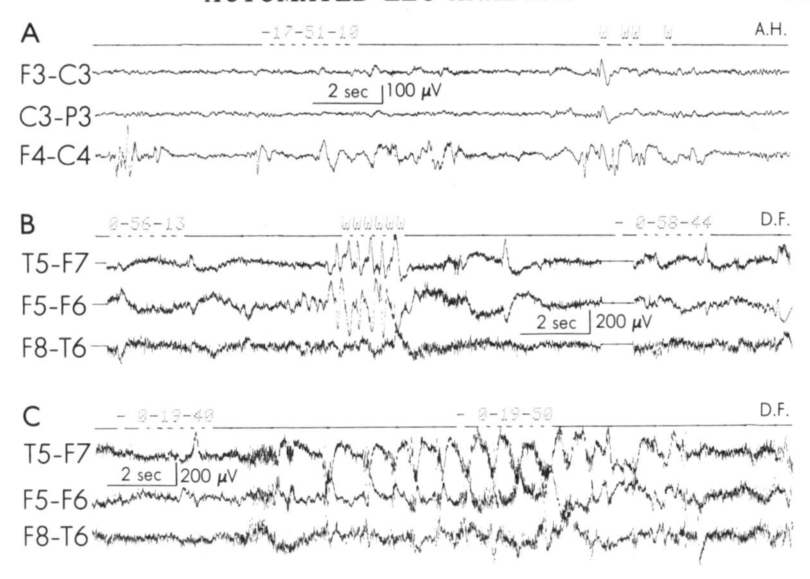

FIG. 4. A few examples of the numerous artifacts that resemble in some way a spike-and-wave pattern; automatic methods ideally should be able to identify them as artifacts. In the method of Koffler and Gotman (16) examples **A** and **B** were detected as bursts, but **C** was not.

Practical Use of Spike-Wave Detection

Given the above discussion, one may wonder whether there is any possible practical use of automatic detection methods. Automatic methods are used more and more frequently in long-term nonambulatory monitoring, typically cable telemetry recordings (19); in this situation, on-line analysis is adequate, and there is no advantage or need for analysis at 20 or 60 times the recording speed. Current computer systems can, therefore, adequately perform the on-line detection; they also make false detections because of artifacts and other transients. Nevertheless, they are useful as an assistant, because they are capable of rejecting, with reasonable accuracy, large sections of EEG that do not include epileptiform transients; in this way, they greatly shorten the time required to review long monitoring sessions.

Ambulatory monitoring devices are usually equipped with fast-review systems; this is the way by which the review time is shortened. Automatic methods could further reduce this time by eliminating large sections that, with a high probability, do not include bursts of spike and wave; this may amount to 90 or 95% of the recording. Suspicious sections must then be reviewed, and the observer must decide whether detections are valid. Such an assistance from automatic methods will become more and more useful as the number of channels in ambulatory recordings increases. This is due to the increasing difficulty of performing a fast review with a high number of channels: It is more difficult with eight than with four; review of a 16-channel recording at 60 or even 20 times the recording speed would be very difficult, particularly if one is interested in events that are not generalized.

AUTOMATIC SLEEP STAGING

An important use of portable EEG equipment is the recording of sleep outside the traditional hospital sleep laboratory, for instance, at home or in a familiar environment. Sleep staging is a long and tedious operation that, similarly to spike-and-wave detection, has been the object of many automation attempts. Their success has not been much greater, although there is, at present, a commercial device for automatic sleep staging of ambulatory cassette recordings. In many ways, sleep staging suffers from the same difficulties as spike-and-wave detection: It is difficult to use sophisticated algorithms when analysis has to proceed at 20 or 60 times the recording speed; there is a significant level of disagreement among sleep-staging experts, particularly when dealing with pathologic sleep; finally, the standard definition of sleep stages (20) is relatively well suited to visual interpretation but cannot be exactly imitated by automatic methods. It is, therefore, to be expected that results from automatic analysis and from visual analysis will differ to some extent.

A review of methods for automatic sleep staging and analysis of sleep data has been published recently (7); in that review, no mention is made of systems specifically designed for ambulatory recordings. To date, there are no articles describing a complete sleep-staging system for ambulatory recordings. Burr and Stefan (13) present the analysis of one channel from a cassette recording, with spike-and-wave detection and the calculation of a low-frequency index giving information on sleep; this is performed on a standard minicomputer. A commercial system (Medilog Sleep Stager, Oxford Instruments) uses special-purpose hardware and a microprocessor to perform sleep staging: It detects rapid eye movements, EMG levels, activity in the alpha and delta bands, spindles, and some artifacts and then assigns sections of recording to different stages according to criteria based on those of Rechtschaffen and Kales (20).

Three evaluations of this commercial system have been done. Crawford (21) compared automatic and traditional methods in 20 subjects and found a level of agreement varying between 74 and 89%; agreement was best in Stages 2 and 4 and worst in Stage 1 and REM, both being often mistaken for wakefulness.

Höller and Riemer (22) compared the automatic system to visual analysis in four recordings. They concluded that the automatically scored sleep onset time was always shorter in the automatic analysis; they attribute this to the difference in the definition of sleep onset, which is not the standard one in the machine; they also found that REM was sometimes mistakenly classified as wakefulness or Stage 1, particularly REM epochs not including eye movements. Nevertheless, they stress that all REM periods were detected by the automatic system. An example of the comparison between visual and automatic analysis is shown in Fig. 5.

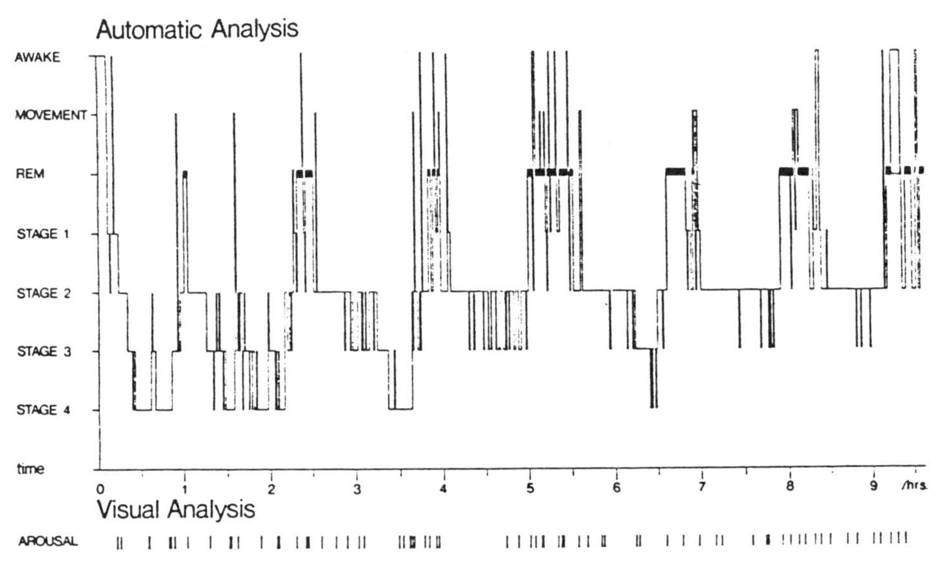

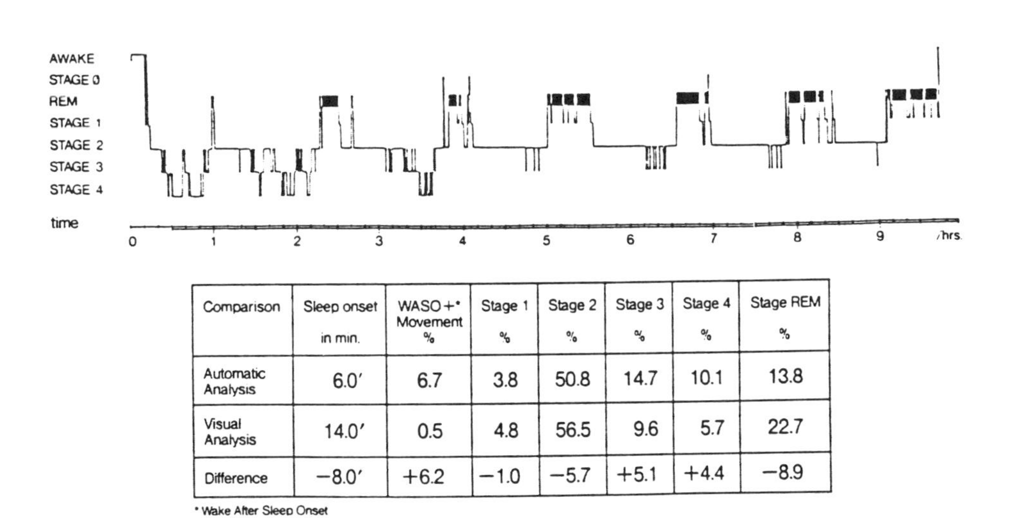

Comparison	Sleep onset in min.	WASO+* Movement %	Stage 1 %	Stage 2 %	Stage 3 %	Stage 4 %	Stage REM %
Automatic Analysis	6.0′	6.7	3.8	50.8	14.7	10.1	13.8
Visual Analysis	14.0′	0.5	4.8	56.5	9.6	5.7	22.7
Difference	−8.0′	+6.2	−1.0	−5.7	+5.1	+4.4	−8.9

* Wake After Sleep Onset

FIG. 5. Comparison of visual and automatic sleep staging. **Upper graph** is from automatic analysis and **lower graph** is from visual analysis. The automatic analysis preserves the basic cyclicity and detects all REM periods; it attributes too many epochs to Stages 3 and 4 and too few to Stages 1, 2, and REM. Not shown in the table is also excessive fragmentation (number of stage shifts) indicated by the automatic analysis when compared with visual scoring. (From Höller and Riemer, ref. 22.)

Ferri et al. (23) compared the automatic analysis to the classification of four tracings by nine groups of human readers. They stress that the variability between human readers was such that comparisons between automatic staging and only one or two readers can give results that may not be widely applicable. They underline one problem with the automatic system, as did Höller and Riemer (22): The starting point of the analysis cannot be determined with accuracy; this renders difficult the comparison with visual analysis and causes repeated automatic analyses of the same data to show slightly different results. Ferri et al. also found that the automatic scoring system tended to mix wakefulness, Stage 1, and REM and to give too high a number of stage shifts. They indicate that large errors in the determination of sleep-onset latency appear to have been partly corrected in a later version of the program.

It is clear that an automatic system cannot perform perfectly, since inter-reader differences preclude the definition of "perfection." A more modest role could be one similar to that discussed for the detection of epileptiform events: a system to assist in sleep staging. The system could offer its classification for rapid review, and the human interpreter could make corrections where he felt they were required. Another use of an automatic system could be in particular circumstances in which its validity has been established: If the object of study is the amount of Stages 3 and 4 during the night and if the automatic system has been shown to be effective for these factors, then it can be used safely.

Although it is important to compare systematically human interpretation to computer-analysis results, use of the automatic system should not necessarily be slaved to such a comparison: The computer can perform consistently its own classification, which may not be exactly the same as that performed by the human but which may have its own validity. It is not inconceivable that an alternate definition of sleep stages would be of an operational nature: Sleep stages could be defined as classes detected by a particular automatic-detection procedure. Such a classification is not necessarily more arbitrary than the traditional one; it would also lead to more consistent results than visual interpretation.

CONCLUSION

The preferred method for reviewing data from long-term ambulatory recordings is at present the fast visual-review system. It is an efficient system, particularly if recordings are limited to eight channels. It allows the easy detection of prominent epileptiform transients; sleep staging can also be performed. Computer-analysis methods have not reached the stage where they can replace visual review. We have discussed their abilities and weaknesses. At present, and for the near future, computer methods can be best used to assist in visual review rather than to replace it. During the past 20 years, ever since computer analysis has been applied to electroencephalography, a large effort has been made at developing methods that could replace the electroencephalographer and at comparing their performance to the human observer. The human analysis is an empirical process that has significant interindividual variability, and perfect agreement between man and machine analysis is, therefore, an elusive goal.

If the aim of computer analysis is restated in terms of assistance to visual analysis, then practical application is feasible. The complete review of a 24-hr recording for the identification of epileptiform events can be replaced by the selective review of sections marked as "possibly interesting" by the computer. These include true epileptiform events, if present, as well as a variety of false detections, which the human observer has to discard. Present computer analysis is quite capable of ensuring that very few true epileptiform events are missed. Such a selective review is much less tedious than the complete review and allows a more careful analysis of interesting events.

In the context of sleep staging, a "sleep staging assistant" may be a more appropriate tool than a "sleep stager." We have seen that the accuracy of automatic sleep-staging systems varies with subjects and with stages of sleep; most important, its level of agreement with human scorers varies highly because of differences between individual scorers. A sleep staging assistant could perform a tentative classification and propose it to the human scorer; on a fast-review system, the scorer could simply accept it in most cases and modify it when in disagreement.

REFERENCES

1. Gotman J. Automatic recognition of interictal spikes. In: Gotman J, Ives JR, Gloor P, eds. *Long-term monitoring in epilepsy*. Amsterdam: Elsevier, 1985;93–114.
2. Gotman J. Seizure recognition and analysis. In: Gotman J, Ives JR, Gloor P, eds. *Long-term monitoring in epilepsy*. Amsterdam: Elsevier, 1985;133–145.
3. Gotman J. Computer analysis of EEG in epilepsy. In: Lopes da Silva FH, Storm van Leeuwen W, Rémond A, eds. *Handbook of electroencephalography and clinical neurophysiology,* vol 2. New York: Elsevier, 1986;171–204.
4. Frost Jr JD. Automatic recognition and characterization of epileptiform discharges in the human EEG. *J Clin Neurophysiol* 1985;2(3):231–249.
5. Principe JC, Smith JR. Automatic detection of spike-and-wave bursts. In: Gotman J, Ives JR, Gloor P, eds. *Long-term monitoring in epilepsy*. Amsterdam: Elsevier, 1985;115–131.
6. Ktonas PY. Automated spike and sharp wave (SSW) detection. In: Gevins A, Rémond A, eds. *Handbook of electroencephalography and clinical neurophysiology,* vol 1. Amsterdam: Elsevier, 1987;211–241.
7. Smith JR. Automated analysis of sleep EEG data. In: Lopes da Silva FH, Storm van Leeuwen W, Rémond A, eds. *Handbook of electroencephalography and clinical neurophysiology,* vol 2. New York: Elsevier, 1986;131–147.
8. Carrie JRG, Frost JD. Clinical evaluation of a method for quantification of generalized spike and wave by computer. *Comput Biomed* 1977;10:449–457.
9. Gevins A, Blackburn, J, Dedon, M. Very accurate computer recognition of three per second generalized spike-and-wave discharges. In: Wada JA, Penry JK, eds. *Advances in epileptology. The Xth Epilepsy International Symposium.* New York: Raven Press, 1980;121–128.
10. Principe JC, Smith JR. Microcomputer-based system for the detection and quantification of petit mal epilepsy. *Comput Biol Med* 1982;12(2):87–95.
11. Quy RJ, Fitch P, Willison RG. High-speed automatic analysis of EEG spike and wave activity using an analogue detection and microcomputer plotting system. *Electroencephalogr Clin*

Neurophysiol 1980;49:187–189.

12. Whisler JW, ReMine WJ, Leppik LE, et al. Machine detection of spike-wave activity in the EEG and its accuracy compared with visual interpretation. *Electroencephalogr Clin Neurophysiol* 1982;54:541–551.
13. Burr W, Stefan H. Computerized analysis of epileptic activity and sleep in mobile long-term EEG monitoring. *Eur Neurol* 1986;25(suppl 2):61–65.
14. Mony L, Pasquier C. Un système d'analyse automatique pour enregistrements ambulatoires. *Rev EEG Neurophysiol* 1982;12:332–336.
15. Jayakar P. Rule-based graded analysis of ambulatory cassette EEGs. Ph.D. thesis, University of Manitoba, 1987.
16. Koffler DJ, Gotman J. Automatic detection of spike-and-wave bursts in ambulatory EEG recordings. *Electroencephalogr Clin Neurophysiol* 1985;61:165–180.
17. Gotman J, Ives JR, Gloor P. Automatic recognition of interictal epileptic activity in prolonged EEG recordings. *Electroencephalogr Clin Neurophysiol* 1979;46:510–520.
18. Gotman J. Automatic recognition of epileptic seizures in the EEG. *Electroencephalogr Clin Neurophysiol* 1982;54:530–540.
19. Gotman J, Ives JR, Gloor P, et al. Long-term monitoring at the Montreal Neurological Institute. In: Gotman J, Ives JR, Gloor P, eds. *Long-term monitoring in epilepsy*. Amsterdam: Elsevier, 1985;327–340.
20. Rechtschaffen A, Kales A. *A manual of standardized terminology, techniques and scoring system for sleep stages of human subjects.* Washington D.C.: Public Health Service, US Government Printing Office, 1968.
21. Crawford C. Sleep recording in the home with automatic analysis of results. *Eur Neurol* 1986; 25(suppl 2):30–35.
22. Höller L, Riemer H. Comparison of visual analysis and automatic sleep stage scoring (Oxford Medilog 9000 system). *Eur Neurol* 1986;25(suppl 2):36–45.
23. Ferri R, Ferri P, Colognola RM, et al. Scoring del sonno umano normale: analisi della variabilita' della lettura visiva e confronto con un metodo di lettura automatico. *Rivista Italiana di EEG E Neurofisiologia Clinica* 1987;10:77–107.

Ambulatory EEG Monitoring,
edited by John S. Ebersole.
Raven Press, Ltd., New York © 1989

7

Clinical Utility of Cassette EEG in Adult Seizure Disorders

John S. Ebersole

Department of Neurology, Yale University School of Medicine, New Haven, Connecticut 06510

The evaluation of disorders with paroxysmal symptoms and signs has long posed problems for physicians who commonly see the afflicted patients after the episode, when the exam may be normal and the historical account is less than crystal clear. The workup of patients with suspected seizure disorders has relied on EEG for diagnostic support. Although traditional laboratory EEG provides one of the few ways to measure cerebral function, its deficiency in temporal sampling is all too evident when these patients are studied. A half-hour view of brain electrical activity out of a 24-hr day leaves much to be desired when searching for intermittent interictal markers of epilepsy and even less frequent ictal events. For this reason, long-term EEG monitoring has evolved in specialized epilepsy centers over the past 15 years and has become a much sought after form of evaluation, despite the fact that patients are commonly hospitalized for days to weeks in the process.

Intensive inpatient monitoring now represents the ultimate standard with which all other forms of epilepsy evaluation are compared, but it has inherent disadvantages of required hospitalization, confinement to monitoring rooms, and an unnatural setting. Just as unfortunate is a lack of availability to all but a few patients with seizure disorders. Epilepsy centers in the United States cater principally to patients with chronic intractable seizures, who may be appropriate for surgical therapy. A much larger population of patients, who require monitoring for initial diagnosis or classification of their type of epilepsy or who need an assessment of the effects of a modification in their antiepileptic drug regimen, seldom has the opportunity to benefit from long-term monitoring.

Approximately 15 years ago, clinical trials began with portable tape recorders that would eventually provide a solution for the unfilled diagnostic need in epilepsy evaluation. Several technological developments were necessary to allow the logical extension of Holter ECG technique to EEG. These included multichannel capability, preamplification of signals three orders of magnitude smaller than ECG, and a means of efficiently analyzing all the data once recorded. One by one, these obstacles were overcome (1,2). Less than 10 years ago, the first commercial ambulatory cassette EEG systems appeared. They offered physicians a means of monitoring for prolonged periods the EEG of patients who could be totally ambulatory, both within a hospital setting, but, more important, as outpatients in their normal environment. For the first time, long-term EEG data could be conveniently gathered, easily stored, and efficiently analyzed. As a consequence, widespread availability became possible.

There was initially much skepticism when the first 4-channel systems were introduced, since it seemed a step backward from 16-channel laboratory EEGs. Gradually the expansionist mentality—that more channels are always better—was overcome. Physicians began to realize that fewer channels may be better if the data are more likely to contain the desired information. Methodology was refined to ensure quality recordings over an entire day and under the most adverse conditions (3). Protocols to enhance diagnostic yield and to analyze the cassette records efficiently were developed (4,5). Computer programs and systems were created that could detect epileptiform discharges automatically and mark them for a confirmatory review by the electroencephalographer (6).

A second generation of continuous recorders with eight data channels brought with it many technological advances and improved analysis features. A major result of the increased number of channels was the capability for greater precision in differentiating abnormal EEG features from the artifacts so abundant in the records of ambulatory patients. Additionally, a broader range of studies could be performed, in which multiple physiologic measures were monitored in addition to EEG. At approximately the same time, a separate line of cassette EEG technology also developed, which emphasized spatial resolution by means of an increase in channel numbers to 16, and, most recently, 24, at the expense of continuous recording (1,7). These epoch or event recorders provide an accuracy of EEG topography that is superior to other forms of cassette EEG and is felt by some to be sufficient for selecting candidates for epilepsy surgery (8).

From the inception of ambulatory EEG, the evaluation of seizure disorders has been its principal use. It remains the foremost indication for cassette EEG today. Within this category is not only the diagnosis of epilepsy, which is probably the single most often addressed clinical problem, but also the characterization of seizure type once diagnosed and the quantification of seizures or epileptiform discharges. Within a few years after ambulatory EEG equipment became available, numerous clinical investigations had documented its usefulness in the differential diagnosis of epilepsy (9–22). Diagnostic yield superior to routine EEG recordings was reported in nearly every instance as well.

The clinical utility of ambulatory EEG spans the gamut in both seizure types, from generalized to partial, and in patient age, from premature neonate to the elderly. The small, unobtrusive size of a cassette EEG recorder, coupled with its long-term monitoring capability, has made it an attractive method for recording from neonates in newborn intensive care units (23–27). It has been a particular boon in monitoring the EEG of children, who have a high incidence of seizure disorders, but who also often do not tolerate prolonged inpatient recording (28).

DIFFERENTIAL DIAGNOSIS OF EPILEPSY

In adults and adolescents, the principal use for ambulatory EEG is in diagnosis of seizure disorders or, more often, in the differentiation of seizure disorders from other medical conditions with paroxysmal features. In one clinical series, 75% of patient referrals for ambulatory EEG were for attacks of uncertain origin (29) in which diagnostic clarification was sought. Such patients may present several diagnostic dilemmas. 1. Do they have epilepsy, or are their spells related to noncerebral organic disease? 2. Are their episodes pseudoseizures and the manifestation of psychiatric disturbance? 3. Should the patient be treated with anticonvulsants or, just as important, should the patient who is on anticonvulsants inappropriately be taken off them? 4. Is the development of new spells in a patient with previously well-controlled epilepsy related to breakthrough ictal phenomena or some other episodic dysfunction? 5. If there has been only one attack historically, is there evidence of intermittent epileptiform EEG abnormalities that might suggest the potential for recurrence? In each instance, long-term recording of EEG is needed to document whether the patient's episodes are seizures. When this is not achievable, the presence of appropriate interictal epileptiform abnormalities may lend support to an otherwise tentative clinical diagnosis.

Generalized Epilepsies

Early investigations with ambulatory EEG were directed principally at the diagnosis of generalized, particularly spike-wave, epilepsies. This emphasis was related to several factors. First, the nonconvulsive types of generalized epilepsy were difficult to follow clinically, since there was little or no behavioral manifestation of the attacks. A means of efficiently detecting and then monitoring spike-wave discharges was sorely needed. Second, the electrographic patterns of the abnormalities were so distinctive that they could be easily recognized with three or four channels of EEG. Even skeptical electroencephalographers agreed that these features should be adequately detected with limited montages. Indeed, several studies soon documented the ease with which 3-Hz spike and wave episodes could be identified and differentiated from activity artifact (9,30). The regular and rhythmic patterns of the generalized epilepsies were also the most promising place to develop automated means of analyzing recorded data (31–37).

Certain symptoms raise the specter of a generalized seizure disorder. Among the more common is episodic loss of awareness or consciousness. In this category, staring spells are a typical complaint, and although absence seizures are more likely a problem in children (see ref. 28), spike-wave paroxysms with clinical accompaniments are not uncommon in adolescents and adults. As reviewed in Chapter 13 (38), a high percentage of patients reporting staring spells have epileptiform features on their ambulatory EEGs, and a significant portion of these are generalized spike-wave discharges. Involuntary movements or myoclonic jerks, as a sign, are associated with a lesser yield but, nonetheless, one worth pursuing diagnostically. Although the utility of ambulatory EEG has been extended greatly beyond absence and other generalized seizures, cassette recordings remain the most efficient means of identifying and, as discussed later, of characterizing and quantifying paroxysms of spike-wave activity.

Ambulatory EEG can also be useful in distinguishing between primary generalized and secondary generalized epilepsy in patients with tonic-clonic seizures. Cassette recordings in the former often show characteristic spike-wave or polyspike-wave features interictally. This distinction is important, since those with secondary etiologies may need further diagnostic evaluation, while those with a primary or idiopathic etiology may benefit from a different drug regimen that is aimed at the elimination of both the convulsive and nonconvulsive aspects of their seizure disorder. Prolonged runs of spike-wave during wakefulness may be disruptive to the patient's cognition, even though specific absences are not noticed by him. These are most easily documented via ambulatory EEG. In practice, patients with tonic-clonic seizures of idiopathic etiology, who are not doing well cognitively, could benefit from cassette monitoring to rule out nonconvulsive spike-wave paroxysms.

Partial Epilepsies

In the adult population, partial seizures, simple or complex, are commonly in the differential diagnosis of attacks of uncertain nature. Utility in this regard is clearly important, since many of the patients who would logically be referred for ambulatory EEG, possessing perhaps an atypical history and a normal or equivocal routine EEG, would be more likely to have a partial epilepsy. However, some electroencephalographers were initially skeptical of the usefulness of 3- or 4-channel ambulatory EEG in the evaluation of partial seizure disorders. Establishing among physicians confidence in the ability of cassette EEG to provide this diagnostic information required proving that partial seizures and focal interictal transients could be confidently identified and differentiated from the multitude of artifacts that were so abundant in EEG recordings of active patients. In addition, being able to record and analyze other physiologic measures would be essential in diagnosing disease that was not epilepsy.

Ives and Woods (39) demonstrated the feasibility of cassette monitoring for lateralized ictal discharges; however, it was our laboratory (40–45) that specifically addressed the problem of adapting ambulatory EEG to partial seizure disorders. Three-channel montages, designed to maximize the detection of common focal, as well as generalized, epileptiform features, were developed (4,40). Controlled studies of this approach versus 8- or 16-channel cable telemetry showed a respectable relative yield (77 and 93%) for ambulatory EEG in the identification of epileptiform abnormalities (42,43). Detection of seizures was 100% for those both generalized and focal, and false-positive errors were at an acceptable level. Identification of epileptiform abnormalities, both interictal and ictal, was increased by ambulatory EEG over routine EEG by a factor of 1.5 to 2.5 (42,43). The ability of the electroencephalographer to differentiate abnormalities from artifacts and normal transients on rapid video review was found to be a greater limiting factor than the restricted number of data channels (41,46). Most important, the capability of routinely identifying focal as well as generalized epileptiform features was confirmed.

In an analysis of clinical usefulness relative to the referral questions for patients with principally partial epilepsy, 24 hr of ambulatory EEG was found to provide as much positive or negative information as did intensive inpatient monitoring in 60% of diagnostic admissions. The additional information obtained through video monitoring of behavior and the ability to withdraw antiepileptic medications under medical observation and monitor the patients for days thereafter provided the advantage that intensive inpatient monitoring had over ambulatory EEG (43). It was not the superiority of EEG recording that made the difference.

The evaluation of partial epilepsies benefited from the introduction of 8-channel ambulatory EEG systems, but it was not simply that more abnormalities were identified. During the intensive monitoring of 30 patients by means of cable telemetry EEG, simultaneous 3- and 8-channel ambulatory EEG recordings were also obtained in a recent study (45). Blinded interpretations of the cassette tapes were compared to those of the 8- or 16-channel cable-telemetry records. Analyses of both tapes produced a nearly comparable yield in the detection of interictal and ictal EEG features (93% and 100%, respectively). Only in detailed characterization of epileptiform events were eight channels shown to be superior to three. However, 8-channel recordings clearly had an advantage in allowing better differentiation of true abnormalities from artifacts and in so doing yielded a reduced number of false-positive errors.

This may also explain the high rate of uninterpretable ambulatory EEGs (27%) accompanying clinical attacks noted by Blumhardt et al. (47), who used a 4-channel recorder with only two channels of EEG, versus essentially no uninterpretable ambulatory EEGs during attacks noted by Powell et al. (29), who used an 8-channel recorder and a full complement of EEG channels. Better ability to differentiate real abnormalities from artifacts is the most significant advantage of 8-channel over 3- to 4-channel ambulatory EEG. Eight channels provide an increased level of confidence with which an interpreter can make decisions regarding the nature of suspicious paroxysms. Since false-positive errors in diagnosis are often more damaging to the patient than false-negative impressions, this precision is important.

Overall Yield in Epilepsy Diagnosis

The utility of ambulatory cassette EEG, like any other diagnostic test, is dependent on the appropriateness of the question asked and the likelihood of answering the question, even if appropriate. Rates for recording the attacks or spells in question by means of ambulatory EEG vary dramatically with the clinical frequency of these episodes, as would be expected. A 77% success was achieved in patients with one or more seizures daily (10), whereas only 16% of unselected patients had spells recorded (22). A 50% capture rate could be attained in patients who had only one attack per week by allowing at least 3 days for monitoring each of them (29).

Similarly, the yield for documenting epileptiform abnormalities is quite variable in the literature and is most likely due to different patient populations. Reports of ambulatory EEG use in unselected patients have suggested a positive yield of evidence to support a diagnosis in the range of 10 to 15% (18,48). Of attacks recorded in several series, the proportion that were identifiable as seizures has ranged from 23 to 73% (11,16).

Several years ago, we reviewed our experience with 500 consecutive patients, age 2 months to 82 years, undergoing ambulatory EEG for the first time (44). Seizures, interictal epileptiform abnormalities, or both were detected in 87 of the tapes, or 17.4%. Among these, there was a 64% increase in the yield of interictal epileptiform abnormalities and a 21-fold increase in seizure recording with ambulatory EEG, as compared with laboratory EEGs. Failure to detect epileptiform abnormalities on ambulatory EEG after their demonstration on routine EEG was seen in a few patients with photoconvulsive responses or initiation of anticonvulsant medication between the two studies.

Our experience has now grown to include cassette recordings of approximately 2100 patients (38). Most were 24 hr in duration. The overall yield of epileptiform findings has remained nearly the same, 15.4%; actual seizures were recorded in nearly 6%. Clinical events similar to those for which the patient was referred were noted in the diary of 36% of the patients, and over 11% of these recordings contained symptom-related seizures. The yield of evidence (ictal or interictal) in support of a diagnosis of epilepsy varied considerably when selected populations were analyzed. When the referring physician had already made a clinical diagnosis of epilepsy, the likelihood that a cassette recording would contain confirmatory abnormalities increased to 39%. Certain symptoms or signs were associated with a relatively high yield of epileptiform EEG abnormalities, e.g., involuntary motor activity, 24%; episodic loss of contact,

25%, while others were related to low yields, e.g., dizziness, 2%; anxiety or panic, 6%. Interestingly, over half of the patients who referred to an episode as a "seizure," had an accompanying electrographic ictal discharge.

In another recent study comparing ambulatory EEG to preceding laboratory EEGs (29), 50% of patients had clinical attacks while being monitored by cassette recorder and 35% of these were, in fact, seizures. Of note, 25% of patients being evaluated for attacks of unknown origin, who had seizures recorded, had completely normal routine EEGs. More specifically, one-third of patients found to have absence seizures during ambulatory monitoring had no spike-wave discharges during routine EEG with hyperventilation; 56% of patients with partial seizures recorded had no epileptiform abnormalities on baseline studies. Overall, the ambulatory EEG yield for definite epileptiform abnormalities (ictal plus interictal) was 10 times that of laboratory EEG recording.

Epilepsy versus Syncope and Dizziness

Paroxysmal loss of consciousness or syncope and spells of dizziness are very common diagnostic problems. Ambulatory EEG provides a means of monitoring both ECG and EEG long enough to be likely to record an episode (see ref. 49). Several studies have shown that this form of combined monitoring can be useful in clarifying the etiology of the patient's complaint, particularly if it is cardiac arrhythmia (16,22,50–53). A predominantly cardiac yield is to be expected, given the relative infrequency with which epilepsy was uncovered in a large series of patients presenting with syncope (54).

Early studies with combined ambulatory EEG/ECG demonstrated that the yield in unselected populations is rather low, even for cardiac arrhythmias. In fact, of 113 patients studied in four studies, only eight or approximately 7% showed cardiac abnormalities (10,16,22,55). Recently, Keilson and Magrill reviewed their extensive series of 8-channel combined EEG and ECG recordings (49). Of 422 patients with complaints of syncope, dizziness, or faints, approximately 10% had significant cardiac arrhythmias detected. Although the majority of these patients were over 60 years old, and thus fell into a subpopulation with an expected increased incidence of arrhythmias, 2% of younger patients, who may not have had Holter monitoring routinely, also had significant cardiac rhythm disturbances.

Finding epileptiform EEG abnormalities as support for a diagnosis of epilepsy among patients with these complaints is quite uncommon and has ranged in two recent reviews from 5% to less than 1% (38,49). If patients with a prior history of seizures are removed from the former investigation, only 2% possess epileptiform EEGs. Complaint-related seizures have been documented only rarely. Ambulatory EEG in these patients seems most useful as a source of reassurance that the episodes are not a manifestation of epilepsy.

ECG abnormalities may accompany seizures (47). In most instances, these consist of ictal tachycardia and, at times, abrupt changes in rate rather than dangerous rhythm disturbances. In Keilson and Magrill's (49) recent analysis of 96 seizures greater than 20 sec' duration in 36 patients, 97% of the ictal episodes were accompanied by tachycardia, but no ectopia or conduction defects were observed. The relationship between seizures and heart-rate changes has led some to postulate that the increased incidence of sudden death among people with seizure disorders is related to cardiac arrhythmias and that patients with this potential may be discovered by ECG screening. The former assumption seems less likely and the latter unworkable on the basis of ambulatory EEG/ECG data, which show that the prevalence of cardiac arrhythmias among known epileptics is no greater than among nonepileptics (52,53).

Arrhythmogenic or vasovagal syncope, which results in a loss of consciousness, may be accompanied by convulsive movements. Among patients with this syndrome is a small population with a familial abnormality of cardiac conduction that results in a long QT interval. These patients, who are mostly young, are at high risk for serious life-threatening arrhythmias, particularly with exercise. Patients with possible convulsive syncope might benefit greatly from combined EEG/ECG monitoring (49), since the long QT syndrome can be medically treated if diagnosed.

Given the above review, it would seem reasonable to recommend simultaneous ECG monitoring in all patients who are referred for ambulatory EEG if they are over 50 to 60 years old. The case for ECG monitoring in younger individuals is less strong. The yield is small, but not inconsequential, when considering the ease with which it is done and the minimal loss of EEG data by doing so. In younger patients with cardiac symptoms and certainly in those with a history of relatives who died following exercise or supposed seizures, ECG monitoring is clearly warranted.

Seizures versus Pseudoseizures

It is not uncommon for clinicians to be faced with the problem of differentiating between bona fide seizures and psychogenic or pseudoseizures, be they conversion reactions or outright malingering. Ambulatory cassette EEG can be useful in this regard, if its limitations are known and appropriate discretion is observed in interpreting the results. Certainly the long-term recording capability of cassette EEG increases the likelihood of recording both real as well as unreal seizures; however, the fact that the patient is ambulatory makes it less likely that the episode will be observed by professionals trained in this differentiation. This is the liability of cassette EEG that must be borne in mind when considering pseudoseizure diagnosis.

Ambulatory EEG is of greatest help when it confirms the diagnosis of epilepsy by demonstrating that an attack was a seizure. Several investigations have demonstrated its utility in clarifying the epileptic nature of behavior that was considered to be a manifestation of psychiatric disease (9,13,17,21,56). The bizarre presentations of patients with extratemporal, "frontal lobe" epilepsy are particularly troublesome in this regard. Cassette EEG has been shown to be of value in making the correct diagnosis (57). When an attack is not recorded, circumstantial evidence may be provided by identifying interictal abnormalities appropriate for the type of seizure disorder being considered.

Most alterations of behavior or awareness that are questioned as being pseudoseizures involve motor activity, often mimicking that of a major motor convulsion. In these instances, ambulatory EEG can, at times, be diagnostic. Primary or secondarily generalized ictal discharge can easily be recognized during tape analysis, even when accompanied by muscle and movement artifact. In convulsive seizures that are more subtle electrographically, an electrodecremental onset and postictal slowing lend support for an ictus in an intervening period obscured by muscle artifact, as do appropriate interictal abnormalities in other portions of the record. The appearance of normal alpha activity immediately following a supposed generalized convulsion in which the other elements of ictal activity were not present suggests pseudoseizure. The same is true for an episode of apparent total loss of consciousness during which no ambulatory EEG changes are observed.

The situation is more complicated when the attack in question is similar to a partial seizure in which there has been only an alteration of consciousness. The absence of a detectable ambulatory EEG correlate may make the episodes more likely to be functional, but the lack of EEG change cannot rule out the possibility of partial seizures with no surface EEG manifestations. This is particularly true of simple partial seizures. Objective behavioral, as well as EEG, monitoring is extremely valuable in the diagnosis of pseudoseizures. Video recording of behavior combined with ambulatory EEG can provide this documentation (see ref. 58) and is discussed below under the heading of characterization of seizures.

In the case of psychiatric disorders that have no paroxysmal features, the yield for detecting underlying epilepsy has been very low and, in one investigation, zero (44). Cassette EEG monitoring may, however, be useful in identifying and quantitating disturbances in sleep architecture, particularly REM onset latency, that purportedly are observed in patients with depression and that may resolve with drug treatment (see ref. 59).

Cassette EEG Monitoring in Emergency Situations

Most indications for cassette EEG are based on its ambulatory feature. A less emphasized, though equally useful, aspect is the ease with which EEG recording can be obtained in nearly any situation. This may be particularly advantageous in acute hospital settings, such as in emergency rooms and intensive care units, when patients have suspected seizures during the night, on weekends, or at other times when routine EEG may not be available. Cassette EEG is, however, infrequently initiated outside traditional workday hours, since collodion-applied electrodes are routinely used for outpatients and placement of these requires the expertise of trained technologists. The recent introduction of small, self-adhering electrodes, intended for nerve conduction studies, has provided an alternative, when used on bare skin in a subhairline montage (60). This technique, combined with the simplicity of the cassette recorder, has made it possible for nontechnical personnel, such as neurology housestaff, to institute EEG monitoring in nonambulatory patients in less than 10 min.

In a recent investigation (61), 25 patients were recorded with cassette EEG for 16 to 24 hr using a 5-channel subhairline montage and self-adhering electrodes following a supposed seizure(s). Interpretations of these tapes were compared with those of standard portable or laboratory EEGs of eight and 16 channels, respectively, and of half-hr duration, which were obtained whenever possible, usually the next morning. Although both types of EEG were abnormal in 80+% of patients, epileptiform features (definite sharp waves, spikes, or ictal discharges) were documented in 48% of cassette recordings, but in only 24% of routine studies. More important, seizures were recorded in 24% of patients via cassette EEG but in none with routine EEG.

These results underscore the utility of EEG monitoring immediately following supposed seizures and verify that this can be accomplished by means of cassette EEG recordings. Self-adhering electrodes used in a subhairline montage make this type of monitoring practical in emergency and off-hours settings, when trained personnel may not be available. This technique is not suitable, however, for long-term EEG monitoring in ambulatory outpatients, since the electrodes are not as secure or stable as those applied with collodion, and a standard 7- or 8-channel montage provides better spatial resolution.

CLASSIFICATION/CHARACTERIZATION OF SEIZURES

The clinical utility of ambulatory EEG goes beyond the diagnosis of seizure disorders to include the classification of seizure types and the characterization of associated EEG abnormalities, both ictal and interictal. Even in patients previously confirmed to have epilepsy, questions arise the answers to which are most effectively sought by long-term EEG monitoring and most conveniently obtained by cassette EEG. For example, among those patient whose epilepsy is not well controlled, have their seizures been properly classified? Are they of multiple or mixed types? Do they represent atypical primary generalized spike-wave epilepsy, or are they partial seizures with complex symptomatology?

This distinction between nonconvulsive spike-wave and partial seizures may be extremely difficult to perceive by clinical criteria, yet it is one of the few that can necessitate a major change in drug regimen. Accordingly, proper classification of nonconvulsive seizures is essential. Ambulatory EEG is an efficient means of obtaining the necessary information, preferably by recording the habitual attacks but, if not, at least by recording the typical interictal activity. Finding lateralized sharp waves from the temporal regions would certainly favor a different diagnosis than would finding generalized spike-wave or polyspike-wave discharges. Both are commonly absent in routine EEG recordings, whereas both are frequently present, if at all, during sleep and the latter also on morning awakening. Recording at these times is the forte of cassette EEG.

Other EEG features characterized by ambulatory recordings may play a useful, if not essential, role in patient management. These include distinguishing primary from secondarily generalized convulsive seizures. Medication regimens are similar, but further evaluation of the patient may be indicated in the case of symptomatic epilepsy arising from a localized origin. The search for etiologies is aided when it can be determined that the patient's seizures are consistently of focal versus generalized onset and the interictal features are appropriately focal versus bilateral.

As noted previously, a major reason why intensive inpatient monitoring provides more information than outpatient ambulatory EEG monitoring is the ability with the former to evaluate seizure-associated behavior as recorded on video tape. Comparisons of the diagnostic yields of the two techniques have demonstrated the crucial role of behavioral observation in differential diagnosis (43). Video information can be an important complement to EEG data in characterizing a patient's epilepsy.

New video technology and inexpensive portable cameras and recorders have made the combination of ambulatory EEG and video recording of behavior an attractive and easily accomplished alternative to traditional intensive monitoring. Such a mobile monitoring setup can be readily moved to wherever it is needed within the hospital or clinic. Outpatient recordings can be performed in physicians' offices, or even hotel rooms and patients' homes. To the extent that patients are willing or able to stay within view of the camera, valuable information can be gathered. The only technical necessity is that the cassette EEG tape and the video tape of patient behavior are synchronized so that temporal correlations can be made. This is most easily done by adding a time-code generator to the video recorder system and synchronizing it to the cassette recorder time code at the beginning of a monitoring session. A video record of the patient allows a more accurate classification of seizure types, is useful in confirming the artifactual versus epileptiform nature of suspicious EEG paroxysms, and may help differentiate pseudoseizures (58).

A supposed disadvantage of cassette EEG is the lessened spatial resolution that comes from a reduced number of channels. As pointed out earlier, this limitation does not significantly interfere with detecting ictal or interictal EEG abnormalities and thus does not adversely influence diagnosis. Distinguishing real abnormalities from artifacts is aided by additional channels, but this benefit would probably suffer diminishing returns with ever-increasing channel numbers. Once the distinction between partial and generalized epilepsy is made, and it is determined that the abnormalities are unilateral or bilateral, dependent or independent, there is little more to be gained clinically by EEG characterization, unless precise localization is sought in order to consider epilepsy surgery. In this instance, more than eight channels are routinely required, and combinations of surface and invasive electrodes are commonly employed. Of the presently available cassette EEG recording systems, only the 16- to 24-channel epoch recorder affords this much spatial sampling capability (see ref. 8). The disadvantage of its restricted recording time has been significantly lessened with the recent inclusion of a portable computer with detection programs for seizures and spikes, which can automatically select those epochs of EEG likely to contain significant abnormalities.

Continuous recorders, particularly those of 8-channel design, can also be usefully employed before inpatient presurgical EEG evaluation by providing continuous records of the patient's habitual seizures and interictal abnormalities. Patients with consistently lateralized seizures and interictal transients would more likely be excellent surgical candidates and thus might be able to have shortened and simpler inpatient monitoring. Those patients with documented inconsistent or bilateral focal features from cassette records would also benefit, since it would be known beforehand that a more comprehensive inpatient evaluation will be necessary.

Finally, ambulatory EEG may be used to characterize the relationship of seizures to specific precipitating circumstances or stimuli (62,63). This may be particularly worthwhile if attacks appear related to environmental or social influences that cannot readily be duplicated in an inpatient epilepsy center. It is a common experience that patients, who report numerous recent seizures, cease to have them when hospitalized for monitoring (64). Seizure patterns may also be periodic and fluctuate with hormonal or sleep-wakefulness cycles. Attacks that are principally nocturnal or occur on morning awakening are easily characterized by outpatient ambulatory EEG, whereas they are seldom recorded by routine EEG.

Catamenial epilepsy is also conveniently studied with cassette EEG. Recording patients before and during their menses is much easier to arrange on an outpatient basis than trying to schedule in advance an inpatient hospitalization, particularly when considering the variability of such biological rhythms. Few epilepsy centers have the flexibility of admitting patients on demand whenever a flurry of seizures arises. Ambulatory EEG provides the capability of taking advantage of such situations and gathering information that may not otherwise be obtained by predetermined scheduling of monitoring times.

There has also been much interest of late in the relationship between epileptiform discharges and the sleep-waking cycle. Although this type of information was traditionally obtained via inpatient monitoring, cassette EEG has now been employed by several investigators (65,66). These data not only are useful in those patients with nocturnal seizures, but also may be important in understanding the basic mechanisms of epilepsy and how it is modulated by sleep.

QUANTIFICATION OF SEIZURES OR EPILEPTIFORM DISCHARGES

A third major area of clinical utility for cassette EEG is in the quantification of seizures and/or interictal discharges. Convulsive seizures are apparent either to patient or observer or to both. Unless simple or complex partial seizures are very frequent, and subtle enough to be missed, innumeration by ambulatory EEG is unlikely to be more effective than traditional seizure counts. The same is not true for nonconvulsive seizures. Behavioral manifestations may be minimal or absent. In the case of absence seizures, the patient may not even know that he is having them, let alone know how many are occurring or how long each is. Several studies using cassette EEG have documented the inaccuracy of patient and observer reports concerning the number and duration of absence attacks (67,68). Accordingly, there is little way by history alone for the neurologist to know how effective his treatment of these seizures is or if it needs to be altered.

Spike-waves of absence epilepsy can be reduced in number or even eliminated by appropriate antiepileptic drugs. Therapy can be titrated on an individual basis by following the amount of abnormal activity in the EEG. Unfortunately, a consistent effect of major anticonvulsants on focal or nonspike-wave generalized discharges has not been demonstrated; effectiveness of therapy cannot be judged, therefore, by the number of remaining epileptiform features. In terms of both seizures and interictal events, quantification by ambulatory EEG has its greatest use in monitoring the course of nonconvulsive seizure disorders.

Spike-wave or polyspike-wave discharges are among the easiest patterns to recognize in rapid review of cassette EEG. Detection is commonly accomplished by the characteristic audio signal generated by these patterns, and counting the number of paroxysms can be done at the highest rate of review. Quantifying the total duration of spike-wave activity requires additional time but can be reliably performed from ambulatory tapes. Evaluation of the primary generalized epilepsies is the principal situation where 4-channel ambulatory EEG recorders continue to have utility nearly equal to 8-channel recorders.

In times past, intermittent laboratory EEGs have sufficed for following patients with nonconvulsive, particularly absence, epilepsy. The variability in the number of spike-wave paroxysms per unit time over the course of a day, documented by inpatient monitoring and now by ambulatory EEG (62,69), readily proves the inadequacy of a short EEG sample, when trying to take measure of overall drug effectiveness. Long-term EEG affords a more accurate assessment of the need to alter therapy, and this can most easily be done via cassette recordings (70–72).

A recent study comparing the efficacy of once- versus twice-daily valproate is a good example of how cassette EEG documentation can be used to custom-tailor a drug regimen (73). Patients had ambulatory recordings before and up to nine times during the initiation of therapy. Considerable variation in drug doses necessary to reduce and to abolish discharges was found among the patients. Individualizing therapy permitted several patients to achieve complete control at doses as low as 15 mg/kg, rather than at the mean of 22 mg/kg, thus minimizing side effects. Other patients required considerably more drug in order to eliminate prolonged paroxysms during wakefulness that were not clinically recognized.

Quantitative studies using ambulatory EEG data have made a number of interesting and useful observations concerning spike-wave epilepsy. Spike-wave paroxysms are more frequent on morning awakening and at sleep onset than at other times during the day (71,73). Partial treatment did not alter this temporal distribution or mean duration of paroxysms but did reduce the total duration of spike-wave activity. In addition, there is not a close relationship between the fluctuation of the serum concentration of valproate and the amount of spike-wave activity during the day (74).

REFERENCES

1. Ives JR. Evolution of ambulatory cassette EEG. In: Ebersole JS, ed. *Ambulatory EEG monitoring.* New York: Raven Press, 1989;1–12.
2. Sams MW. Recording and playback instrumentation for ambulatory monitoring. In: Ebersole JS, ed. *Ambulatory EEG monitoring.* New York: Raven Press, 1989;13–26.
3. Clenny SL. The technique of cassette EEG recording. In: Ebersole JS, ed. *Ambulatory EEG monitoring.* New York: Raven, 1989;27–50.
4. Ebersole JS. Montage design for cassette EEG. In: Ebersole JS, ed. *Ambulatory EEG monitoring.* New York: Raven Press, 1989;51–68.
5. Ebersole JS. Audio/video analysis of cassette EEG. In: Ebersole JS, ed. *Ambulatory EEG monitoring.* New York: Raven Press, 1989;69–96.
6. Gotman J. Automated analysis of ambulatory EEG recordings. In: Ebersole JS, ed. *Ambulatory EEG monitoring.* New York: Raven Press, 1989;97–110.
7. Ives JR. A completely ambulatory 16-channel cassette recording system. In: Stefan H, Burr W, eds. *Mobile long-term EEG monitoring: proceedings of the MLE symposium, Bonn, May 1982.* New York: Fischer, 1982;205–217.
8. Ives JR, Schomer DL, Blume HW. Presurgical evaluation with cassette EEG. In: Ebersole JS, ed. *Ambulatory EEG monitoring.* New York: Raven Press, 1988;
9. Stores G. Ambulatory EEG monitoring in neuropsychiatric patients using the Oxford Medilog 4-24 recorder with visual play-back display. In: Stott FD, Raftery EB, Goulding L, eds. *ISAM 1979: proceedings of the third international symposium of ambulatory monitoring.* London: Academic Press, 1980;399–406.
10. Davidson DLW, Fleming AMM, Kettles A. Use of ambulatory EEG monitoring in a neurological service. In: Dam M, Gram L, Penry JK, eds. *Advances in epileptology: XIIth epilepsy international symposium.* New York: Raven Press, 1981;319–321.
11. Ives JR, Hausser C, Woods JF, et al. Contributions of 4-channel cassette EEG monitoring to differential diagnosis of paroxysmal attacks. In: Dam M, Gram L, Penry JK, eds. *Advances in epileptology: XIIth epilepsy international symposium.* New York: Raven Press, 1981;329–336.
12. Oxley J, Roberts M, Dana-Haeri J, et al. Evaluation of prolonged 4-channel EEG-taped recordings and serum prolactin levels in the diagnosis of epileptic and nonepileptic seizures. In: Dam M, Gram L, Penry JK, eds. *Advances in epileptology: XIIth epilepsy international symposium.* New York: Raven Press, 1981;343–355.

13. Stores G. Differential diagnosis of seizures: psychiatric aspects. In: Dam M, Gram L, Penry JK, eds. *Advances in epileptology: XIIth epilepsy international symposium.* New York: Raven Press, 1981;259–263.
14. Callaghan N, McCarthy N. Twenty-four hour EEG monitoring in patients with normal, routine EEG findings. In: Dam M, Gram L, Penry JK, eds. *Advances in epileptology: XIIth epilepsy international symposium.* New York: Raven Press, 1981;357–360.
15. Ramsay RE, Hershkowitz A. 24-hour ambulatory EEG: a clinical appraisal. *Electroencephalogr Clin Neurophysiol* 1981;51:20.
16. Callaghan N, McCarthy N. Ambulatory EEG monitoring in fainting attacks with normal routine and sleep EEG records. In: Stefan H, Burr W, eds. *Mobile long-term EEG monitoring: proceedings of the MLE symposium, Bonn, May 1982.* New York: Fischer, 1982;61–65.
17. Oxley J, Roberts M. The role of prolonged ambulatory monitoring in the diagnosis of nonepileptic fits in a population of patients with epilepsy. In: Stott FD, Wright SL, Raftery EB, et al., eds. *ISAM 1981: proceedings of the fourth international symposium on ambulatory monitoring.* London: Academic Press, 1982;195–202.
18. Ramsay RE. Clinical usefulness of ambulatory EEG monitoring of the neurological patient. In: Stott FD, Wright SL, Raftery EB, et al., eds. *ISAM 1981: proceedings of the fourth international symposium on ambulatory monitoring.* London: Academic Press, 1982;234–243.
19. Stores G, Brankin P, Crawford C. Aspects of differential diagnosis using ambulatory EEG monitoring. In: Stefan H, Burr W, eds. *Mobile long-term EEG monitoring: proceedings of the MLE symposium, Bonn, May 1982.* New York: Fischer, 1982;55–60.
20. Zschoske ST, Hunger J, Alexopoulos T. Gain of information using mobile EEG long-term monitoring. In: Stefan H, Burr W, eds. *Mobile long-term EEG monitoring: proceedings of the MLE symposium, Bonn, May 1982.* New York: Fischer, 1982;19–28.
21. Forrest GC, Crawford C. Ambulatory monitoring and child psychiatry. In: Stott FD, Wright SL, Raftery EB, et al., eds. *ISAM 1981: proceedings of the fourth international symposium on ambulatory monitoring.* London: Academic Press, 1982;157–161.
22. Blumhardt LD, Oozeer R. Simultaneous ambulatory monitoring of the EEG and ECG in patients with unexplained transient disturbances of consciousness. In: Stott FD, Wright SL, Raftery EB, et al., eds. *ISAM 1981: proceedings of the fourth international symposium on ambulatory monitoring.* London: Academic Press, 1982;171–182.
23. Eyre J, Crawford C. Prolonged electroencephalographic recording in neonates. In: Stott FD, Wright SL, Raftery EB, et al., eds. *ISAM 1981: proceedings of the fourth international symposium on ambulatory monitoring.* London: Academic Press, 1982;143–150.
24. Eyre JA, Oozeer RC, Wilkinson AR. Diagnosis of neonatal seizures by continuous recording and rapid analysis of the electroencephalogram. *Arch Dis Child* 1983;58:785–790.
25. Eyre J. Clinical utility in neonatal seizure disorders. In: Ebersole JS, ed. *Ambulatory EEG monitoring.* New York: Raven Press, 1989;141–156.
26. Bridgers SL, Ebersole JS, Ment, LR et al. Cassette EEG in the evaluation of neonatal seizures. *Arch Neurol* 1986;43:49–51.
27. Bridgers SL, Ment LR, Ebersole JS, et al. Cassette EEG recordings of neonates with apneic episodes. *Ped Neurol* 1985;1:219–222.
28. Stores G, Bergel N. Clinical utility in childhood seizure disorders. In: Ebersole JS, ed. *Ambulatory EEG monitoring.* New York: Raven Press, 1989;129–140.
29. Powell TE, Harding GFA, Jeavons PM. Ambulatory EEG monitoring: a preliminary follow-up study. In: Ross E, Chadwick D, Crawford R, eds. *Epilepsy in young people.* London: J Wiley and Sons, 1987;131–139.
30. Quy RJ, Fitch P, Willison RG, Gilliatt RW. Electroencephalographic monitoring in patients with absence seizures. In: Wada JA, Penry JK, eds. *Advances in epileptology: the Xth epilepsy international symposium.* New York: Raven Press, 1980;69–72.
31. Quy RJ, Fitch P, Willison RG. High-speed automatic analysis of EEG spike and wave activity using an analogue detection and microcomputer plotting system. *Electroencephalogr Clin Neurophysiol* 1980;49:187–189.
32. Burr W, Stefan H, Penin H. Spike-wave analysis in 24-hour EEG: comparison between conventional and computerized methods. In: Dam M, Gram L, Penry JK, eds. *Advances in epileptology: XIIth epilepsy international symposium.* New York: Raven Press, 1981;275–286.
33. Zetterlund B, Bromster O. A system for quantification of spike and wave episodes in 24-hour tape recordings of EEG. In: Dam M, Gram L, Penry JK, eds. *Advances in epileptology: XIIth*

epilepsy international symposium. New York: Raven Press, 1981;361–364.
34. Bailey C. Evaluation of a spike and wave processor for use in long-term ambulatory EEG monitoring. In: Stott FD, Wright SL, Raftery EB, et al., eds. *ISAM 1981: proceedings of the fourth international symposium on ambulatory monitoring.* London: Academic Press, 1982;203–207.
35. Von Albert HH. Efficacy of non-computerized spike-wave analysis in long-term EEG. In: Stefan H, Burr W, eds. *Mobile long-term EEG monitoring: proceedings of the MLE symposium, Bonn, May 1982.* New York: Fischer, 1982;245–252.
36. Zetterlund B. Quantification of spike and wave episodes in 24-hour tape recordings of EEG. In: Stefan H, Burr W, eds. *Mobile long-term EEG monitoring: proceedings of the MLE symposium, Bonn, May 1982.* New York: Fischer, 1982;237–244.
37. Koffler DJ, Gotman J. Automatic detection of spike-and-wave bursts in ambulatory EEG recordings. *Electroencephalogr Clin Neurophysiol* 1985;61:165–180.
38. Bridgers SL. Evaluation of episodes of altered awareness or behavior. In: Ebersole JS, ed. *Ambulatory EEG monitoring.* New York: Raven Press, 1989;217–230.
39. Ives JR, Woods JF. A study of 100 patients with focal epilepsy using a 4-channel ambulatory cassette recorder. In: Stott FD, Raftery EB, Goulding L, eds. *ISAM 1979: proceedings of the third international symposium of ambulatory monitoring.* London: Academic Press, 1980;383–392.
40. Leroy RF, Ebersole JS. An evaluation of ambulatory, cassette EEG monitoring. I. Montage design. *Neurology (Cleve)* 1983;33:1–7.
41. Ebersole JS, Leroy RF. An evaluation of ambulatory, cassette EEG monitoring. II. Detection of interictal abnormalities. *Neurology (Cleve)* 1983;33:8–18.
42. Ebersole JS, Leroy RF. Evaluation of ambulatory, cassette EEG monitoring. III. Diagnostic accuracy compared to intensive inpatient EEG monitoring. *Neurology (Cleve)* 1983;33:853–860.
43. Bridgers SL, Ebersole JS. The clinical utility of ambulatory cassette EEG. *Neurology (Cleve)* 1985;35:166–173.
44. Bridgers SL, Ebersole JS. Ambulatory cassette EEG in clinical practice: experience with 500 patients. *Neurology (Cleve)* 1985;35:1767–1768.
45. Ebersole JS, Bridgers SL. Direct comparison of 3 and 8-channel ambulatory cassette EEG with intensive inpatient monitoring. *Neurology (Cleve)* 1985;35:846–854.
46. Ebersole JS, Bridgers SL, Silva CG. Differentiation of epileptiform abnormalities from normal transients and artifacts on ambulatory cassette EEG. *Am J EEG Technol* 1983;23:113–125.
47. Blumhardt LD, Smith PEM, Owen L. Electroencephalographic accompaniments of temporal lobe epileptic seizures. *Lancet* 1986; May 10:1051–1056.
48. Green J, Scales D, Nealis J, et al. Clinical utility of ambulatory EEG monitoring. *Clin EEG* 1980;11:173–179.
49. Keilson MJ, Magrill JP. Simultaneous ambulatory cassette EEG/ECG monitoring. In: Ebersole JS, ed. *Ambulatory EEG monitoring.* New York: Raven Press, 1989;171–194.
50. Lai C, Ziegler DK. Syncope problem solved by continuous ambulatory simultaneous EEG/EKG recording. *Neurology (NY)* 1981;31:1152–1154.
51. Graf M, Brunner G, Weber H, et al. Simultaneous long-term recording of EEG and ECG in "syncope" patients. In: Stefan H, Burr W, eds. *Mobile long-term EEG monitoring: proceedings of the MLE symposium, Bonn, May 1982.* New York: Fischer, 1982;67–75.
52. Keilson MJ, Magrill JP, Hauser WA, et al. Electrocardiographic abnormalities in patients with epilepsy. *Epilepsia* 1984;25:645.
53. Keilson MJ, Hauser WA, Magrill JP, et al. ECG abnormalities in patients with epilepsy. *Neurology (Cleve)* 1987;37:1624–1626.
54. Kapoor WN, Karpf M, Wieand S, et al. A prospective evaluation and follow-up of patients with syncope. *N Eng J Med* 1983;309:197–204.
55. Docherty TB. Ambulatory EEG monitoring in routine clinical practice. *J Electrophysiol Tech* 1981;7:141–158.
56. Smith EBO. The value of prolonged EEG monitoring to the clinician in a psychiatric liaison service. In: Stott FD, Wright SL, Raftery EB, et al., eds. *ISAM 1981: proceedings of the fourth international symposium on ambulatory monitoring.* London: Academic Press, 1982;162–168.
57. Stores G. Comparison of video and ambulatory (cassette) monitoring in the investigation of attacks in children. In: Palu C, Pessina AC, eds. *Proceedings of the fifth international symposium on ambulatory monitoring, Padua.* Padova: Cleup, 1986;633–638.

58. Leroy RF, Rao KK, Voth BJ. Intensive neurodiagnostic monitoring in epilepsy using ambulatory cassette EEG with simultaneous video recording. In: Ebersole JS, ed. *Ambulatory EEG monitoring.* New York: Raven Press, 1989;157–170.
59. Marsh GR, McCall WV. Sleep disturbances in psychiatric disease. In: Ebersole JS, ed. *Ambulatory EEG monitoring.* New York: Raven Press, 1989;231–348.
60. Bridgers SL, Ebersole JS. EEG outside the hairline: detection of epileptiform abnormalities. *Neurology (Cleve)* 1988;38:146–149.
61. Ebersole JS, Bridgers SL. Cassette EEG monitoring in the emergency room and intensive care unit. *J Clin Neurophysiol* 1987;4:213.
62. Stores G. Patterns of occurrence of seizure discharge. In: Stefan H, Burr W, eds. *Mobile long-term EEG monitoring: proceedings of the MLE symposium, Bonn, May 1982.* New York: Fischer, 1982;115–120.
63. Stores G, Lwin R. Precipitating factors and seizure activity. In: Stott FD, Wright SL, Raftery EB, et al., eds. *ISAM 1981: proceedings of the fourth international symposium on ambulatory monitoring.* London: Academic Press, 1982;183–188.
64. Riley TL, Porter RJ, White BG, et al. The hospital experience and seizure control. *Neurology* 1981;31:912–915.
65. Declerck AC. Interaction sleep and epilepsy. *Eur Neurol* 1986;25(suppl 2):117–127.
66. Monge-Strauss MF, Mikol F. Interest of 8-channel 24 hour cassette recorder for long-term EEG monitoring of ambulatory epileptic patients. *Rev EEG Neurophysiol* 1985;14:309–318.
67. Penry JK. Behavioral correlates of generalized spike and wave discharges in the electroencephalogram. In: Brazier MAB, ed. *Epilepsy, its phenomena in man.* New York: Academic Press, 1973;171–188.
68. Blomquist HK, Zetterlund B. Evaluation of treatment in typical absence seizures: the roles of long-term EEG monitoring and ethosuximide. *Acta Paediat Scand* 1985;74:409–415.
69. Woods I, Ives J, Gloor P. Prolonged EEG recording in patients with generalized epilepsy. *Electroencephalogr Clin Neurophysiol* 1975;39:295.
70. Milligan N, Richens A. Ambulatory monitoring of the EEG in the assessment of anti-epileptic drugs. In: Stott FD, Wright SL, Raftery EB, et al., eds. *ISAM 1981: proceedings of the fourth international symposium on ambulatory monitoring.* London: Academic Press, 1982;224–233.
71. Burr W, Stefan H, Kuhnen C, et al. Effect of valproic acid treatment on spike wave discharge patterns during sleep and wakefulness. *Neuropsychobiology* 1983;10:56–59.
72. Stefan H, Burr W, Fichsel H, et al. Intensive follow-up monitoring in patients with once daily administration of sodium valproate. *Epilepsia* 1984;25:152–160.
73. Powell TE, Harding GFA. Twenty-four hour ambulatory EEG monitoring: development and applications. *J Med Eng Tech* 1986;10:229–238.
74. Burr W, Froescher W, Hoffman F, et al. Lack of significant correlation between circadian profiles of valproic acid serum levels and epileptiform electroencephalographic activity. *Ther Drug Mon* 1984;6:179–181.

Ambulatory EEG Monitoring,
edited by John S. Ebersole.
Raven Press, Ltd., New York © 1989

8

Clinical Utility of Cassette EEG in Childhood Seizure Disorders

Gregory Stores and Nicolette Bergel

University of Oxford Department of Psychiatry, and Special Centre for Children with Epilepsy, and Oxford Regional Paediatric EEG Unit, Park Hospital for Children, Headington, Oxford OX3 7LQ England

Cassette recording has formed a substantial and valued part of our own paediatric EEG service since our first involvement in 1976 in the clinical evaluation of a prototype commercial 4-channel system (1). The early development of the Medilog recorder by Stott and its adaptation for EEG recording have been described by Ives in Chapter 1. Our own enthusiastic adoption of this type of EEG recording procedure was based on the undeniable way in which it met a need to be able to record for long periods outside the hospital setting, if necessary. This greatly increased the chances of identifying directly the physiologic accompaniments of attacks. In this way, recognition of epileptic attacks could be made with much more assurance than the results of conventional interictal recordings allowed and on a wider scale than video/EEG monitoring, the use of which still remains limited to relatively few special inpatient units. The unobtrusive nature of the recording system, when fitted carefully, was a specially valuable feature, in that it permitted long recordings to be carried out in real-life situations without embarrassment to the child or its parents.

Claims that the 4-channel system could be used effectively to detect seizure disorders and to demonstrate lateralisation of seizure discharge (2) met with a sceptical response from at least some of the electrographic orthodoxy. The main reason was concern about the limited information provided by this system, especially as one of the four available channels was usually sacrificed in order to record time and to mark clinical events. It is interesting that subsequent systematic evaluation by Ebersole and Bridgers (3) vindicated the initial belief that cassette recording, even in this relatively rudimentary form, was an important and clinically valuable advance in investigatory procedures.

The development of a commercially available 8-channel system seems to have allayed many of the early misgivings, and cassette recording is now widely employed, at least for adult patients. A paradox appears to persist in that the procedure is relatively little employed with younger patients, although it is possible that the opportunities and need to use cassette recording are greater in children than in adults. A reason for supposing this is that there are very few published reports of its use in paediatric practice. In addition, a survey of the procedure in the UK (Crawford, *unpublished*) pointed clearly to its limited use with children, even in some EEG departments who employed it regularly in older age groups.

If this impression that cassette recording is underused in children is correct, many opportunities are being lost in paediatrics and child psychiatry to diagnose attacks accurately, to clarify the nature of childhood seizures, to demonstrate the patterns of occurrence of seizures in relation to environmental circumstances or drug treatment, and to assess the effects of seizure discharge on the child's neuropsychiatric state. In addition to these main clinical applications in paediatric electroencephalography, cassette recording lends itself very readily to the study of more specific aspects of the epilepsies, as described later. It is the main purpose of this chapter to review the range of clinical uses of ambulatory cassette monitoring in children beyond the neonatal period. First, however, it is appropriate to consider some of the practical aspects of carrying out the cassette recordings compared with older patients.

CASSETTE RECORDING IN CHILDREN

Some special considerations are necessary when investigating children, especially where outpatient recordings are required.

Preparation

It is important to explain to parents exactly what is involved before they come to the EEG department so that, on arrival, they are not unduly anxious or confused about the procedure. If the parents are anxious, the child may also be unsettled, creating difficulties in application of the recording equipment and failure on the parents' part to listen to or understand instructions.

It is useful to send out an explanatory letter before the date of the appointment and invite parents to telephone if they have any questions. Anxieties are usually caused by worry about the child's tolerance of the system, fear that the equipment will be broken, concern about teasing by classmates, or the suggestion to others that the child has something wrong with his brain. As it is our practice always to include one channel of ECG in the recording, explanations and reassurance may be needed as to why the child's heart signals are being recorded. It is time well spent talking to parents at length if they telephone with queries. A further cause for concern can be failure by the referring physician to explain the need for the recording. It is not helpful if the first the family hears about the recording is an appointment from the EEG department.

For practical purposes, recordings are restricted to children having at least three attacks a week, assuming it is the nature of their attacks that is in question. This is explained in the initial letter to parents, who are specifically asked to inform the department if the frequency of their child's attacks has lessened by the time an appointment is received. Special arrangements may be necessary if a child's seizures occur in clusters or if they suddenly recur.

Preliminary Standard Recording

Because of the variability of children's EEG at different ages, standard recordings are always carried out before the cassette recording. This can be of considerable help in interpreting the tape and may also suggest modifications of cassette montage, if necessary. Although studies have been performed in adults concerning electrode placement in relation to the most likely location of seizure sources (4), no such guides exist as yet for children.

Fitting the Recorder

Because children can be very active, it is necessary to attach the electrodes firmly and equally firmly to attach a knot in the electrode lead about 3 cm from the electrode. The knot takes any accidental strain. In addition, the leads are secured to the scalp as necessary and fixed together at the nape of the neck. They should be hidden as far as possible; older children are usually very pleased to see how well they can be concealed. Especially with small children, it is necessary to avoid rushing the attachment procedure, allowing time to play and make it fun as much as possible. It is helpful to invite parents into the recording room when electrodes are being applied in order to demonstrate and explain certain points and answer questions in a relaxed manner.

Most children wear the recorder on a belt around their waist, but in small children an improvised backpack, such as a small rucksack, is more comfortable. It is also sensible to coil up and stick together all the spare cable during the day so that it is out of reach of small inquisitive hands. It is suggested that the recorder is placed under the child's pillow at night. Parents may need reassurance that the child will not become entangled in the leads during sleep.

Infrequently, mischievous, disturbed, or retarded children will pull off the electrodes, unplug the leads, or take out the batteries. If this is thought likely to happen, both the recorder and case can be secured with sticky tape. Occasionally, older children will deliberately tamper with electrodes. It can help to invite their cooperation, showing them that touching an electrode causes artifact. Usually, older children enjoy the responsibility and like to change tapes and batteries themselves.

The Recording Period

To increase the likelihood of recording preferably more than one attack, it is our own practice to record for 48 or 72 hr. Most families do not need to come back to the EEG department each day. They are provided with an illustrated manual explaining exactly how to change the tapes and batteries and re-jelly the electrodes. Problems do not often arise, but parents are encouraged to telephone the department if difficulties do occur.

Observation Sheets

Parents are asked to complete an observation sheet during the recording period in detail. This is not meant to be a minute-by-minute account, but information is specially required on such aspects as crying, tantrums, watching television, eating, and brushing teeth and whether the child is drowsy or alert. The importance of pressing the button when an attack occurs is also stressed to parents, as well as noting on the sheet that they have done so. This is an important way of avoiding confusion caused by the child or his friends pressing the button for fun!

In our experience with children of all ages, levels of intelligence, and types of behaviour, cassette recorders are tolerated very well even when parents are convinced that they will not be. Useful recordings can be made in almost all cases if the technicians have confidence that this is possible and allow sufficient time to put the above guidelines into practice.

DIFFERENTIAL DIAGNOSIS OF ATTACKS

Episodic changes in behaviour are probably more commonly encountered in children than in adults and can be a source of confusion and concern. Jeavons (5) has demonstrated the frequency with which epilepsy is misdiagnosed in children. This is partly the result of professional misconceptions about the nature of these disorders. Allied to this, there is the common failure to undertake a detailed appraisal of the nature of the attacks and the circumstances in which they occur. By these means a correct diagnosis can possibly be achieved in most cases, provided the characteristic features of different types of epileptic and nonepileptic attacks are appreciated (6).

In young or retarded children, however, subjective phenomena cannot be communicated adequately, and sometimes, even in older children, careful clinical enquiry will still leave the diagnosis in doubt. In these circumstances,

EEGs of the correct type can be helpful. The attacks in question are more likely to occur during the course of long-term monitoring than during brief conventional recordings, providing direct information about the physiological changes accompanying the episodes. Thereby, it may be possible to avoid the unhelpful and possibly misleading findings of many conventional interictal recordings (7).

By restricting the use of ambulatory monitoring to children whose attacks have previously been well documented clinically, and that are occurring at least several times a week, a high degree of diagnostic success seems possible (8,9). In our own experience, this success rate is comparable to that of selective inpatient video/EEG monitoring (10). In the absence of video details of the attacks, heavy reliance has to be placed on the observation sheets completed by parents, teachers, or nurses during the monitoring period. Detailed accounts about the episodes should make it possible to know whether the attacks recorded are of the type in question or different episodes that may coexist. The need for accurate observation is obvious on reflection, but without explicit instruction and perhaps practise (as described later) only perfunctory accounts may be provided.

In our own series, results of ambulatory monitoring have been more informative in children with a past history of epilepsy and new attacks of an uncertain nature than in those children with episodes of disturbed behaviour and no past history of definite epilepsy. The former group have been much more likely to have attacks during the recording period and to show positive EEG changes indicating that the episodes are a new manifestation of their seizure disorder (11). This difference has been consistent despite our reluctance to accept for ambulatory monitoring most children referred because of aggressive outbursts, on the grounds that this is a very unusual ictal manifestation. Nevertheless, there have been important examples of strange episodes shown to be epileptic in nature in children without a past history of seizure disorder, perhaps most notably cases of complex partial seizures of frontal lobe origin (12).

The implications of the absence of EEG changes at the time of patients' attacks have been debated widely since the early development of ambulatory monitoring. The absence of scalp-recorded EEG accompaniments in a high proportion of simple partial seizures is well documented (13). Clearly, negative findings do not exclude the possibility of epilepsy. In our own series, a diagnosis of "nonepilepsy" has only been made from a combination of such negative EEG findings and clinical information to suggest that the attacks are other than epileptic in type. In such cases, the diagnosis of nonepilepsy must be provisional and subject to revision in the light of subsequent events. Unfortunately, in most EEG services, such follow-up is not easily achieved in any systematic way.

In a modest study of our own (Stores and Styles, *unpublished*), 26 children, whose attacks had been diagnosed as nonepileptic partly on the basis of negative findings during ambulatory monitoring, were followed up. The attacks were considered to be psychological in nature in most cases. The age of these children ranged from 4 to 16 years; most were females and half had a past history of epilepsy. Follow-up over a period of between 1 and 5 years showed that in none had subsequent findings suggested the need to rediagnose the attacks as epileptic, providing some vindication of the conclusion based largely on negative EEG results. Interestingly, however, in half the series, the rate of the attacks had remained or had increased over the intervening period.

The overall impression from our own experience and that of others (14,15) is that ambulatory monitoring can make a very important contribution to the diagnosis of childhood attacks of an uncertain nature if used in conjunction with careful neurological and, in some cases, psychiatric appraisal. The procedure can lead to a more definite conclusion and programme of care than the often unhelpful results of perhaps repeated conventional EEG recordings between attacks.

PARTICULAR TYPES OF SEIZURE DISORDER

In our own department, special interest has developed in recent times in two particular types of epileptic disorder in children for which the use of ambulatory monitoring can be particularly appropriate: nonconvulsive status epilepticus and complex partial seizures of frontal lobe origin.

Various types of nonconvulsive status epilepticus are encountered in children (16). Their recognition and treatment are of importance not only to the child's immediate well-being but possible long-term neurological and intellectual condition. Unfortunately, these forms of epilepsy are often misdiagnosed or not recognised at all for three main reasons: lack of familiarity with the condition, its largely behavioural manifestations causing confusion with psychiatric states, and its very subtle nature in some patients. While clinical awareness and careful description are again the main ways in which nonconvulsive status epilepticus can be recognised, at least in its more dramatic forms, ambulatory monitoring can be a valuable means of detecting its intermittent occurrence (17).

Complex partial seizures originating in the frontal lobe have been the subject of increasing reports in recent years, highlighting again the risk of misdiagnosis because of the unusual and sometimes bizarre nature of the attacks. Most accounts have been concerned with adult patients for whom intracranial EEG recordings have been advocated, at least where surgical intervention is considered, because of the generally unhelpful nature of scalp-recorded EEGs (18).

Two recent reports (12,19) have demonstrated the occurrence of such attacks in children, misdiagnosis being a prominent feature in these cases. Our own preliminary findings suggest that ambulatory monitoring during attacks, with montages that emphasise frontal and prefrontal placements, can be a valuable noninvasive means of identifying frontal seizure discharge in these cases.

CLASSIFICATION OF SEIZURES

Intensive EEG monitoring, especially combined video/EEG recording, has been an invaluable means of collecting information for careful clinical scrutiny on which to base accurate classification of seizure types. Ambulatory monitoring is capable of making a contribution to this important exercise, especially where it is not feasible to perform video monitoring on a large scale.

The studies just quoted concerning the use of ambulatory monitoring in children with frontal lobe seizures hint at the possibility of more widespread use of the procedure for this purpose, particularly where intracranial monitoring is not justifiable. In such cases, there is the need to distinguish them from complex partial seizures of temporal lobe origin or indeed other extratemporal sources.

Apart from the practical importance of this distinction in the case of the individual patient, the prospect exists of achieving clearer delineation of the nature and consequences of different epileptic syndromes. Plouin (20) has reported cassette studies of children with West syndrome, the results of which provide another example of the way in which subcategories of epileptic disorders can be defined on the basis of their different pathophysiology.

PATTERNS OF SEIZURE OCCURRENCE

The identification of the distribution of seizure discharge over time can be important both clinically and theoretically. On the practical front, it is obviously valuable to demonstrate that the patient's seizures occur consistently or, conversely, are less likely to happen in certain circumstances. It might be possible to use such findings to alter the patient's physical or emotional environment to supplement at least the use of antiepileptic drug treatment.

Ambulatory monitoring lends itself well to the investigation of such phenomena and provides a practical alternative to the ideal of prolonged direct behavioural observation. Sato et al. (21) showed how ambulatory monitoring can be used to demonstrate consistent patterns of seizure occurrence in children with epilepsy encountering different experiences and environments in hospital and at home. These studies confirmed the impression that seizure frequency often increases in situations that the child finds stressful or during periods of inactivity. In another study, also concerned with patterns of seizure occurrence in children with epilepsy (22), stress, anxiety, and (unusually) physical activity were shown to be associated in individual cases with an increase of seizure discharge. In another case from the same series, a clear relationship to mealtimes of striking changes in seizure discharge was evident, although not mediated by changes in blood-sugar levels.

Children in this same study were all subject to absence seizures and as such appeared to be a homogeneous group. However, 24-hr monitoring revealed pronounced differences in the occurrence of seizure discharge in relation to the sleep/wake cycle. While most children showed maximal discharge in the awake state, others showed the converse, and in a small subgroup, seizure discharge was equally distributed between the awake and asleep parts of the 24-hr periods of recording. Such differences could suggest a physiological basis for further subgrouping the types of seizure disorder investigated. Perhaps this is another example of the possible use of ambulatory-monitoring findings in the classification of seizures.

ANTIEPILEPTIC DRUG EVALUATION

Some of Ives' earlier reports on the clinical usefulness of ambulatory monitoring included references to attempts to assess objectively response to antiepileptic treatment (23). Other reports of this application of the procedure, sometimes with outpatients, have followed (24). The value of ambulatory monitoring in the investigation of nonconvulsive status epilepticus, described earlier, extends to the assessment of response to treatment of recurrent bouts of status, which is often a difficult task, especially when the clinical manifestations are not obvious. In studies of short, discrete seizures, some patients have shown marked day-to-day fluctuations in the occurrence of seizure activity irrespective of treatment. Extended periods may be necessary, therefore, when evaluating treatments in this way and possibly an attempt to standardise environmental factors during repeated assessments and different drug conditions (25).

Studies of the type described have been limited to generalised forms of epilepsy, especially absence epilepsy, mainly because of the close correlation between electrographic and clinical events in this form of seizure disorder (26) but also because of the relative ease with which generalised spike-wave activity can be recognised and quantified, including the use of automated analysis systems (27). The use of ambulatory monitoring for evaluation of antiepileptic treatment of partial seizures has received little attention, largely because of the wide variety of electrographic accompaniments of such seizures, which make fully automated analysis an unlikely possibility. Other forms of assisted analysis of cassette tapes ('logging systems') can, however, take some of the tedium out of the analysis procedure.

LEARNING AND BEHAVIOUR PROBLEMS

These problems are commonly described in children with epilepsy. Many factors have been associated with their development (28). These include some of the conditions already described, the evaluation of which can be aided by ambulatory monitoring. In particular, this procedure can be helpful in identifying and quantifying the different types of seizure discharge with possible psychological effects.

Seizure activity known from observations of the patient to have been accompanied by clinical manifestations is obviously important. However, supposedly asymptomatic seizure discharge can sometimes be shown by special testing to have subtle clinical accompaniments (29). In the case of generalised spike-wave discharge, certain features of its distribution and morphology are associated with behavioural impairment, although exceptions to these general tendencies are encountered. Recent reports suggest that even brief or isolated discharges can sometimes have clinical significance (30). In some patients the eradication from the EEG of such discharges appears to be associated with behavioural improvement, for example, in learning ability. Such reports raise the possibility that antiepileptic drug treatment might need to be increased beyond the point at which clinically recognised seizures are suppressed in order to remove residual EEG discharges. Ambulatory monitoring is the only practical way at present of carrying out the assessments required in such circumstances.

There is increasing interest in the possible significance for psychological development of electrical status during sleep (31), with recent attempts to relate the development and persistence of this phenomenon to subsequent psychological development (32). It remains an open question at present whether attempts to suppress this asymptomatic form of EEG activity are justified. Ambulatory monitoring is again an eminently suitable means of collecting electrographic information on this point.

Finally, the possibility has started to be investigated that abnormalities of sleep structure associated with epilepsy or its treatment might cause adverse effect on behaviour. Zaiwalla and Stores (33) found that abnormalities of sleep and arousal were reported by parents significantly more often in epileptic children compared with controls and that there was a strong statistical association between these abnormalities and disturbed behaviour. Zaiwalla (34) has carried out overnight sleep recordings at home by means of cassette to identify the physiological correlates of 'poor quality' sleep of children with epilepsy. In some cases, profuse seizure discharge during sleep was identified; in others, long-duration arousals were more frequent than in control children. These findings suggest that subtle sleep disorders might exist in some children with epilepsy sufficient to affect their psychological functioning during the day.

CONCLUSIONS

Ambulatory monitoring has been a significant advance in clinical electroencephalography, allowing information to be collected in a way that would have been very difficult, if not impossible, by conventional means. Further refinements will, no doubt, extend its clinical usefulness still further.

Advocacy of the use of ambulatory monitoring has been partly an educational process insofar as discussion of its various clinical applications has inevitably promoted consideration of wider aspects of the care of patients with epilepsy beyond initial diagnosis. This is perhaps especially so in the case of children, where this form of investigation can be relevant to such issues as precipitating factors within the family and at school, and the possible influence of subtle effects of seizure discharge on learning and behaviour. The procedure's potential for helping with such issues remains relatively unexplored at the present time.

REFERENCES

1. Stores G, Hennion T, Quy RJ. EEG ambulatory monitoring system with visual play-back display. In: Wada JA, Penry JK, eds. *Advances in epileptology. The Xth epilepsy international symposium.* New York: Raven Press, 1980;89–94.
2. Stores G. Ambulatory EEG monitoring in the diagnosis of epilepsy. In: Parsonage MJ, ed. *Aspects of epilepsy. Res Clin Forums* 1980;2:141–148.
3. Ebersole JS, Bridgers, SL. Direct comparison of 3 and 8 channel ambulatory cassette EEG with intensive inpatient monitoring. *Neurology (Cleve)* 1983;35:846–854.
4. Leroy RF, Ebersole JS. An evaluation of ambulatory cassette monitoring. I. Montage design. *Neurology (Cleve)* 1983;33:1–7.
5. Jeavons PM. Non epileptic attacks in childhood. In: Rose FC, ed. *Research progress in epilepsy.* London: Pitman, 1983;224–230.
6. Pedley TA. Differential diagnosis of episodic symptoms. *Epilepsia* 1983;24(suppl 1):531–544.
7. Kellaway P. Intensive monitoring in infants and children. In: Gumnit RJ, ed. *Advances in neurology, vol 46: Intensive neurodiagnostic monitoring.* New York: Raven Press, 1986;127–137.
8. Forrest GC, Crawford C. Ambulatory monitoring and child psychiatry. In: Stott FD, Wright SL, Raftery EB, et al., eds. *ISAM 1981: Proceedings of the fourth international symposium on ambulatory monitoring.* London: Academic Press, 1982;157–161.
9. Stores G. Clinical and EEG evaluation of seizures and seizure-like disorders. *J Am Child Psychiatry* 1985;24:10–16.
10. Stores G. Comparison of video and ambulatory (cassette) monitoring in the investigation of attacks in children. In: Dal Palu C, Pessina AC, eds. *ISAM 1985: Proceedings of the fifth international symposium on ambulatory monitoring.* Padova: Cleup, 1986;633–638.
11. Stores G. Ambulatory diagnostic monitoring of seizures in children. In: Gumnit RJ, ed. *Advances in neurology, vol 46: Intensive neurodiagnostic monitoring.* New York: Raven Press, 1986;157–167.
12. Stores G, Zaiwalla Z. Misdiagnosis of frontal lobe complex partial seizures in children. *Proceedings of the 17th epilepsy international congress,* Jerusalem, 1987 (in press).
13. Ives JR, Woods JF. A study of 100 patients with focal epilepsy using a four-channel ambulatory cassette recorder. In: Stott FD, Raftery EB, Goulding L, eds. *ISAM 1979: Proceedings of the third international symposium on ambulatory monitoring.* London: Academic Press, 1980;383–392.
14. Bachman, DS. 24 hour ambulatory electroencephalographic monitoring in paediatrics. *Clin Electroencephalogr* 1984;15:164–166.
15. Plouin P, Jalin C, Bour F, et al. Value of ambulatory monitoring in children with epilepsy. Presentation to 1st international conference in ambulatory monitoring in epilepsy and sleep disorders, Telfs, 1986.
16. Stores G. Nonconvulsive status epilepticus in children. In: Pedley TA, Meldrum BS, eds. *Recent advances in epilepsy 3.* Edinburgh: Churchill Livingstone, 1986;295–310.
17. Zaiwalla Z. Cassette EEG monitoring in nonconvulsive status epilepticus. Presentation to Northern European epilepsy meeting, York, 1986.
18. Williamson PD, Spencer SS. Clinical and EEG features of complex partial seizures of extra temporal origin. *Epilepsia* 1986;27(suppl 2):546–563.
19. Numata Y, Yagi K, Seino M. Frontal automatisms. Presentation to the 16th epilepsy international congress, Hamburg, 1985.
20. Plouin P. 24 hour cassette recordings in West syndrome: diagnostic and prognostic implications. Presentation to 2nd international conference on ambulatory monitoring in epilepsy and sleep disorders, Telfs, 1987.
21. Sato S, Penry JK, Dreifuss FE. Electroencephalographic monitoring of generalised spike wave

paroxysms in the hospital and at home. In: Kellaway P, Petersen I, eds. *Quantitative analytic studies in epilepsy.* New York: Raven Press, 1976;237–251.
22. Stores G, Lwin R. Precipitating factors and seizure activity. In: Stott FD, Wright SL, Raftery EB, et al., eds. *ISAM 1981: Proceedings of the fourth international symposium on ambulatory monitoring.* London: Academic Press, 1982;183–188.
23. Ives JR, Woods JF. Four channel 24 hour cassette recorder for long term EEG monitoring of ambulatory patients. *Electroencephalogr Clin Neurophysiol* 1975;39:88–92.
24. Burr W, Stefan H, Kuhnen C, et al. Effects of valproic acid treatment on spike-wave discharge patterns during sleep and wakefulness. *Neuropsychobiology* 1983;10:56–59.
25. Milligan, N, Richens A. Ambulatory monitoring of the EEG in the assessment of anti-epileptic drugs. In: Stott FD, Wright SL, Raftery EB, et al., eds. *ISAM 1981: Proceedings of the fourth international symposium on ambulatory monitoring.* London: Academic Press, 1982;224–233.
26. Kellaway P, Saltzberg B, Frost Jr, JD. Relationship between clinical state, ictal and interictal EEG discharges, and serum drug levels: generalized epilepsy/ethosuximide. *Neurology* 1979;29:559.
27. Bailey C. Evaluation of a spike and wave processor for use in long-term ambulatory EEG monitoring. In: Stott FD, Wright SL, Raftery EB, et al., eds. *ISAM 1981: Proceedings of the fourth international symposium on ambulatory monitoring.* London: Academic Press, 1982;203–207.
28. Stores G. Learning and emotional problems in children with epilepsy. In: Reynolds EH, Trimble MR, eds. *Epilepsy and psychiatry.* Edinburgh: Churchill Livingstone, 1981;33–48.
29. Stores G. Effects on learning of 'subclinical' seizure discharge. In: Aldencamp AP, Alpherts WCJ, Meinardi H, et al., eds. *Education and epilepsy.* Amsterdam: Swets and Zeitlinger 1987;14–20.
30. Aarts JHP, Binnie CD, Smit AM, et al. Selective cognitive impairment during focal and generalised epileptiform EEG activity. *Brain* 1984;107:293–308.
31. Tassinari CA, Dravet C, Roger J. Encephalopathy related to electrical status epilepticus during slow sleep. *Electroencephalogr Clin Neurophysiol* 1977;43:529–530.
32. Morikawa T. Clinical relevance of continuous spike-wave during slow wave sleep or 'electrical status epilepticus sleep (ESES)'. Proceedings of the 17th epilepsy international congress, Jerusalem, 1987 (in press).
33. Zaiwalla Z, Stores G. Sleep disorders and quality of sleep in children with epilepsy. Presentation to the 17th epilepsy international congress, Jerusalem, 1987.
34. Zaiwalla Z. Sleep and arousal disorders in childhood epilepsy. *Electroencephalogr Clin Neurophysiol* (in press).

Ambulatory EEG Monitoring,
edited by John S. Ebersole.
Raven Press, Ltd., New York © 1989

9

Clinical Utility of Cassette EEG in Neonatal Seizure Disorders

Janet A. Eyre

Department of Child Health, The Medical School, Framlington Place, Newcastle Upon Tyne NE2 4HH England

The diagnosis of seizure in the newborn infant is important not only because seizure may be the presenting symptom of a neurological or metabolic disorder, but also because there is a strong association between seizures in the neonatal period and permanent handicap in the survivors (1). The pathogenesis of brain damage as a consequence of repeated seizures has been attributed to neuronal necrosis secondary to increased neuronal energy requirement in the presence of the hypoxaemia that may accompany the motor activity of a seizure. In his studies in animals, however, Wasterlain found that seizures during the neonatal period (induced by indirect electroconvulsive shock, flurothyl, bicuculline, or fever) inhibit brain DNA synthesis, permanently reduce the number of brain cells and brain size, and delay behavioural milestones even in animals adequately ventilated and oxygenated throughout the seizures. Similar defects were not found in studies of mature animals. These studies using an animal model suggest that the poor prognosis associated with neonatal seizures may not be solely a consequence of the underlying illness, but that the neonatal brain is susceptible to permanent damage as a consequence of seizure (2–7). The diagnosis of seizure will, therefore, not only allow the identification of a baby at high risk of subsequent handicap, but early treatment may decrease the high incidence of associated morbidity.

Seizures in the newborn are difficult to diagnose because the clinical signs manifest and the waveforms of the electroencephalographic activity are different from those in older children and adults. Generalised tonic clonic seizures are rare in newborn babies (8,9); the clinical manifestations of seizure are most commonly atypical and subtle (10–13). Thus Dreyfus-Brisac and Monod (14), utilising cinematography with the electroencephalogram, showed that blinking, nystagmus, vasomotor instability, apnoea, and changes in muscle tone were commonly the only manifestation of electroencephalographic seizure activity.

All these signs also occur frequently in ill newborn infants who are not seizing, thus making it impossible to diagnose seizures on clinical signs alone.

Subclinical seizures have also been reported in the newborn infant (12,13,15), and seizures have been recorded in very sick infants paralysed to facilitate artificial ventilation (16,17). For these reasons, the diagnosis of seizure from clinical signs in the newborn may be very difficult, and even status epilepticus may be missed (18,19). The spike-and-wave pattern typical of seizure activity in older children is rarely, if ever, seen in the newborn infant. Neonatal electroencephalographic seizure activity takes two basic forms—either the sudden onset of rhythmical sharp or slow waves (Fig. 1) or the paroxysmal appearance of rhythmic activity of a single frequency within the alpha or theta frequencies (Fig. 2)(20). Although different from the pattern of seizure activity recorded in older children and adults, the neonatal patterns of electroencephalographic seizure activity are easily recognised, thus making the EEG very useful in making or confirming a diagnosis of seizure.

The difficulty in making a clinical diagnosis of seizure and the increasing use of paralysis to facilitate artificial ventilation in those babies at most risk of seizing indicate a need to monitor continuously the EEG of very sick babies receiving intensive care. It is in the monitoring of the EEG of the sick newborn within the intensive care unit that we have found the cassette recording of the EEG is most valuable in the neonatal period.

METHODS

There are major problems associated with making a prolonged record of a standard EEG in a neonatal intensive care nursery. First, the record is subject to artefact during nursing and medical procedures; second, electrical interference poses appreciable difficulties; and, finally, the recorder is large and may obstruct access. Such an obstruction can be life threatening when providing intensive care to a very ill baby.

Cassette recording of the EEG offers particular advantages in the intensive care nursery; the recorder is small and, therefore, can lie beside the baby either in an incubator or on the bed under an overhead heater (Fig. 3). It is battery powered, which almost eliminates the problems associated with electrical artefact. Scalp-mounted preamplifiers significantly reduce electrical and movement artefact (Fig. 4). The data are stored on cassette tapes, and automated replay allows the EEG to be reviewed and analysed in a manageable time period.

There are, however, two principal disadvantages of using cassette EEG. First, the absence of a technician continuously noting down the recording conditions makes the recognition of artefacts difficult. Some rhythmical artefacts can be confused easily with seizure activity. The confusion arises most frequently in association with artefact from respiration (see Fig. 1) or the sudden appearance of ECG artefact, particularly during cardiac arrhythmias (see Fig. 5). In order

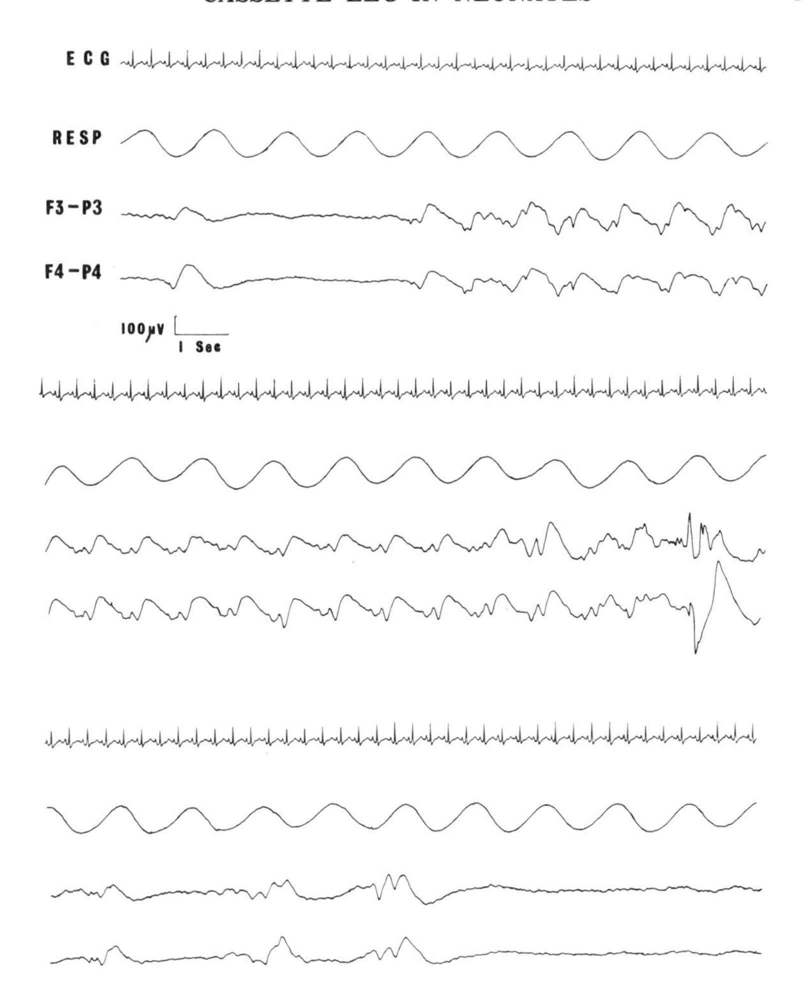

FIG. 1. Baby H 26 wk male age 2d. Seizure discharge with abrupt onset of synchronous and symmetrical rhythmic sharp and slow waves in the right and left channels of the EEG. Note that, in the absence of a record of respiration, the rhythmic slow-wave activity might be considered to be movement artefact from respiration.

to assist in the recognition of these artefacts, we record the ECG and respiration using transthoracic impedance.

The second disadvantage of cassette recording is the limited montage available. There are, however, practical limitations to the number of EEG channels that can be recorded continuously during neonatal intensive care. The disadvantages of limited information obtained from a restricted montage are balanced by a reduction in disturbance to the baby and the minimal interference with nursing care. In addition, the newborn baby, particularly the very preterm

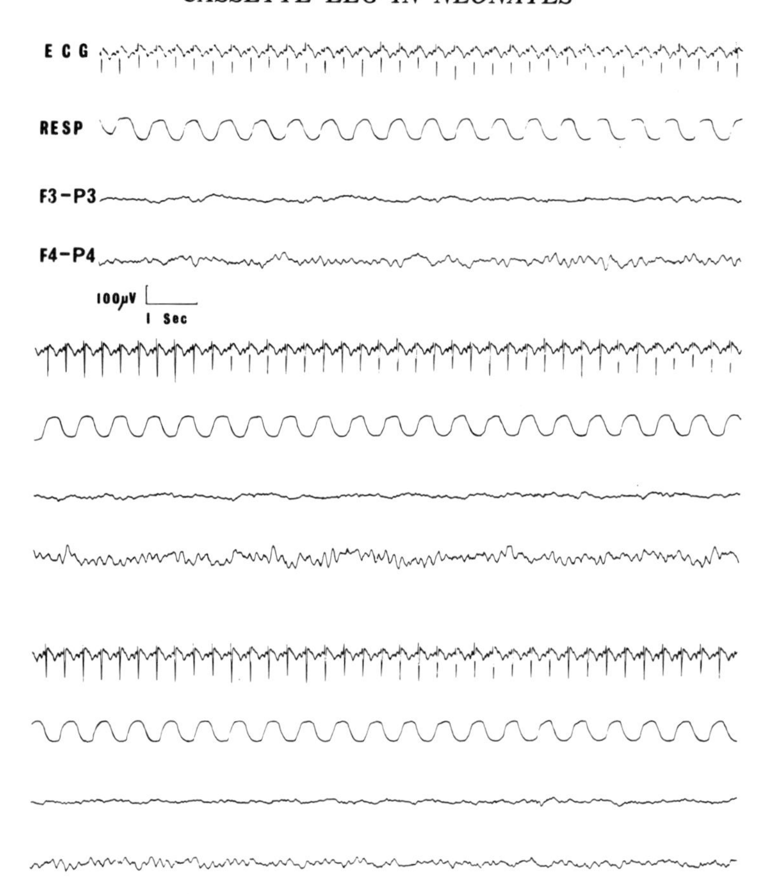

FIG. 2. Baby L 24 wks female age 6 wk. Seizure discharge of rhythmic waves in the theta frequency in the right channel of the EEG.

infant, has a small head; it is important to maintain access to the anterior fontanelle for ultrasound and to scalp vessels for venous or arterial cannulation. For these reasons, we have chosen to record only two channels of EEG, one from the right and one from the left hemisphere. Although some episodes of focal seizure may be missed, we have found that such recordings significantly increase the detection of seizures (see below) and, as such, were very useful for the continuous *monitoring* of the EEG. Such a limited montage, however, cannot be regarded as a substitute for the standard 16-channel diagnostic EEG.

The EEG is recorded using standard silver/silver chloride cup electrodes. The electrodes are fixed to the scalp with collodion, and, after filling with saline jelly, the holes in the electrode are sealed with collodion to prevent evaporation of the conducting jelly in the hot environment of the intensive care unit. To reduce movement artefact, we have chosen to record the EEG from F_3-P_3 and F_4-P_4

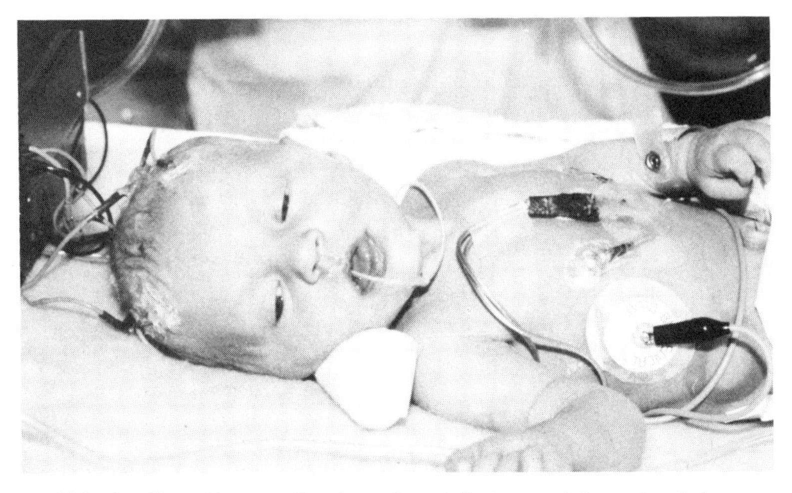

FIG. 3. Cassette recording in preterm infant nursed in an incubator.

because, in these positions, the electrodes do not come into contact with the mattress. To protect the electrodes from displacement during movement, the miniaturised preamplifiers are also fixed to the scalp over the vertex with collodion. Thus, displacement during movement occurs primarily at the scalp/preamplifier junction and not at the EEG electrode. This results in a considerable reduction in movement artefact (Fig. 4), and in our studies artefact from movement obscured less than 10% of any recording.

The time taken to apply the electrodes and the skin-mounted preamplifiers is approximately 20 to 30 min, and we have found that, with care, the application of the electrodes does not disturb the clinical condition of even very sick babies.

During the period of monitoring, we measure the skin-to-electrode impedance at 6 to 8 hourly intervals to ensure it remains below 5 K ohm. When a high impedance is found, the collodion seal over the hole in the electrode is dissolved with acetone and additional jelly injected; the hole is then resealed with collodion. On average, the electrodes need re-siting after 6 days, although, in some babies, we have found that the electrodes did not need re-siting for 16 days or more. At the end of the monitoring period, the electrodes can be removed by gently dissolving the collodion with acetone.

We measure the transthoracic impedance using silver/silver chloride cup electrodes filled with saline jelly, which were attached to the chest with collodion. To minimise artefact from displacement of the electrodes during movement, the patient leads are fixed to the chest wall using adhesive tape and collodion (Fig. 3). The ECG is recorded from silver/silver chloride disposable electrodes.

We have found that the recordings do not interfere with intensive care and recording can continue throughout all nursing and medical procedures, including surgery, because the cassette recorder can be transported with the

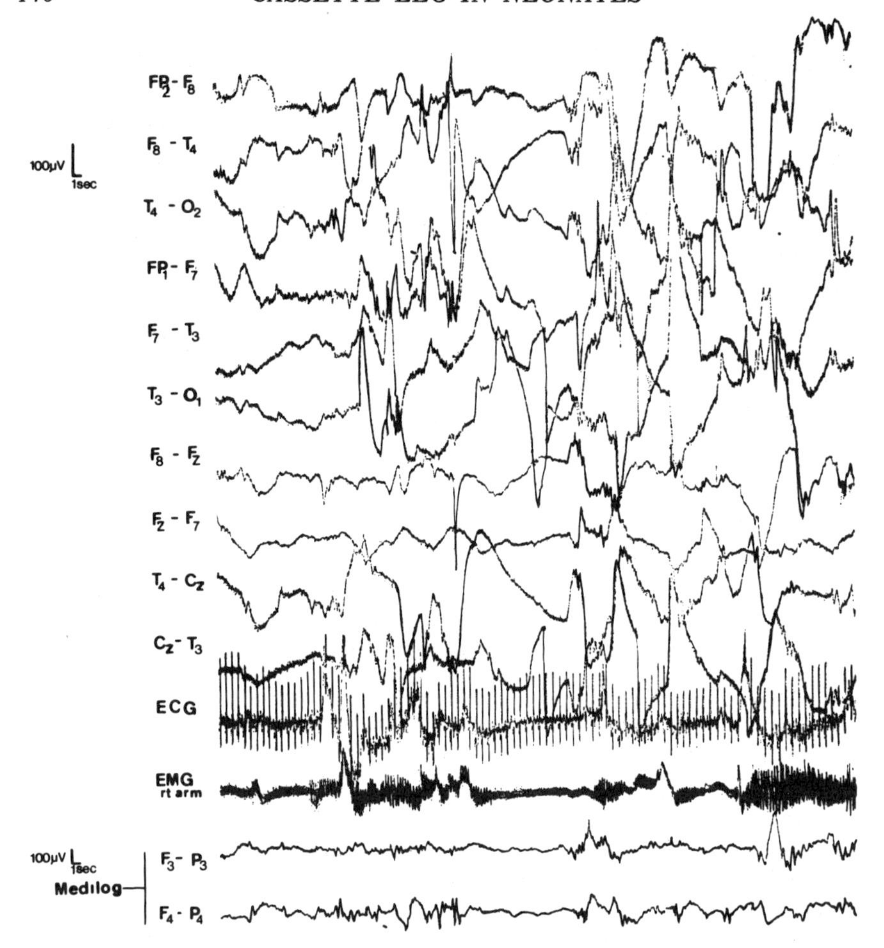

FIG. 4. Movement artefact in a standard 9-channel EEG compared with an artefact-free simultaneously recorded 2-channel cassette EEG from electrodes and preamplifiers attached to the scalp with collodion.

baby if necessary. We find that approximately 30 min of attention per day is necessary to maintain the electrodes.

During the recording, the data can be displayed above the bed on an oscilloscope. The tape record can be reviewed at intervals determined both by the clinical condition of the baby and by the previous findings. We review the recordings on a visual display unit, where the data are presented in a paginated format on a video screen at $\frac{1}{20}$th or $\frac{1}{60}$th of real time; in addition, a copy is made in compressed formation onto paper (Fig. 6). In this way, both electroencephalographic seizure activity can be detected and the number of episodes and the total duration of ictal activity can be calculated. The time taken to analyse a 24-hr

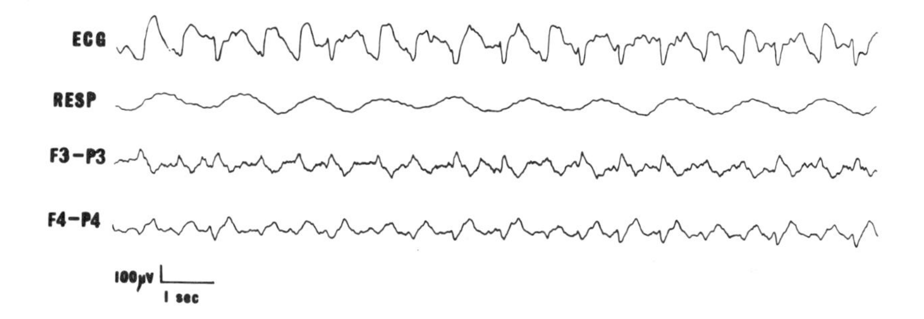

FIG. 5. Baby W 36 wk male age 1d. Rhythmic artefact appearing on both the right and left channels of the EEG from a cardiac arrhythmia.

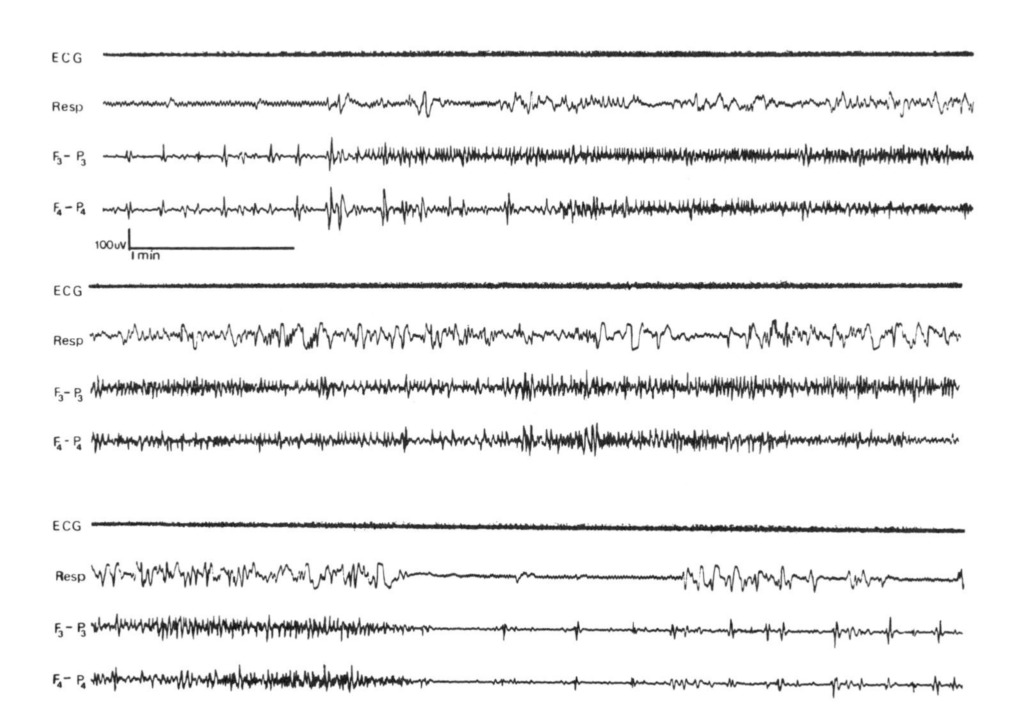

FIG. 6. Baby W 38 wk female age 1d. A compressed record of an ictal episode showing the left-sided onset of a seizure with secondary generalisation to the left hemisphere. The seizure persists for 11.5 min and is followed by a prolonged apnoea.

record varies from 30 min when no abnormality is found to 3 hr for a complicated tape showing EEG abnormalities.

RESULTS

We have assessed the value of monitoring the EEG for the diagnosis of seizure in sick newborn infants receiving intensive care in two studies.

In the first study the value of EEG monitoring in 25 neonates with diagnosed neurological complications was assessed (16). The details concerning these babies are summarised in Table 1. The EEG was monitored continuously throughout the period of their neurological illness, and so the recording period varied from 11 hr to 16 days; the median was 72 hr and the total recording period was 2680 hr.

Electroencephalographic seizure activity was recorded in 20 of 25 babies studied. In 11, clinical signs accompanied some of the seizures; however, there was a high incidence of subclinical seizures in these babies. Four babies were paralysed during the seizure activity; in these and five other babies, there were no clinical signs recognised in association with electroencephalographic seizure activity. Thus, in nine of the 20 babies with seizure, the diagnosis would have been missed without EEG monitoring, and, in a further nine babies, the frequency and duration of the seizures would not have been appreciated by clinical signs alone.

A total of 3619 episodes of electroencephalographic seizure activity were recorded. There was no difference between the EEG recorded during subclinical seizures and those in which there were clinical signs. Three babies had clinically unrecognised status epilepticus for more than 9 hr. In both the right and left channels 2279 (63%) ictal episodes occurred synchronously and symmetrically; 108 (3%) occurred simultaneously but asynchronously in the right and left channels, while 1232 (34%) were recorded in only the right or left channel, Eighty-two percent of the seizure discharges comprised paroxysms of rhythmical sharp or slow waves and 18% comprised paroxysms of rhythmical activity in the alpha or theta frequencies.

For 14 babies, the seizure activity was confined to paroxysmal discharges of rhythmic sharp or slow waves. In five, both paroxysms of rhythmic sharp or slow waves and paroxysmal discharges in the alpha or theta frequency were found, and, in one baby, the seizure activity consisted solely of paroxysmal discharges of rhythmical activity in the alpha or theta frequency.

Seizure activity ceased within 6 hr of the intravenous administration of anticonvulsants in only four babies, although serum values were within accepted therapeutic range in all 20 babies with seizure activity.

The large number of seizures recorded in these 20 babies and the high incidence of subclinical seizures even in those with clinical signs were unexpected findings. These results established the need for EEG monitoring in

TABLE 1. *Clinical details of the 25 babies with recognised neurological complications*

Sex	Gest[a] (w)	Bwgt[b] (g)	Neurological complication	Recording period (hr)	Total seizures (N)	Total seizures Duration (hr)	Clinical signs
F	41	3995	Birth asphyxia	384	667	25.90	Clonic movements
M	41	3440	Birth asphyxia	336	650	39.00	No signs
M	41	2930	Birth asphyxia	48	414	11.50	paralysed
F	40	3230	Birth asphyxia	261	381	20.60	No signs
M	38	2590	Asphyxia	72	241	20.40	Clonic movements
M	38	2840	Birth asphyxia	144	235	7.30	Clonic movements
M	34	2930	Birth asphyxia	11	200	3.70	No signs
M	32	2750	Meningitis	8	192	10.60	Clonic movements
M	27	1190	Asphyxia	120	188	8.10	Paralysed
M	26	1200	ICH[c]	72	147	4.70	Paralysed
M	40	4160	ICH	24	100	5.00	Opisthotonic
F	24	790	Cardiac arrest	24	76	1.30	No signs
F	41	3130	Birth asphyxia	168	55	4.30	Apnoea
M	42	4160	Birth asphyxia	120	45	5.00	Clonic movements
F	40	3390	Birth asphyxia	48	13	1.30	Opisthotonic
F	40	3460	Birth asphyxia	192	10	0.80	Opisthotonic
M	33	1940	Asphyxia	120	2	0.10	No signs
M	38	2550	Birth asphyxia	72	1	0.10	Clonic movements
M	40	3800	Birth asphyxia	48	1	0.03	Paralysed
F	38	2530	Birth asphyxia	24	1	0.20	Opisthotonic
F	41	3880	Birth asphyxia	24	0	0.00	Opisthotonic
M	32	1840	Birth asphyxia	48	0	0.00	Clonic movements
F	27	1020	Birth asphyxia	48	0	0.00	Unconscious
M	26	810	Birth asphyxia	120	0	0.00	Tonic posturing
F	38	2725	Asphyxia	120	0	0.00	Paralysed

[a]Gest, gestation.
[b]Bwgt, birthweight.
[c]ICH, intracranial haemorrhage.

babies with recognised neurological complications; however, it also raised two questions: first, was there a similarly high incidence of subclinical seizures in other babies receiving intensive care in whom neurological complications had not been recognised? Second, does subclinical electroencephalographic seizure activity occur in well babies receiving nursing care only?

In order to answer these questions, we monitored continuously for the first 5 days after birth the EEG of 80 babies selected at random from the 399 children who were admitted to the John Radcliffe Maternity Hospital Special Care Nursery between 1981 and 1983 and who required assisted ventilation from within a few hours after birth (21); these children we observed to be at high risk of neurological complications. In addition, we similarly recorded continuously for the first 5 days after birth the EEG of 25 children who were at low risk of neurological complications; these children were selected from those infants who were well and receiving nursing care for prematurity or were cared for by their mother on the postnatal wards.

In all subjects, the recording began as soon as informed consent was obtained from the parents. The median time to the onset of the recording was 5 hr after birth, with a range of 1 to 12 hr; the recording continued for 5 days or until the baby died.

The children whose EEG was recorded have subsequently been examined at 18 months by an independent observer, who performed a neurological examination and a Griffith's developmental assessment. The details of the children studied and of the remaining 319 children admitted for intensive care over the study period are summarised in Table 2.

There were no clinical signs suggestive of seizures in the 25 well (low-risk) babies, and no electroencephalographic seizure discharges were recorded.

Seizure activity was recorded in 34 (46%) of the 80 babies who were receiving assisted ventilation. There was a high incidence of subclinical electroencephalographic seizure activity; all 34 had episodes of subclinical seizure. In 24 children, clinical signs accompanied some of the electroencephalographic seizures, but, in 10, no clinical signs were noted and the diagnosis of seizure was not made clinically (see Table 3).

The median time to the onset of seizure activity was 14 hr, with a range of 1 to 96 hr. Of the 34 children, 23 (68%) started to seize within 24 hr after birth, and 27 (80%) within 48 hr after birth (see Fig. 7).

Seizures were most frequent and of longest duration on the day of onset of seizure activity and decreased progressively in number and duration (see Fig. 8) with each succeeding day. The median period over which seizure activity occurred was 48 hr. Eight of the 34 children with seizures died within the first 5 days and were still seizing at the time of death. Eight children were still seizing at the end of the first 5 days; for five of these children, seizures began on day 3 or later after birth. Eighteen stopped seizing within the 5 days of recording; 16 of these children had seizures for less than 48 hr.

In total, 2825 ictal episodes were recorded; 1362 (43%) of the episodes of seizure activity had a focal onset and remained confined to one hemisphere, while 1463 (57%) were primarily or became secondarily generalised. Rhythmic sharp and slow waves were recorded in 2702 (95%) of the seizures and rhythmical alpha or theta in 123 (5%).

By 18 months corrected age, 19 of the 105 children studied had died; 82 of the 86 survivors were seen at follow-up by an independent observer. All 25 low-risk infants were well and developmentally and neurologically normal. The outcomes of the 80 high-risk babies are summarised in Table 4. A discriminant analysis showed that both the number of seizures and the total duration of seizure activity were significantly related to outcome.

DISCUSSION

Cassette EEG, which was developed to provide prolonged EEG recording in ambulatory epileptic patients, has proven adaptable to the neonatal intensive care unit, where considerations of space and patient access have limited the application of conventional EEG for long-term monitoring. Continuous cassette recordings of the EEG not only allow the diagnosis of seizure in babies who have been paralysed or who have minimal signs of seizure activity but also have revealed a high incidence of subclinical seizure amongst those babies in whom a clinical diagnosis of seizure has been made.

A review of the published literature shows that most neonatal seizures occur within 3 days after birth; the percentage of seizures reported to occur during this time varies from 43%, as found by Brown and his colleagues, to 86%, as reported by Burke (9,22–24). A continuous record during the first 5 days after

TABLE 2. *Details of the high- and low-risk babies (in whom a continuous 5-day recording of the EEG was made) in comparison to the total population of babies receiving intensive care between 1981 and 1983*

	Sample population		Newborn children
	High risk	Low risk	receiving intensive care
N	80	25	319
Weight	(g)		
Mean + SD	2050 + 1030	2410 + 909	2110 + 935
Median	1740	2210	1850
Range	520–4600	990–4120	490–4840
Gestation	(w)		
Mean + SD	32.7 + 5.16	34.6 + 3.84	32.4 + 4.5
Median	31.5	34	32
Range	26–42	26–42	23–42

There are no significant differences between the 80 babies studied and the 319 remaining children who received intensive care over this period.

TABLE 3. *Details of the high-risk babies with and without electroencephalographic seizure activity*

	No seizure	Seizure
N	46	34
Weight (g)		
Mean + SD	1890 + 990	2210 + 1070
Range	520–4600	850–4160
Gestation (w)		
Mean + SD	32.2 + 4.7	34.2 + 5.6
Range	26–42	26–42
Abnormal clinical signs	8	10
Reason for admission		
Prematurity and hyaline membrane disease	27 (59%)	17 (50%)
Birth asphyxia	12 (26%)	14 (41%)
Infection meningitis	1 (2%)	2 (6%)
other	2 (4%)	1 (3%)
Other	4 (9%)	0

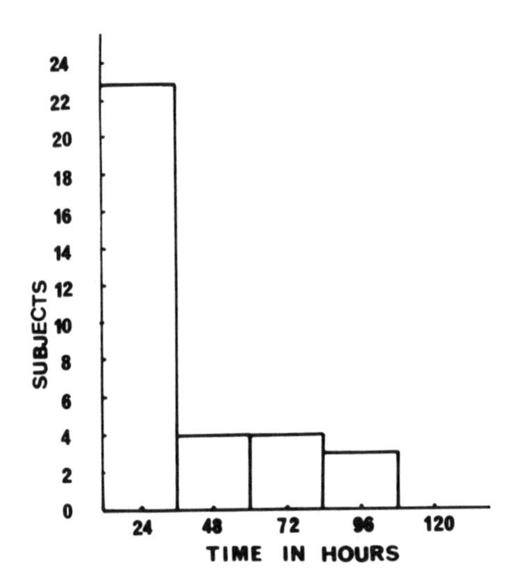

FIG. 7. The time of onset of seizure activity in 34 babies monitored while receiving intensive care during the first 5 days after birth.

birth, or during the immediate period after a neurological complication, therefore, will identify most babies who have neonatal seizures.

The continuous record of the EEG enables quantification of both the number of episodes and the total duration of electroencephalographic seizure activity during the period of monitoring. Because of the association between the number and duration of seizures in the neonatal period and poor outcome, these data can be used, in addition to other factors, to identify babies at high risk of future handicap.

The continuous record of the EEG can also be used to assess the efficacy of

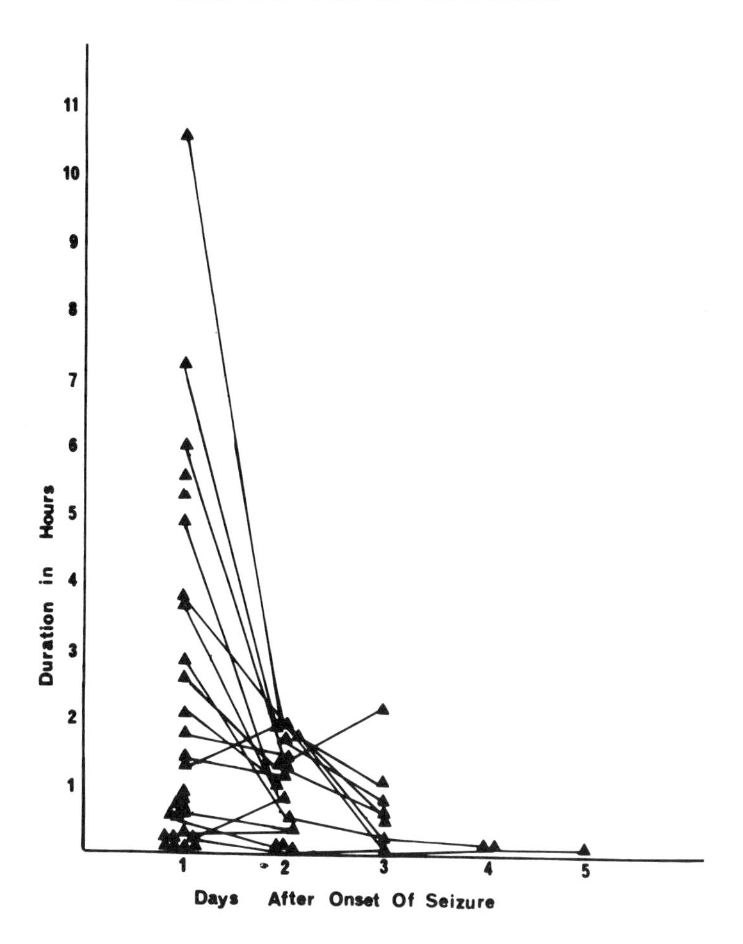

FIG. 8. The total duration of ictal activity in each 24-hr period after the onset of seizure activity in 34 babies monitored while receiving intensive care during the first 5 days after birth.

anticonvulsant therapy. While the aim of the studies described above was not to assess the efficacy of treatment, the unexpectedly high numbers of seizures, despite apparently adequate serum levels of anticonvulsant drugs, suggest that appropriate anticonvulsant therapy for the newborn needs further investigation.

The ability to diagnose seizure in those babies who are paralysed and in those with no or subtle signs of seizure is dependent upon the electroencephalographic finding of seizure activity. Cassette recording of the EEG provides a practical noninvasive method to monitor the EEG in very sick babies receiving intensive care.

TABLE 4. *Details of the outcome of the babies studied*

	No seizure	Seizure	Total duration of ictal activity in min/hr of recording	
	(N)	(N)	Median (min/hr)	Range (min/hr)
Died	4	15	2.71	0.12–20.41
Abnormal	10	10	0.48	0.06– 2.40
Normal	29	8	0.24	0.04– 3.61
Lost to follow-up	3	1	—	—

ACKNOWLEDGEMENTS

I would like to acknowledge the generous support of The National Fund for Research into Crippling Disorders.

REFERENCES

1. Mellits ED, Holden KR, Freeman JM. Neonatal seizures. II. A multivariate analysis of factors associated with outcome. *Peds* 1982;70:177–185.
2. Wasterlain CG, Plum F. Vulnerability of developing rat brain to electroconvulsive seizures. *Arch Neurol* 1973;29:38–45.
3. Wasterlain CG. Inhibition of cerebral protein synthesis by epileptic seizures without motor manifestations. *Neurology (Minneap)* 1974;24:175–180.
4. Wasterlain CG. Mortality and morbidity from serial seizures. An experimental study. *Epilepsia* 1974;15:155–176.
5. Wasterlain CG. Effects of neonatal status epilepticus on rat brain development. *Neurology (Minneap)* 1976;26:975–986.
6. Wasterlain CG. Does anoxemia play a role in the effects of neonatal seizures on brain growth? An experimental study in the rat. *Eur Neurol* 1979;18:222–229.
7. Wasterlain CG. Breakdown of brain polysomes in status epilepticus. *Brain Res* 1972;39:278–284.
8. Craig WS. Convulsive movements occurring in the first ten days of life. *Arch Dis Child* 1960;35:336–340.
9. Harris R, Tizzard JP. The electroencephalogram in neonatal convulsions. *J Ped* 1960;45:501–520.
10. Volpe JJ. Neonatal convulsions. *Clin Perinatol* 1977;2:43–66.
11. Nogan AG. Neonatal seizures: A reappraisal. *Clin Electroencephalogr* 1984;15:133–139.
12. Watanabe K, Hara K, Miyazaki S, et al. Electroclinical studies of seizures in the newborn. *Folia Psychiatr Neurol Jpn* 1977;31:383–392.
13. Rose AL, Lombroso CT. Neonatal seizure states. *Pediatrics* 1970;45:404–445.
14. Dreyfus-Brisac C, Monod N. Electroclinical studies of status epilepticus and convulsions in the newborn. In: Kellaway P, Petersen I, eds. *Neurological and electroencephalographic correlative studies in infancy.* New York: Grune & Stratton, 1964;250–272.
15. Eyre JA, Oozeer RC, Wilkinson AR. Continuous electroencephalographic recording to detect seizures in paralysed newborns. *Br Med J* 1983;286:1017–1018.
16. Eyre JA, Oozeer RC, Wilkinson AR. Diagnosis of neonatal seizure by continuous recording and rapid analysis of the electroencephalogram. *Arch Dis Child* 1983;58:785–790.
17. Staudt F, Roth JG, Engel RC. The usefulness of electroencephalography in curarised newborns. *Electroencephalogr Clin Neurophysiol* 1981;51:205–208.
18. Mora EU, de Alba GO, Garcia DV, et al. Neonatal status epilepticus. I. Clinical aspects. *Clin Electroencephalogr* 1984;15:193–196.

19. Dreyfus-Brisac C, Monad N. Neonatal status epilepticus. *Electroencephalogr Clin Neurophysiol* 1972;5:30–52.
20. Fenichel GM. *Neonatal electroencephalography. Neonatal Neurology.* London, Edinburgh: Churchill Livingstone 1980;235–239.
21. Eyre JA, Chaplais JC, Davies S, et al. Analysis of continuously recorded electroencephalogram may predict outcome at 18 months. *Pediatr Res* 1986;20:1063.
22. Burke JB. The prognostic significance of neonatal convulsions. *Arch Dis Child* 1954;29:342–345.
23. Brown JK, Cockburn F, Forfar JO. Clinical and chemical correlates in convulsions of the newborn. *Lancet* 1972;i:135–139.
24. Knauss TA, Marshall RE. Seizures in a neonatal intensive care unit. *Dev Med Child Neurol* 1977;19:719–728.

Ambulatory EEG Monitoring,
edited by John S. Ebersole.
Raven Press, Ltd., New York © 1989

10

Intensive Neurodiagnostic Monitoring in Epilepsy Using Ambulatory Cassette EEG with Simultaneous Video Recording

Robert F. Leroy, Kalpana K. Rao, and Barbara J. Voth

Department of Neurology, University of Texas, Southwestern Medical Center at Dallas, Dallas, Texas 75235

Simultaneous recording of behavior and EEG activity, called neurodiagnostic monitoring, is often the key to appropriate evaluation of patients whose seizures present difficult diagnostic or therapeutic problems. Unlike most who use combined behavioral and EEG monitoring, we have employed cassette EEG for this purpose (1). Because we are also engaged in more typical neurodiagnostic monitoring employing hard-wired 32-channel EEG monitoring and synchronized video recording, we have been able to evaluate the newer technique within the context of what can be achieved with the more elaborate and sophisticated, yet decidedly less mobile, approach to neurodiagnostic monitoring generally employed by epilepsy centers engaged in presurgical evaluation. In this chapter, we will present our rationale for this use of cassette EEG, review the technique as we have developed it, and present the results of our initial clinical experience with 100 patients.

BACKGROUND

Neurodiagnostic Monitoring

Neurodiagnostic monitoring in epilepsy consists of observing and recording the ictal manifestations of seizures while evaluating the pharmacologic, behavioral, and neurologic state of the patient (2). Conventional seizure diagnosis, in contrast, relies on interictal EEG data and descriptions of ictal behavior provided by untrained and often frightened witnesses.

Because of the requirements for special equipment and experienced personnel, neurodiagnostic monitoring is usually conducted in hospital-based epilepsy referral centers. Neurodiagnostic monitoring requires a laboratory equipped for simultaneous acquisition and storage of EEG data and behavioral data in a form that can be easily reviewed and analyzed (3). The equipment is frequently built into specialized inpatient laboratory rooms. The patient is connected to a multichannel EEG machine, which transmits the EEG to a central control room for permanent storage. Simultaneous with the EEG data acquisition is the observation of the patient's behavior over a closed-circuit video and audio system. Both the EEG and audio-video signals are usually recorded on magnetic media, such as audio tape, video tape, computer disks, or optical disks. A digital clock is used to record a time-and-date signal simultaneously on both the EEG and video records. The EEG and the seizure behavior can then be correlated and examined in detail by the physician.

Four clinical questions important in epilepsy diagnosis and treatment can be answered by neurodiagnostic monitoring (4,5). These are: (a) Are the episodes in question seizures? (b) If so, how frequently do the seizures occur? (c) What type of seizures are occurring? (d) If seizures are of localized onset, from where do they arise?

The first question is answered by the exposure of correlated EEG and behavior recording to scrutiny by experienced and knowledgeable analysts. Neurodiagnostic monitoring circumvents the limitations of patient memory and EEG alone in answering the second question. Patients are often amnestic for ictal events, and untrained observers may fail to recognize subtle ictal phenomena. Particularly in primary generalized epilepsy, interictal epileptiform abnormalities and actual seizures may be quite similar on EEG, with confident differentiation achieved only through correlation of the EEG changes with concomitant behavior.

The third and fourth questions must be answered to guide appropriate therapy. Relatively distinct EEG morphology has been described for many seizure types (6). Changing the seizure type from partial to primary generalized may suggest a change in antiepileptic medication or prevent further investigations into possible surgical treatment. Alternatively, the change of diagnosis from primary generalized seizures to partial seizures raises the question of surgery for medically refractory patients. When surgery is planned, neurodiagnostic monitoring allows correlation of the typical behavioral events with localizing information provided by EEG recording from scalp or intracranial electrodes.

Patients with problem epilepsy have benefited from being studied with intensive neurodiagnostic monitoring. A surprising number of diagnoses, 22% in one series (7), are changed from epilepsy to another disorder manifested by brief paroxysmal abnormal behavior. The type of seizure can be reclassified for more specific drug management and the site of seizure origin documented for surgical treatment. Better classification of the seizures and understanding of the patients have yielded improvement in both seizure control and quality of life (8,9).

Cassette EEG

Cassette EEG recording, also known as 24-hr ambulatory EEG recording, has become an accepted neurodiagnostic tool over the past 10 years (10). Initially configured as a 4-channel EEG system, currently available commercial systems offer either nine or 16 channels for recording data. Electrodes are fixed to the scalp and connected by lead wires to a box containing amplifiers and a cassette tape recorder. The recorder box is small and lightweight, allowing unrestricted patient activity when worn at the waist. The technique uses standard ⅛-in. audiocassette tapes rotating at a slow speed to capture 24 hr of EEG on a single tape. The EEG can be recorded continuously or intermittently (11,12). The mobility of cassette EEG systems has popularized use of the technique in the outpatient setting. Multichannel long-term EEG can be obtained during the patient's routine activities and in the patient's normal environment, increasing the likelihood of recording seizures under typical circumstances.

Several studies have defined the clinical accuracy and utility of cassette EEG recording. Montages have been designed and tested, demonstrating that bipolar montages with as few as three channels sequentially linked from electrodes placed on the scalp at the most active sites for interictal epileptiform abnormalities will adequately record those abnormalities (13–15). With eight channels of EEG, the interictal epileptiform abnormalities may be localized as well as detected (16). Detection of interictal abnormalities has been studied more extensively than detection of seizures. No study has directly compared the accuracy of cassette EEG recording to that of simultaneously obtained multichannel scalp EEG in a large number of patients. However, it is clear that seizures generally can be detected and characterized (15–17).

The development of inpatient neurodiagnostic monitoring centered on cassette EEG rather than standard telemetry has both potential advantages and potential drawbacks. The major advantages are the compact and portable nature of the system and the economic data storage. Problems include the fixed and limited montage and the lack of any on-line monitoring of live data to ensure the adequacy of the study. As might be expected, there are some situations in which the balance of gains and losses is favorable and others in which this is not the case.

THE OPERATING SYSTEM

Equipment

Basic equipment needed for data acquisition consists of a cassette EEG recorder, a portable video camera, and a video tape-recorder system. The video recording system must have some form of time-signal generator that supplies a current time input onto the tape. This is then correlated to the time on the cassette EEG recording. The playback units must allow for simultaneous display of data and the time signal.

Our EEG system is the 9-channel Oxford Medilog 9000 system. The cassette EEG recorder features eight data channels and one channel that codes the clock time. An even marker keyed by the patient or an observer at the time of an event is also present on the ninth channel. Thus, the EEG is synchronized with time and events. The typical electrode interface with the patient is accomplished with 6- to 10-mm tin cup electrodes with central hole for filling with electrode gel. Each electrode, along with a short length of connecting wire, is secured to the scalp with collodion. The electrodes are attached in a prearranged montage following measurement using the International 10-20 System of electrode placement. The electrodes are filled with commercially available electrolyte gel and are regelled every 8 hr.

The montages employed are bipolar sequential channels emphasizing the most probable sites for finding interictal epileptiform abnormalities. The usual montage includes seven channels of EEG and one channel of EKG. Slightly different montages are used for patients in different age groups. The montages are indicated in Table 1.

At the time of the patient setup, the recorder is calibrated by putting an

TABLE 1. *Montages used for 9-channel tape cassette EEG monitoring among different age groups*

Channel	Neonatal[a]	Pediatric[b]	Adult[c]
1	C3-P3	C3-01	F3-P3
2	01-T3	T5-T3	T5-T3
3	T3-FP3	T3-F7	T3-F7
4	Fz-Pz	F7-F8	F7-F8
5	FP4-T4	F8-T4	F8-T4
6	T4-02	T4-T6	T4-T6
7	P4-C4	02-C4	P4-F4
8	EKG	EKG	EKG
9	Time/Event	Time/Event	Time/Event

[a]Ages up to 3 months.
[b]Ages up to 16 years.
[c]Ages above 16 years.

electrical signal of known voltage and duration into each channel and adjusting the amplifier output. Amplifier outputs are monitored during both calibration and biocalibration on an EEG machine to ensure adequate electrode and amplifier function. In order to ensure good recording onto the tape, a sample recording of the EEG is checked on the display monitor prior to completion of the cassette EEG hookup. The cassette recorder's batteries and tapes are changed every 24 hr.

The cassette tapes are reviewed every 24 hr for technical quality and examined for seizures and interictal epileptiform abnormalities. The EEG is viewed on a monitor, which displays both the EEG data and the time of recording. The playback unit allows both rapid review at 20 to 60 times real time and transcription to paper of significant EEG segments. The cassette tapes are retained and stored for archival purposes.

The video system used consists of a camera, a microphone, a video tape recorder, and a time-code generator. Cameras are commercial grade, black-and-white with low light sensitivity to allow recording in a dark room illuminated by only a 60-watt red light bulb. Alternatively, video cameras sensitive to infrared light illuminated by an infrared light generator may be used. The camera lens uses an auto-iris system, which automatically adjusts to the ambient light of the recording locale, usually a patient's room. We have used cameras mounted on a portable cart or permanently mounted on a wall with remotely controlled pan-tilt-zoom capabilities. With either technique, the camera is positioned in such a way that the patient is the target with highest illumination. The camera should not be directed toward a source of light such as a window. The video output is routed through a time-and-date generator, which adds these to the video signal. The video signal is then recorded onto a videocassette recorder (VCR). We have used two half-inch VHS format VCRs. A time-lapse format recorder allows recording for 24 hr without changing the cassette. A second VCR system features a standard four-head VHS VCR, which allows 6 to 8 hr of recording per cassette. A microphone is connected to the VCR for audio recording. Finally, the output signal from the VCR is connected to a video monitor for focusing of the camera and confirming proper video-system function. All of this equipment can be mounted compactly on a portable cart or mounted permanently within a laboratory.

Abnormal behavioral events recorded on the video tape are edited for further review and archival storage. The EEG technologist can transfer the segment of video signal to a second edit tape using two VCRs linked in series with or without editing features. The original video tape is saved prior to reuse until the cassette EEG record has been reviewed for unsuspected events.

Patient Management and Data Analysis

Neurodiagnostic monitoring with cassette EEG and video is performed in an inpatient hospital setting. The patient is admitted and informed consent obtained both for video taping of behavior and for antiepileptic drug withdrawal to promote seizures. The consent form discusses the risks involved with neurodiagnostic monitoring such as aspiration pneumonia, fractures, status epilepticus, and other seizure-related injuries. The patient is restricted to bedrest both for better video recording and for patient safety during seizures.

The EEG technologist applies the electrodes and sets up the cassette EEG and video systems for simultaneous recording. The clocks on the cassette EEG recorder and the video equipment are synchronized. At the start of the study, standard physician's orders specify times for electrodes to be regelled and times for cassette tapes, batteries, and video tapes to be changed. These tasks may be performed by either the EEG technology staff or the nursing staff. The patient, nursing staff, and visitors are instructed to push the event marker on the cassette EEG recorder and make a notation in a diary at the time of any apparent seizures or episodes of behavioral alteration.

Daily physician's orders may include decrease or withdrawal of antiepileptic medication or institution of sleep deprivation. These maneuvers, particularly antiepileptic drug withdrawal, may be necessary to precipitate seizures in the hospital. This puts the patient at risk for status epilepticus and is one reason for the patient's being hospitalized during monitoring.

Another reason for hospitalization is to promote skilled neurologic evaluation by hospital staff during and after apparent seizures. Diagnostic procedures such as computerized axial tomography (CAT) scan or magnetic resonance imaging (MRI) scan, which require the patient to be off camera, are delayed until neurodiagnostic monitoring is completed and medication restarted. Other evaluations, such as neuropsychological testing or psychiatric consultation, can take place in the patient's room during neurodiagnostic monitoring. These tests, which require long periods of patient test performance under observation, can be helpful during monitoring, both because of the enhanced opportunity to witness subtle behavioral changes and because of the resultant stress, which may precipitate seizures or other abnormal behaviors.

Data analysis is performed throughout the neurodiagnostic monitoring study. At any time that an event needs to be reviewed, the tape can be removed and replaced while interpretation is performed. At the end of each 24-hr period, the EEG data are reviewed for seizures and interictal EEG abnormalities. If an abnormal event is seen on the EEG, the corresponding video-tape segment is viewed, edited, and retained for archival purposes. If the EEG shows no change and a clinical event occurred according to the patient or witnesses, the appropriate video segment is reviewed and retained for archival purposes.

Ictal EEG changes have a definite morphology, which differs according to the type of seizure. Ictal EEG changes are observed in all absence (18) and generalized tonic-clonic seizures (19). Most complex partial seizures (20) and many elementary partial seizures (19) have accompanying EEG manifestations, but extra caution must be used in correlating these seizure types with scalp EEG. Partial seizures, especially elementary partial seizures, have been reported to occur without scalp EEG manifestations (19). The behavioral manifestations of the seizure must be taken into account when the EEG is equivocal. The seizure must be analyzed within the clinical context of the possible seizure type. For example, the patient reporting sensory episodes unaccompanied by EEG evidence of seizure may have similar episodes occurring as the auras of complex partial seizures, with clear-cut EEG manifestations. Also, the clinician's practical experience must be used in these situations where maximum observational data are available.

The neurodiagnostic monitoring study is stopped when a typical event has occurred or some limiting factor makes further recording impossible. One particular limitation may be the tolerance of the patient's scalp for the electrodes. After many days of monitoring, the study must be stopped or injury to the scalp will occur from the electrodes and their collodion attachment. Since hospitalization cannot be continued indefinitely for most patients, some will be discharged without witnessed seizures or behavioral events.

If an event cannot be elicited during the neurodiagnostic monitoring period, the EEG may still be helpful if new interictal epileptiform abnormalities are observed after medication withdrawal. If a diagnosis of pseudoseizures is suspected and no clinical events occur off all medications, neurodiagnostic monitoring is continued for a sufficient period of time to make it unlikely that the patient will enter status epilepticus if the diagnosis of pseudoseizures is incorrect. If the patient has a documented pseudoseizure on antiepileptic medication and also does not have interictal epileptiform abnormalities on EEG, then the monitoring is continued during medication withdrawal. At the conclusion of the monitoring study, if the final diagnosis of the problem behaviors is not epilepsy, then appropriate evaluation of the new diagnosis is initiated.

CLINICAL REVIEW

Material

Our experience using cassette EEG with video monitoring at two adjoining hospitals affiliated with the University of Texas Southwestern Medical Center at Dallas is the basis of this retrospective analysis.

At Children's Medical Center of Dallas, cassette EEG and video was the only available technique for neurodiagnostic monitoring and was used for all patients. A cassette EEG playback unit was not available for immediate tape review. Therefore, calibration and biocalibration were done through an EEG machine without direct tape review. Video monitoring was always portable and performed in the patient's hospital room. Parents and nurses together maintained a clinical diary and helped maintain the system by changing tapes and regelling the electrodes. Review of the data was performed in our other laboratory.

This second site was Parkland Memorial Hospital, where monitoring was conducted primarily at the Epilepsy Treatment Center laboratory. The Parkland unit is equipped with hard-wired, multichannel EEG and built-in video recording equipment. However, the more portable cassette EEG and video system is used on many patients who are not considered epilepsy surgery candidates. The diagnostic problem in patients undergoing neurodiagnostic monitoring with cassette EEG and video was often differentiation of apparent pseudoseizures from real seizures. When available, one of the permanent monitoring rooms in the Epilepsy Treatment Center with fixed audio-video equipment was used in association with the cassette EEG recorder. Otherwise, a portable cart-mounted video system similar to that employed at Children's Medical Center was transported to the patient's regular hospital room. The equipment was maintained through the joint efforts of the EEG technical staff and the nursing staff. The cassette EEG and video playback units at Parkland were used for review of recordings from both hospitals.

For this review, results of daily monitoring have been analyzed on 100 patients undergoing a total of 257 days of neurodiagnostic evaluation using cassette EEG and video recording. Patients ranged in age from 1 month to 64 years. Nearly half were age 16 and under. The overall age distribution is indicated in Table 2.

Overwhelmingly, these patients were referred for neurodiagnostic monitoring to confirm or exclude a diagnosis of epilepsy. The question of whether seizures could account for specific abnormal behavior was asked in 82% of the studies. The question of what type of seizures were occurring was asked in 10% of the studies. Questions of seizure localization and frequency each accounted for 4% of the studies. There was no notable difference in the frequency with which any of these diagnostic questions were asked in the adult and pediatric populations.

The duration of monitoring depended on several factors, as indicated in Table 3. Patients were monitored for as long as 8 days, although 30 studies were only 1 day in duration and 88 lasted 4 days or less. There was a tendency for pediatric monitoring studies to be shorter in duration, with 21 of 44 (48%) lasting only 1 day while only nine of 56 adult studies, or 16%, lasted only 1 day. The studies asking specific questions about known seizures (i.e., type, quantity, or localization) were shorter in duration, with none lasting longer than 4 days. When the question was whether the symptomatic behavior was epileptic, the studies extended for longer periods.

TABLE 2. *Ages of patients undergoing TC/EEG seizure monitoring*

Patient age in years	Numbers of patients
< 1	7
1–3	2
3–6	9
6–12	14
12–20	12
20–40	36
40–60	18
> 60	2

Results

Clinical questions were successfully answered in 68 of the 100 patients. A breakdown of the overall results is presented in Table 4. When the clinical question involved type of seizure, localization of seizure focus, or frequency of seizures, 17 of 18 patients had successful studies. Among patients studied for the question of whether seizures were occurring, 51 of 82, or 62%, had the question answered. The clinical question was answered almost always by the occurrence of an episode or episodes of abnormal behavior, with or without EEG evidence of seizure activity. In only two studies was the question answered by the occurrence of interictal epileptiform abnormalities. In both of these patients, a previously undetected 3-Hz spike-and-wave pattern compatible with the diagnosis of primary generalized epilepsy was detected during neurodiagnostic monitoring. One study was considered compatible with the existence of a seizure disorder on the basis of the video record of behavior, although the EEG was not diagnostic.

Of the 32 patients for whom the clinical question could not be answered, 26 did not have any episodes of abnormal behavior during neurodiagnostic monitoring. For the other six patients, there was a mismatch between the behavior and the EEG observations. In two patients, the abnormal behavior observed was not the behavior being questioned. One patient appeared to have a seizure behaviorally without accompanying EEG changes, so that no diagnosis was made. Another patient exhibited abnormal behavior in association with EEG changes, which could have been explained by ischemia or seizure. Two other patients reported subjective sensory symptoms without EEG change and were considered study failures. Of the patients considered study failures, 31 underwent neurodiagnostic monitoring in order to confirm or exclude the diagnosis of epilepsy. The number of monitoring days for these unsuccessful studies was not notably different from the duration of successful studies.

The diagnosis was changed from possible epilepsy to a diagnosis other than epilepsy in 36 of 82 patients, or 44%, on the basis of definite abnormal studies, as indicated in Table 5. The diagnosis was confirmed as epilepsy in 15 of 82 patients, or 18%, with definite abnormal studies. The most common discharge diagnosis in the nonepileptic patients was psychogenic seizures (17 patients). Also observed were sleep disorders (3 patients), movement disorders (7 patients), infantile apnea (2 patients), hyperventilation syndrome (1 patient), prescription drug abuse (1 patient), nonepileptic syncope (1 patient), autism (1 patient), learning disorder (1 patient), and eye fluttering (1 patient). Among patients who did not have a definite diagnosis due to lack of observed events, 20 of 31 were considered at discharge to have pseudoseizures on clinical grounds. Other diagnoses suspected at discharge include infantile apnea (3 patients), migraine syndrome (1 patient), nonepileptic syncope (2 patients), sleep disorder (1 patient), insulinoma (1 patient), and epilepsy (2 patients).

Two specific situations, infantile apnea and syncope, are worth noting when the clinical question is one of whether seizures are occurring. Five babies were evaluated for apneic episodes possibly related to seizure activity. Two of the children had apneic episodes during neurodiagnostic monitoring and neither episode was seizure-related. Also, three patients were evaluated for syncope. None was documented to have seizures, and none was found to have a cardiac arrhythmia during neurodiagnostic monitoring. These clinical situations are often encountered, but the yield of neurodiagnostic monitoring in either is probably low. Further experience is required.

Seizures occurred in 22 of 100 patients studied, and these represented 67% of the 33 patients considered to have epilepsy on completion of neurodiagnostic monitoring. It was possible to classify the type of seizures in all of these patients. Seven patients were found to have primary generalized seizures, and 15 were found to have partial seizures. When the clinical question was specifically what

TABLE 3. *Number of days of monitoring among different age groups*

Days of monitoring	All ages	Pediatric[a]	Adult[b]
1	30	21	9
2	29	11	18
3	18	6	12
4	11	2	9
5	5	0	5
6	2	1	1
7	3	3	0
8	2	0	2
Total studied	100	44	56

[a]Ages 16 years or less.
[b]Greater than 16 years of age.

TABLE 4. *Summary of clinical questions and study results*

Clinical question	Behavior event	Ictal EEG	Question answered	Number of patients
Seizures	Yes	Yes	Yes	15
Seizures	Yes	No	Yes	36
Seizures	No	No	No	31
Seizure type	Yes	Yes	Yes	8
Seizure type	No	No	Yes[a]	2
Seizure focus	Yes	Yes	Yes	3
Seizure focus	Yes	No	No	1
Seizure frequency	Yes	Yes	Yes	2
Seizure frequency	No	No	Yes	2

[a]Interictal EEG consistent with primary generalized seizures.

type of seizures were occurring (N = 10), 100% successful classification was possible. The focality of seizure onset was successfully ascertained in three of four patients for whom this was the clinical issue. The single failure occurred when seizures evident on video could not be correlated with specific EEG changes. These seizures were later confirmed by depth-electrode study to be real and of frontal lobe origin.

DISCUSSION

We have used cassette EEG recording with simultaneous video recording for neurodiagnostic monitoring in 100 patients. This sample includes infants, children, and adults with a variety of problems possibly related to epilepsy. During the time period when these 100 patients were monitored using cassette EEG, over 400 patients were tested with neurodiagnostic monitoring in our laboratories. Clinical problems in the larger group included medically refractory seizures, misdiagnosis of seizure type, antiepileptic drug toxicity, and behavioral disturbances related to underlying brain damage. Sleep disorders, migraine syndrome, drug abuse, movement disorders, hyperventilation syndrome, and psychogenic seizures with various psychiatric diagnoses were all encountered in patients previously diagnosed as epileptic. Similar problems of differential diagnosis were observed in the smaller sample, for whom we used the cassette EEG technique.

The choice of neurodiagnostic monitoring technique used at our laboratories depends on the clinical question asked. If the patient is referred as a candidate for epilepsy surgery, we use the permanently established monitoring facilities in our Epilepsy Treatment Center, with hard-wired cable telemetry capable of handling 32 channels of EEG and exact synchronization of EEG and video recording of behavior. If the patient is being evaluated to confirm or deny the

TABLE 5. *Discharge diagnosis following seizure monitoring in patients admitted to differentiate seizures*

Study results	Discharge diagnosis	Number of patients
Negative	Psychogenic seizures	20
Abnormal	Psychogenic seizures	17
Abnormal	Seizures	15
Negative	Unchanged	11
Abnormal	Movement disorders	7
Abnormal	Sleep disorders	3
Abnormal	Infantile apnea	2
Abnormal	Syncope	2
Abnormal	Hyperventilation	1
Abnormal	Drug abuse	1
Abnormal	Autism	1
Abnormal	Learning disorder	1
Abnormal	Eye fluttering	1

diagnosis of epilepsy, we now prefer to use the cassette EEG technique with simultaneous video recording of behavior. Because of the limited number of channels, and resultant limited spatial resolution, we do not ordinarily use this technique when the clinical question is localization of a seizure focus. Also, we have not often used the inpatient setting for evaluation of the frequency of seizures, since hospitalization itself has been shown to result in a reduction in seizure frequency. To quantify the number of seizures occurring, we usually employ cassette EEG on an ambulatory outpatient basis to get a better idea of the true frequency, unless the patient is amnestic for the events. Thus, the patients tested in our series were not a representative sample of patients with problem epilepsy, although we feel that our experience clearly indicates the potential utility of neurodiagnostic monitoring based on cassette EEG.

The clinical question was successfully answered by 68% of the studies performed, relying on actual behavioral events, ictal EEG abnormalities, and interictal EEG abnormalities. This actually underestimates the success rate of the technique, for another 20% of patients were felt clinically to be experiencing pseudoseizures but did not have events after antiepileptic drug withdrawal. This 88% yield attests to the high degree of clinical utility this type of testing can bring to the differential diagnosis of epilepsy.

The most frequent clinical problem was documentation of the existence of seizures. When this is the diagnostic issue, it is necessary to persist in the study until the patient has the typical abnormal behavioral event. This can be accomplished with the patient as an outpatient or as an inpatient, but inpatient monitoring provides the physician with critical video data and the use of specific activation tools. The interictal data are insufficient in most instances to document that seizures are the cause of abnormal behavior, since patients with epilepsy may also be experiencing nonepileptic behavioral events. The use of sleep deprivation, hyperventilation, and antiepileptic drug withdrawal as activating procedures may promote seizures. Under such circumstances, 68% of our patients had typical events while being monitored. The most frequent length of stay was 1 to 2 days, but the duration of monitoring did extend up to 8 days when necessary. In the 20% of patients with no clinical or EEG events following prolonged monitoring with activating procedures, it was felt that the diagnosis of epilepsy was unlikely.

Our experience demonstrates that the cassette EEG technique is easily used in pediatric patients with problem epilepsy. The same general questions were encountered in the 44 of our patients who were 16 years old or younger as in the adult population. One difference from the adult group was a shorter average duration of monitoring. We made no attempt to determine what the prehospitalization seizure frequency was, and this may account for the differences in duration. There were no problems that were specific to the pediatric age group.

Although there were occasions when the EEG equipment malfunctioned with resultant loss of a single day's monitoring, there were no complete study failures due to equipment problems. We did not review formally the occurrence of single-channel or electrode failure. Subjectively, however, these were commonly encountered. One of the weaknesses of cassette EEG is that there is no ongoing display of the EEG so that equipment malfunction will not be detected until after completion of the day's monitoring. As a safeguard, we encourage twice-daily checks of the tape to ensure successful recording. Of course, this requires examination of the tape in the playback unit. The most common reasons for channel loss were electrode disconnection and lead wire breakage. The video equipment failures were limited to late tape changes.

CONCLUSIONS

Neurodiagnostic monitoring using cassette EEG has significant utility, as demonstrated by our experience. It is a technique that is readily available for development by the neurologist interested in epilepsy, with minimal capital and personnel investment. The cassette EEG recording system can be set up and maintained by EEG technical staff during the day and by regular ward personnel with minimal training during evening and night hours. The video system is inexpensive, portable, and easily maintained by hospital ward staff. The study results can be analyzed by the EEG technical staff and by the electroencephalographer on a timely basis. In addition, the cassette EEG recorders are available for outpatient ambulatory EEG studies when not being used for inpatient seizure studies.

An area for future development is the use of cassette EEG recorders with home video equipment for outpatient neurodiagnostic monitoring. Although this is attractive as a way to minimize hospitalization, potential problems may limit its use. In particular, there is the risk of status epilepticus during antiepileptic drug withdrawal. In addition, problems with reliable control of the patient's position on camera can be anticipated. However, selected patients such as those with pediatric apnea and those with frequent abnormal behaviors on medication may be candidates for this type of testing. Furthermore, the incorporation of simultaneous video recording into cassette EEG recording for sleep problems might well increase the yield in that rapidly developing area of cassette EEG use.

REFERENCES

1. Leroy RF, Rao KK, Voth BJ, et al. Ambulatory EEG with simultaneous video monitoring for problem epilepsy. *Epilepsia* 1986;27:633.
2. Gumnit RJ. *Intensive neurodiagnostic monitoring. Advances in Neurology.* New York: Raven Press, 1987.
3. Ives JR, Thompson CL, Gloor P. Seizure monitoring: a new tool in electroencephalography. *Electroencephalogr Clin Neurophysiol* 1976;41:422–427.
4. Engel Jr, J. A practical guide for routine EEG studies in epilepsy. *J Clin Neurophysiol* 1984;1:143–157.
5. Engel Jr, J, Crandall PH, Rausch R. The partial epilepsies. In: Rosenberg RN, Grossman RG, Schochet S, et al., eds. *The clinical neurosciences,* vol 2. New York: Churchill Livingstone, 1983;1349–1380.
6. League Against Epilepsy. Proposal for revised clinical and electroencephalographic classification of epileptic seizures. *Epilepsia* 1981;22:489–501.
7. Mattson RH. Value of intensive monitoring. In: Wada JA, Penry JK, eds. *Advances in epileptology. The Xth epilepsy international symposium.* New York: Raven Press, 1980;43–51.
8. Porter RJ, Penry JK, Lacy JR. Diagnostic and therapeutic reevaluation of patients with intractable epilepsy. *Neurology (Minneap)* 1977;27:1006–1011.
9. Porter RJ, Theodore WH, Schulman EA. Intensive monitoring of intractable epilepsy: a two year followup. In: Dam M, Gram L, Penry JK, eds. *Advances in epileptology: XIIth epilepsy international symposium.* New York: Raven Press, 1981;265–268.
10. Ebersole JS. Ambulatory EEG monitoring. In: Aminoff MJ, ed. *Electrodiagnosis in clinical neurology.* New York: Churchill Livingstone, 1986;125–148.
11. Ebersole JS, Bridgers SL. Performance evaluation of an 8 channel ambulatory cassette EEG system. *XVth Epilepsy International Symposium Abstracts,* Washington 1983;476.
12. Ives JR. A completely ambulatory 16-channel cassette recording system. In: Stefan H, Burr W, eds. *Mobile long-term EEG monitoring: proceedings of the MLE symposium, Bonn, May 1982.* New York: Fischer, 1982;205–217.
13. Leroy RF, Ebersole JS. An evaluation of ambulatory, cassette EEG monitoring. I. Montage design. *Neurology (Cleve)* 1983;33:1–7.
14. Ebersole JS, Leroy RF. An evaluation of ambulatory, cassette EEG monitoring. II. Detection of interictal abnormalities. *Neurology* 1983;33:8–18.
15. Ebersole JS, Leroy RF. An evaluation of ambulatory, cassette EEG monitoring. III. Diagnostic accuracy compared to intensive inpatient EEG monitoring. *Neurology* 1983;33:853–860.
16. Ebersole JS, Bridgers SL. Direct comparison of 3 and 8-channel ambulatory cassette EEG with intensive inpatient monitoring. *Neurology (Cleve)* 1985;35:846–854.
17. Aminoff MJ, Goodin DS, Berg BO, et al. Ambulatory EEG recordings in epileptic and nonepileptic children. *Neurology* 1988;38:558–562.
18. Penry JK, Porter RJ, Dreifuss FE. Simultaneous recording of absence seizures with video tape and electroencephalography. A study of 374 seizures in 48 patients. *Brain* 1975;98:427–440.
19. Gastaut H, Broughton R. *Epileptic seizures.* Springfield: Charles C Thomas, 1972.
20. Delgado-Escueta AV. Epileptogenic paroxysms: modern approaches and clinical correlations. *Neurology (NY)* 1979;29:1014–1022.

Ambulatory EEG Monitoring,
edited by John S. Ebersole.
Raven Press, Ltd., New York © 1989

11

Simultaneous Ambulatory Cassette EEG/ECG Monitoring

Marshall J. Keilson* and Jason P. Magrill**

**Division of Neurology, Maimonides Medical Center, Brooklyn, New York 11219; and **Neuro-Monitoring Inc. Lynbrook, New York 11563*

Prolonged electrocardiographic (ECG) monitoring has been a standard feature of cardiac evaluation for over two decades. In contrast, long-term monitoring of electroencephalographic (EEG) activity has become possible only more recently and has been performed mainly on inpatients at specialized centers. With the advent of ambulatory cassette EEG (AEEG), and especially the newer 8-channel recorders, neurologists are now able to obtain simultaneous EEG/ECG for prolonged periods on outpatients. Thus, in situations where either cerebral or cardiac abnormalities could be implicated as the primary cause of a patient's symptoms, both can be monitored. Such recordings may be helpful both during the event as well as during asymptomatic periods.

These new monitoring techniques are useful in both research and clinical areas, only some of which have been explored thus far. We will review the clinical applications of simultaneous EEG/ECG monitoring, as well as discuss the technique used to obtain such recordings.

CLINICAL APPLICATIONS

The clinical utility of AEEG has been demonstrated in earlier chapters in this volume. As will be elaborated later, the addition of simultaneous cardiac monitoring is technically feasible with only a minimum of time and effort. Thus, the questions are (a) in what situations is this effort worthwhile? and (b) what gain can be expected?

Syncope

Uncomplicated syncope is a common cause of outpatient evaluation and hospital admission in all age groups. Often routine history and physical and laboratory examinations (metabolic studies, ECG, EEG, etc.) are unrevealing. There are numerous potential causes of syncope with and without heart disease, which have been reviewed elsewhere (1–3). In this section, we shall focus on those aspects of syncope that relate to the neurologic practitioner and specifically those aspects that touch on simultaneous monitoring.

In 1957, Gastaut wrote that "the differential diagnosis between syncope and epilepsy is extremely important and not always easy" (4). Thirty years later, this same difficulty persists, and neurologists are often consulted on patients with episodic syncope. Presenting symptoms may include pallor, diaphoresis, nausea, nonspecific dizziness, and a feeling of "closing in" associated with loss of consciousness. The clinical description alone may not always clarify the underlying etiology. This is especially true when syncope is associated with convulsive activity. In some cases, the search for a cerebral abnormality may delay correct diagnosis or even lead to inappropriate treatment with anticonvulsant medication (5–9).

"Holter" ECG monitoring is recognized as an indispensable part of the syncope evaluation. Several reports document the usefulness of this procedure in patients with transient neurologic symptoms, including syncope (7,10–14). Until recently, EEG studies of syncope used conventional EEG equipment and monitored patients only for limited periods. Routine EEGs have generally been unrevealing (1,3). Syncope has also been provoked during monitoring by various methods, including ocular compression, in the hope of clarifying the underlying cause (4,15–17).

Following the introduction of simultaneous EEG/ECG monitoring by means of cassette recorders, several studies have reported on its application in these patients (18–22). A case reported by Lai and Zeigler is widely quoted as an example of how these difficult cases can be solved with simultaneous monitoring (22). Although their patient did manifest some "twitching of facial muscles" during his syncopal spells, which might have suggested convulsive etiology, he also was known to suffer from significant cardiac disease. Documenting cardiac abnormalities was not, therefore, unexpected.

It is not clear from the literature how valuable combined monitoring is in terms of uncovering epilepsy instead of cardiac disease. An early study by Graf et al. reported on 22 patients with "syncope" that was not defined (20). Only two channels of EEG were monitored along with one for ECG and one as a time marker. Three patients suffered "attacks," one of which was a generalized seizure. In eight patients, cardiac arrhythmias were detected that required treatment. The overall value of this study may be limited, however, as the authors acknowledged that EEG findings were "not fully interpretable" due to the limited number of channels. They correctly concluded that, with more EEG channels, this modality may more appropriately be applied in the differential diagnosis of spontaneous attacks.

In the same volume, a study by Callaghan and McCarthy reported on 48 inpatients, who previously had normal EEGs and normal metabolic studies (19). All patients had experienced "episodes of loss of consciousness." Monitoring was performed with three channels of EEG and one channel of ECG. Of 16 patients who carried a clinical diagnosis of "syncope," six were found to have "epilepsy," whereas in only five was a cardiac basis detected. Unfortunately, no further information is provided as to how the diagnosis of epilepsy was made. Simultaneous testing was again recommended in patients with loss of consciousness, when "more routine tests have failed to establish a diagnosis." However, in a more recent review of 500 patients who had AEEG, 67 of whom were evaluated for syncope, near syncope, or episodic dizziness, only one had an epileptiform abnormality detected on their recording (18).

These latter results are remarkably similar to our own findings (21). In addition to uncomplicated syncope, we included patients who experienced recurrent dizziness or a "faint feeling." Patients were monitored with seven channels of EEG and one channel of ECG for a minimum of 21 hr. ECG activity was analyzed independently from the EEG channels. Arrhythmias were classified as negative, low-risk, or high-risk, based on historical potential for sudden death. High-risk arrhythmias are listed in Table 1. Low-risk and negative studies were combined for comparison with high-risk arrhythmias. We studied a total of 422 patients with age range of 6 to 88 (mean, 46). In only one patient was a newly discovered epileptiform abnormality found, and this was exclusively interictal.

Alternatively, nearly 10%, 40 patients, were found to have significant cardiac arrhythmias. Most of these patients were over 60 years old (see Table 2). Although the yield was lower in younger patients, the inconvenience imposed by the addition of the ECG channel is minor when compared with the possibility of documenting a high-risk cardiac arrhythmia. In addition, any positive cardiac diagnosis in patients under 60 has increased significance, since it is less likely that they would have necessarily undergone standard Holter monitoring.

TABLE 1. *High-risk cardiac arrhythmias*

Ventricular couplets
Ventricular tachycardia
Severe bradycardia (HR < 35/m)
Prolonged sinus pause
Prolonged supraventricular tachycardia
2° AV Block-Mobitz II
Premature ventricular beats $> 10/1000$
(generally associated with bigeminy and trigeminy)

TABLE 2. *Cardiac arrhythmias in patients with syncope*

Age	High risk (%)	Neg/Low risk (%)	Total
0–19	1 (1.6)	63 (98.4)	64
20–39	3 (2.4)	121 (97.6)	124
40–59	4 (4.3)	89 (95.7)	93
≥ 60	32 (22.7)	109 (77.3)	141
	40 (9.4)	382 (90.6)	422

Illustrative Cases

Case 1. A 16-year-old male underwent AEEG/ECG for evaluation of dizziness and syncope. AEEG was negative, but the modified Holter ECG channel demonstrated sinus bradycardia in the high 30s during wakefulness and as low as 31 during sleep.

Case 2. A 32-year-old male with syncope had a normal AEEG, but a ventricular triplet detected on the ECG channel (Fig. 1).

Based on our series, we draw the following conclusions. (a) The yield for diagnosing epilepsy by means of AEEG monitoring in patients with uncomplicated syncope or dizziness is extremely low. (b) If an AEEG is to be performed, including simultaneous ECG is logical in all age groups and necessary in older patients.

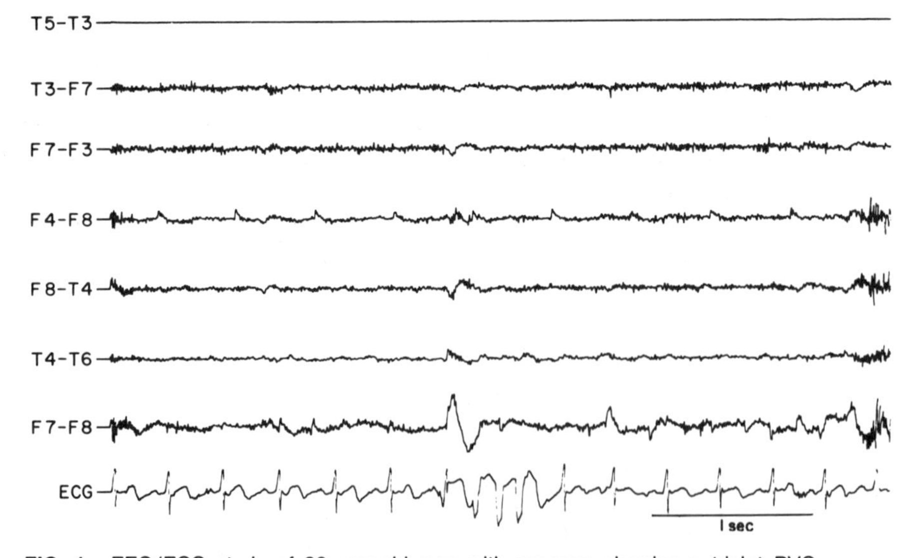

FIG. 1. EEG/ECG study of 32-year-old man with syncope showing a triplet PVC.

Arrhythmias Presenting as Seizures

In addition to syncope, other neurologic symptoms can be associated with cardiac arrhythmias. These include vestibular episodes, transient confusion, psychoses, and focal or other transient ischemic attack (TIA)-like symptoms. Frank seizures are also known on occasion to be of cardiogenic origin. Nonetheless, in the face of a convulsive seizure, a cardiac cause is often not investigated or even considered.

The literature in this regard consists mainly of case reports of patients with known or suspected epilepsy, where a cardiac etiology was fortuitously detected by simultaneous routine EEG/ECG or by prolonged Holter monitoring (5,6,9,13,23,24). In some cases, patients sustained generalized convulsive episodes, while other patients experienced symptoms that were more suggestive of complex partial seizures (9,23). Several reports include patients who carried a long-standing diagnosis of epilepsy and were treated, often unsuccessfully, with various anticonvulsants (5,6,8,9).

Most of the reported cases of arrhythmogenic seizures were associated with bradycardia or asystole (5,6,9,23,24). The results of pacemaker insertion in these patients were often dramatic and potentially life-saving (25). In fact, one author suggests that a "rapid increase" in the number of pacemaker implantations may be indicated in patients with cerebral symptoms (26). Other incriminated cardiac abnormalities have included mitral valve prolapse and excessive vagal response to external stimuli (6,9,24,27). Reports of the latter emphasize the need to maximize the use of technology by reproducing the circumstances that precipitated the patient's symptoms.

The importance of ECG monitoring in cardiac diagnosis is well recognized, but its value in the elucidation of transient neurologic symptoms and especially suspected epilepsy has been underemphasized. Several reports document its essential role in the diagnosis of these conditions (7,10,11,13). In one study of attacks of unclear etiology, 32% of patients were found to have "significant arrhythmias" (14). These authors further noted that one-third of those with epileptic attacks "often manifested significant arrhythmias." They concluded that the seizures were likely to be of cardiac origin. Another report suggested that perhaps as many as 20% of patients referred with "suspected epilepsy" have cardiac arrhythmias as the underlying cause (7). Such percentages will obviously vary greatly depending on referral patterns.

One might speculate that the scarcity of case reports with documented cardiogenic seizures is in part due to the underuse of prolonged monitoring in patients presenting with neurologic complaints. The recent availability of 8-channel recording systems for prolonged, simultaneous EEG/ECG will facilitate large-scale, long-term prospective studies in these patients.

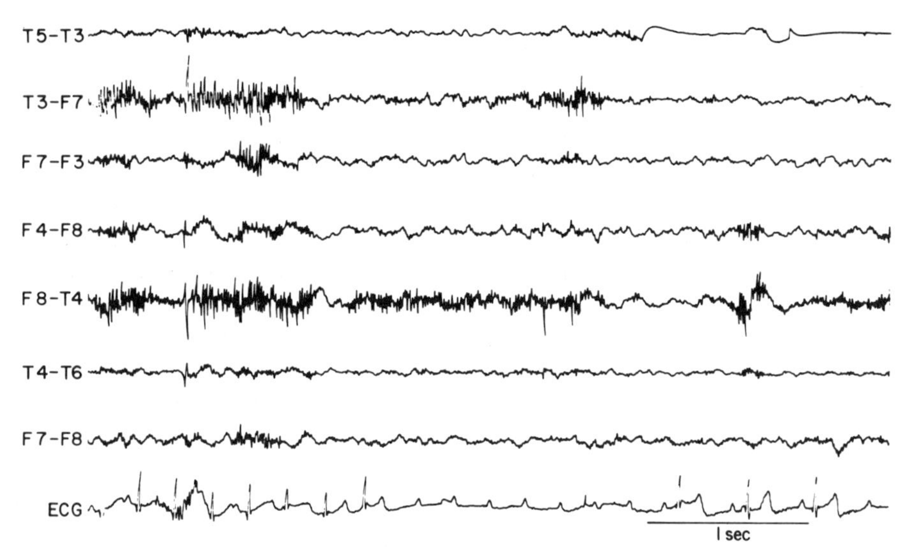

FIG. 2. EEG/ECG study of 6-year-old during a nocturnal period of unresponsiveness showing a 9:1 AV block.

Illustrative Case

Case 3. A 6-year-old experienced spells of uncertain etiology associated with shaking of her extremities. The patient had a negative workup including routine EEG. While being monitored at home with AEEG, the patient, while asleep, had the sudden onset of screaming followed by unresponsiveness for a brief time. Cassette monitoring showed a normal EEG, but 9:1 atrio-ventricular (AV) block on ECG (Fig. 2). A cardiac etiology had not been suspected in a person this young.

Long Q-T Syndrome

The idiopathic long Q-T syndrome has a tendency to mimic epilepsy. This syndrome may occur in hereditary and sporadic forms. The former can be subdivided into the Jervel Lange-Nielson autosomal recessive variety associated with congenital deafness, and the autosomal dominant Romano-Ward syndrome without deafness. The syndrome may also be associated with other conditions including stroke, myocardial infarction, the use of various drugs, and electrolyte abnormalities. Patients may be asymptomatic, with the abnormality detected only on routine ECG, or they may be symptomatic with various arrhythmias. It has been postulated as a possible cause of sudden death in the younger population (28).

Case histories in the literature document the propensity of individuals with this abnormality to develop highly malignant, often fatal, arrhythmias (29–34).

In some instances, siblings have succumbed to sudden death before the diagnosis was finally made (29). For a neurologist, the most striking feature in these case reports is the frequent clinical presentation of well-described, recurrent generalized convulsions; hence, the frequent mistaken diagnosis of epilepsy. In general, there are no distinguishing clinical features to suggest the true cardiac origin of the seizures.

The case reported by Ballardie is particularly illustrative (29). A 16-year-old girl had suffered three nocturnal grand-mal convulsions over a 1-year period. Two siblings had previously died during early-morning convulsions. Neurologic examination and EEG were normal, but an ECG showed a prolonged Q-T interval. Retrospective review of the ECG of one of the deceased siblings also revealed a prolonged Q-T interval.

Illustrative Case

Case 4. A 20-year-old woman had experienced seven generalized tonic-clonic seizures from the age of 10, all associated with vigorous exercise. During the most recent event, which occurred while running up steps, she experienced hand-tingling associated with rapid respiration, which was immediately followed by loss of consciousness, cyanosis, and generalized tonic-clonic activity of the extremities. There was no family history of either seizures or cardiac disease. The patient underwent AEEG with one channel dedicated to ECG. She was instructed, under supervision, to replicate the activity that had triggered the most recent event. After running up more than 40 steps, the patient suddenly lost consciousness and slid to the floor with clonic jerking of the extremities. EEG showed the development of slowing and eventual loss of background rhythms. The ECG abnormality consisted of ventricular tachycardia evolving into ventricular flutter/fibrillation (Fig. 3). After almost 1 min, ventricular tachycardia reappeared, followed by sinus bradycardia and eventually normal sinus rhythm. The patient was found to have a prolonged Q-T interval. She was placed on propranolol and has not experienced any further episodes.

After recognition of the syndrome, treatment is imperative. Untreated, the mortality is greater than 70% (35). Beta-blockers, chiefly propranolol, are the mainstay of treatment. Mortality can be reduced to 6% with this modality alone (35). Resistant patients can be treated with thoracic sympathectomy (36).

The diagnosis of long Q-T syndrome should be considered in young patients presenting with the new onset convulsive seizures. This is particularly true when the seizures do not respond to anticonvulsants and there is a family history of seizures associated with sudden death. Although uncommon, this is one clinical entity where combined EEG/ECG monitoring not only can be diagnostic, but can be life-saving.

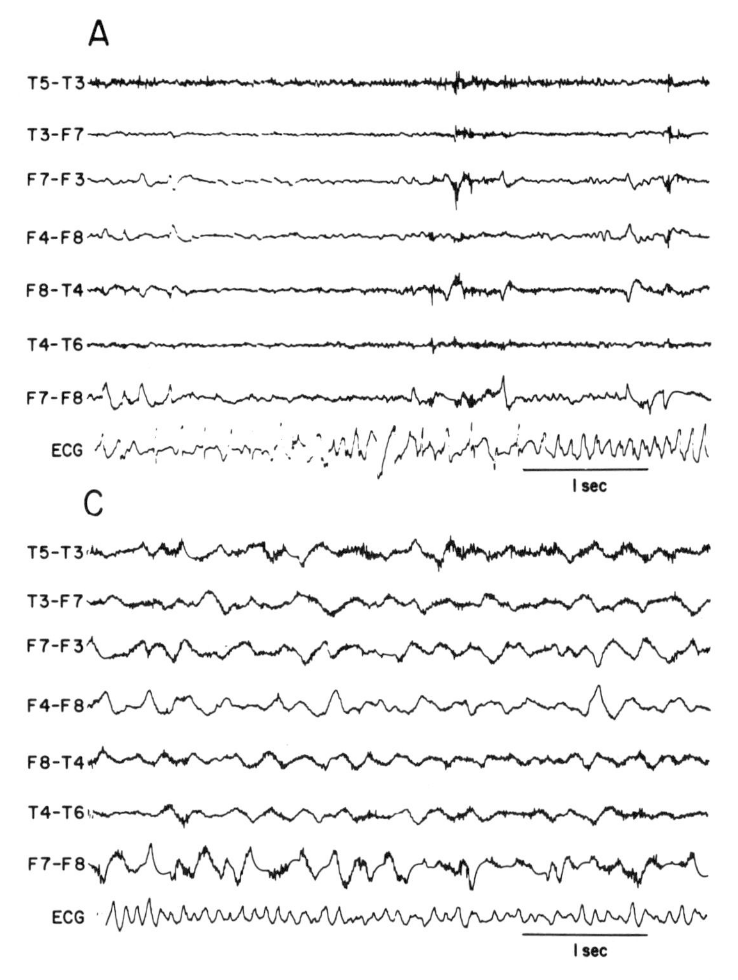

FIG. 3. EEG/ECG study of a symptomatic event in a 20-year-old with exercize-induced loss of consciousness and convulsive activity. Note in sequence on the ECG channel ventricular tachycardia, ventricular flutter-fibrillation, ventricular tachycardia, and a resolution with bradycardia. **A** and **B** are continuous. **C** begins at a 40-sec latency and **D** at an 80-sec latency from onset.

Arrhythmias Associated with Epilepsy

In the course of monitoring patients with a presumed diagnosis of epilepsy, high-risk arrhythmias are occasionally found on ECG, while the EEG is normal. In these instances, where an actual attack is not recorded, it is difficult to determine the extent to which cardiac abnormalities, rather than epilepsy, play an etiologic role.

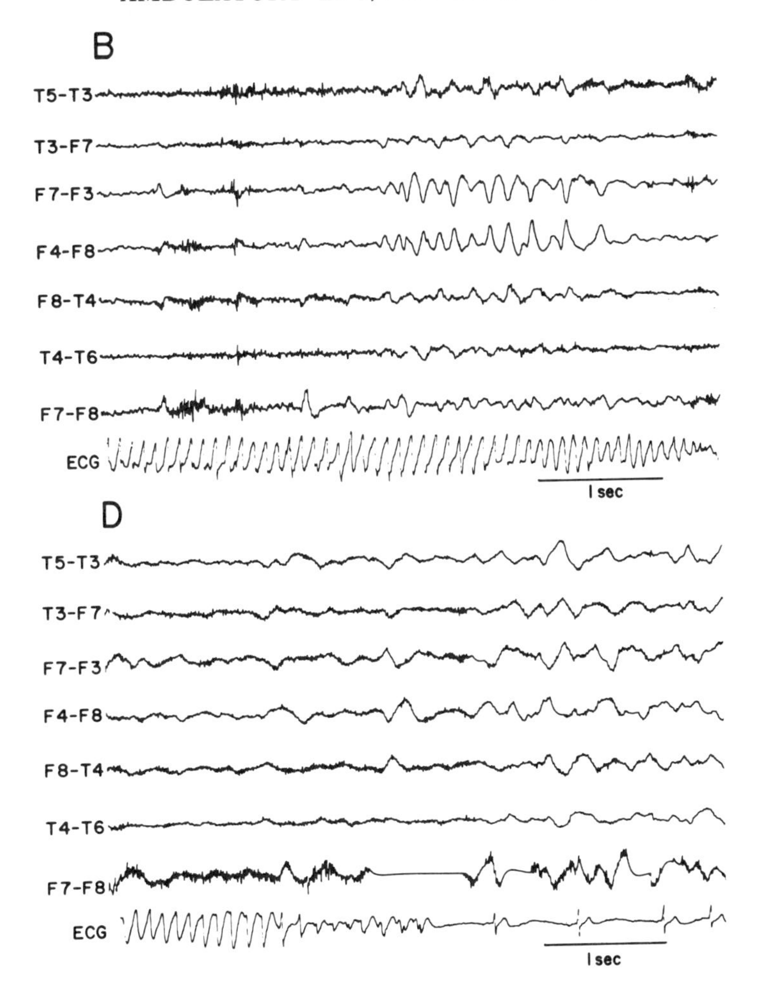

FIG. 3. (*continued*).

Illustrative Cases

Case 5. A 58-year-old man on primidone had a history of episodic memory loss felt to be seizure-related. A 5-beat ventricular paroxysm, seen in Fig. 4, was recorded during monitoring.

Case 6. A 14-year-old girl with a history of a single generalized tonic-clonic seizure underwent prolonged simultaneous monitoring. Tape analysis revealed a normal EEG, but premature ventricular contractions (PVC) at a rate of greater than 10/1000 with periods of bigeminy and trigeminy.

Case 7. A 17-year-old man with episodic fits of rage, thought to be seizures,

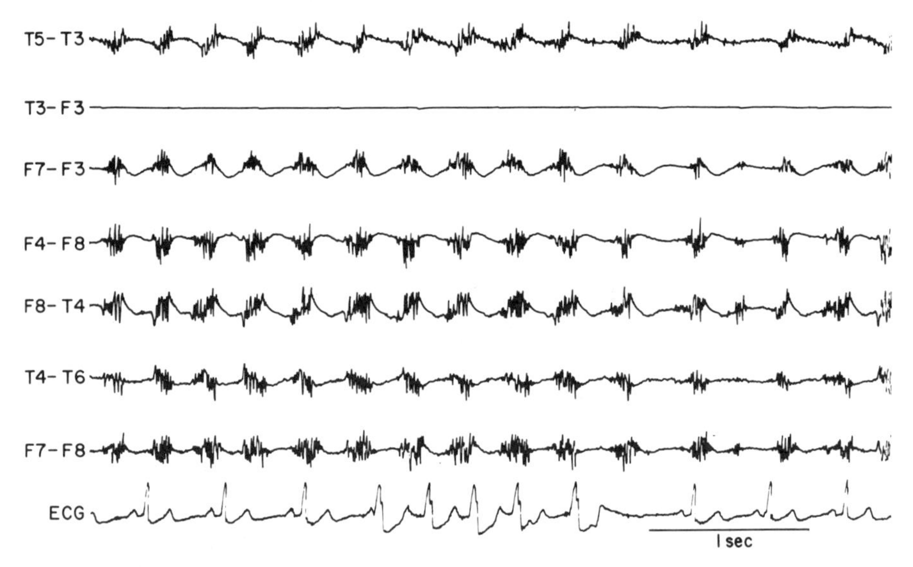

FIG. 4. EEG/ECG study of 58-year-old man with episodic memory loss. Chewing artifact is seen on the EEG channels; ECG shows a run of five PVCs.

had a normal AEEG. The ECG channel revealed ventricular couplets and a 4-beat ventricular paroxysm (Fig. 5).

Neither does finding interictal abnormalities in both ECG and EEG verify the etiology of the patient's attacks. Which one accounts for the patient's symptoms? Definitive diagnosis can be made only by documenting the appropriate abnormality during reported symptoms.

Illustrative Cases

Case 8. A 24-year-old woman with a history of generalized seizures was being treated with carbamazepine and valproate. Simultaneous monitoring showed a highly active left temporal sharp wave focus as well as a ventricular triplet (Fig. 6).

Case 9. An 88-year-old woman with a history of stroke experienced episodes of confusion. AEEG revealed bilateral independent temporal sharp wave foci. The cardiac channel demonstrated PVCs greater than 10/1000, atrial fibrillation, and ventricular couplets.

Case 10. A 12-year-old boy suffered episodic visual difficulties. AEEG showed bifrontal spike-and-wave abnormality, while the simultaneous ECG revealed PVCs greater than 10/1000 and periods of bigeminy and trigeminy.

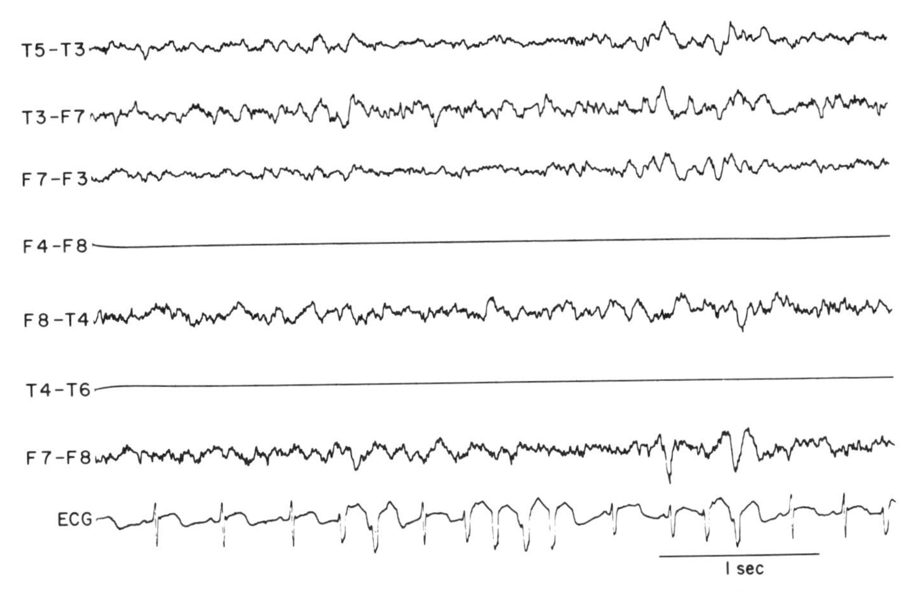

FIG. 5. EEG/ECG study of a 17-year-old man with episodic fits of rage. Channels 4 and 6 were lost due to artifact. ECG shows both PVC couplets and a paroxysm of four PVCs.

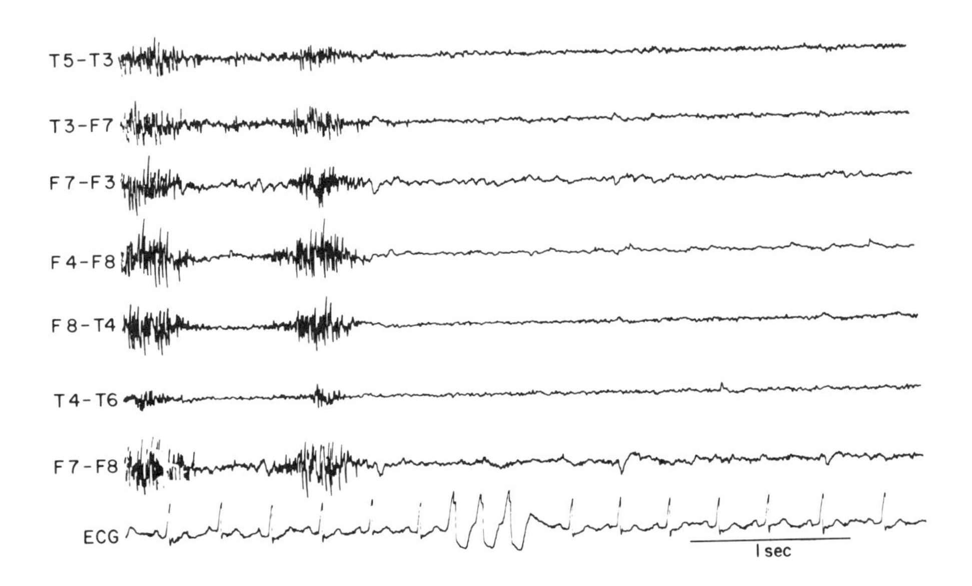

FIG. 6. EEG/ECG study of a 24-year-old with seizures showing a PVC triplet.

TABLE 3. *Cardiac arrhythmias in patients with epilepsy*

Age	High risk (%)	Neg/Low risk (%)	Total
0–19	7 (2.5)	268 (97.5)	275
20–39	4 (1.4)	273 (98.6)	277
40–59	9 (7.3)	115 (92.7)	124
≥ 60	8 (10.3)	70 (89.7)	78
	28 (3.7)	726 (96.3)	754

Epilepsy-Causing Arrhythmias

In the previous sections, we reviewed the causative relationship between primary cardiac arrhythmias and seizures or epilepsy. We shall now examine the converse, seizures as a cause of cardiac arrhythmias. It has been known for more than a century that electrical stimulation of the brain can affect heart rhythm (37). Stimulation of different areas may evoke increased heart rate, decreased heart rate, or various arrhythmias (37). Many disorders of the CNS have been associated with cardiovascular effects, ranging from ECG changes to acute myocardial necrosis (33). Numerous investigations have documented the association between seizure discharge and cardiac arrhythmias (38–56,61). Lathers and Schraeder found autonomic changes, including arrhythmias, even with subconvulsant interictal activity in cats treated with pentylenetetrazol (PTZ) (43,44,52). Pretreatment with phenobarbital did not appear to provide a protective effect (57). Several recent publications review these complex brain-heart interrelationships (58,59).

With the advent of cassette recording, the study of prolonged simultaneous EEG/ECG has been made possible on a large scale. Precise electrical interactions, which can be used to determine cause and effect, are readily studied with this modality. In a clinical study, we reviewed simultaneous AEEG/ECG recordings on 338 consecutive patients with epilepsy (60). The results showed that the incidence of high-risk cardiac arrhythmia was quite low and was comparable to the results of Holter monitoring studies of asymptomatic individuals. This was consistent in all age groups. The study has recently been expanded to include a total of 754 patients. The results are reported in Table 3 and are similar to our previous findings (60). Thus, in this population of patients with epilepsy, the incidence of cardiac arrhythmias is not increased.

If having the clinical diagnosis of epilepsy or having interictal epileptiform discharges on EEG monitoring is not associated with high-risk arrhythmias, then what of the electrographic seizure itself? Various types of cardiac abnormalities have been found during seizures in both experimental and clinical settings. Some clinical reports indicate an associated drop in heart rate or even sinus arrest (40,42,48,61), while others have documented atrial or ventricular arrhythmias (28,38,46,50,55,56,62). The most common finding in both spontaneous and induced seizures is an increased heart rate that was temporally related to the electrographic seizure (38,39,41,45,49,51,53,54,56).

In 1939, Erickson reported the results of ECG monitoring during 54 seizures of various types, spontaneous and induced (39). Cardiac acceleration was the most frequent finding, though in some cases there was no change. In only two attacks was slowing seen, and asystole was not observed. Several studies have reported on PTZ-induced seizures in human subjects (47,53,54,56). Some found an increased heart rate, as well as various arrhythmias (47,56), while others reported observing sinus or supraventricular tachycardias almost exclusively (53,54). Further details regarding the severity of arrhythmias are lacking in these reports.

In a recent series, 12 patients with temporal lobe seizures were monitored simultaneously with video as well as EEG/ECG. All patients demonstrated tachycardia without other significant associated arrhythmias (45). Rossi and Rossi studied 14 patients who had 75 partial seizures while being evaluated for epilepsy surgery (49). Some were studied with implanted electrodes. They found an increase in heart rate in 41 patients (54.6%), bradycardia in five (6.6%), and no change in 29 (38.6%). They did not feel that the heart-rate change was related directly to seizure activity at the epileptogenic focus.

Blumhardt and co-workers recorded 74 electrographic seizures in 25 patients with simultaneous EEG/ECG (38). Using a 4-channel system in which only one channel of EEG was used for each hemisphere (T3-P3, T4-P4), ictal tachycardia was detected in over 90% of events. In eight patients (32%), ictal "arrhythmias" were described, which consisted of irregular, abrupt changes in heart rate mainly toward the end of the seizure. Increased ventricular ectopia was seen in three patients, although it was not quantified.

Our own series included 36 patients, who experienced 96 electrographic seizures (41). All were monitored with 8-channel AEEG, with one channel dedicated to ECG. All EEG studies were reviewed by a board-certified electroencephalographer. ECG was analyzed separately by a trained ECG technician and reviewed by a consultant cardiologist. Only electrographic seizures of at least 20-sec duration were included. Generalized 3-Hz spike-and-wave attacks were excluded. Heart rate was measured 1 min prior to seizure onset and again at its peak rate during the ictus. Tachycardia of varying degrees was almost universal (96.9%). In three seizures, no change was seen, and none was associated with slowing or asystole. Percentage change of heart rate is illustrated in Table 4. The average percentage increase was 59%. A similar number of lateralized seizures ($N=19$) were detected on the left and the right, and both induced the same average percent increase in heart rate, 49%. An average increase of 65% was seen with generalized seizures ($N=58$). No ventricular ectopia or conduction defects were noted. Sinus tachycardia, when present, generally began within 5 sec of the identified seizure onset. The accelerated cardiac rate either gradually slowed following seizure completion or, in some instances, persisted for several minutes thereafter. The type of irregular

TABLE 4. *Percent heart-rate increase during seizures*

% Increase	*N*
0–10	6
11–50	36
51–100	44
> 100	10

rate changes noted by Blumhardt et al. was not found in our series, nor has it been reported by other observers in induced or spontaneous seizures.

Sudden Unexplained Death Among Epileptics

Several reports in the literature have addressed the subject of sudden, unexpected, unexplained death (SUUD) (63–65) among patients with seizure disorders. This phenomenon is of obscure etiology, although some have suggested lethal cardiac arrhythmias as the underlying cause. A rapid heart rate induced by a seizure in patients with preexisting cardiac disease could have serious consequences. The syndrome of SUUD, however, has generally been reported in young, otherwise healthy patients with epilepsy (63–65). Recent preliminary reports suggest that autonomic changes other than heart rate may be an important factor in the pathogenesis of sudden death associated with seizures (66–68).

In a comprehensive review of the subject, Jay and Leestma estimated the incidence of SUUD to be as high as 1/500 to 1/1000 people with epilepsy (64). They concluded that "a careful cardiac workup in epileptic patients may be indicated to identify and treat those at risk." Unfortunately, this may not be practical. Although our data cannot elucidate the cause of SUUD in patients with epilepsy, they do suggest that identifying the population at risk in advance may be difficult (60), since, among epileptics, there was no apparent increase in arrhythmias or no other ECG sign to identify them. The patient who succumbs to SUUD may have experienced his first and final cardiac arrhythmia.

Critique of Miscellaneous Studies of EEG/ECG Monitoring

As is clear from information presented in earlier chapters in this volume, AEEG plays an important role in the diagnostic evaluation of various neurologic problems. It has also been pointed out that, as with any clinical tool, its usefulness is dependent on the indication for the study and the quality of the information obtained. To date, only a handful of studies have reported data from simultaneous EEG/ECG monitoring (69–72). No studies, other than ours, have yet been reported in which the new 8-channel unit was employed. Thus, all the earlier investigations used only three channels of EEG or, in some cases, only two. Our experience in over 3000 8-channel studies suggests that the limited number of EEG channels formerly employed could pose significant problems in drawing useful conclusions regarding EEG abnormalities. This would apply especially to detection of focal seizures and interictal epileptiform changes.

The reports of Graf et al. (20) and Callaghan and McCarthy (19) deal primarily with syncope patients and were discussed above. In 1985, Cull reported on 62 patients (mean age, 35.3) who underwent simultaneous monitoring for "episodes of loss of consciousness or impaired awareness" (71). All records in that study (EEG and ECG) were reviewed by the author himself. No patient was found to have a significant cardiac arrhythmia, and in only five were minor abnormalities of rhythm detected.

In an early report, Blumhardt and Oozeer studied 68 patients with "episodes of disturbed consciousness," and specifically excluded patients with known epilepsy or heart disease (70). Three patients were found to have newly detected cardiac arrhythmias (including one during a reported symptom). Many of their patients experienced symptoms without EEG/ECG abnormalities. This would effectively rule out a cardiac etiology, but not necessarily epilepsy, given the limitations of the 2-channel EEG recordings. Although only a preliminary study, the authors felt the results confirmed the value of simultaneous monitoring. In an expanded study, Blumhardt (69) studied 145 patients. "Significant" arrhythmias associated with reported symptoms occurred in only 2%. Two additional patients with symptomatic arrhythmias were later diagnosed as having epilepsy as well. He concluded that, despite the low yield, "neurologists requesting AEEG monitoring must insist on the inclusion of simultaneous ECG."

In an abstract presented by Nousiaianen et al. (72), 2 to 3% of patients were found to have malignant ECG dysrhythmias when studied with AEEG monitoring. They concluded that simultaneous EEG/ECG monitoring is, in fact, "mandatory."

Our own results in patients with syncope or epilepsy have been presented above. Remaining after these two groups are excluded are a total of 965 additional patients who have had combined recordings with methods similar to those previously outlined for a variety of reasons. Our results, shown in Table 5, are consistent with those of the cardiac literature for the general population. The arrhythmia rates are also similar to those documented in the previous tables for the syncope/dizziness and epilepsy subpopulations. The only exception is that the group of epilepsy patients older than 60 have an arrhythmia rate that is lower than the other groups of similar age. Whether this is related to the "protective" effect of anticonvulsant medication or some other factor is unclear and requires further investigation.

TABLE 5. *Cardiac arrhythmias in nonepilepsy, nonsyncope group*

Age	High risk (%)	Neg/Low risk (%)	Total
0–19	5 (2.0)	244 (98.0)	249
20–39	12 (3.8)	301 (96.2)	313
40–59	17 (8.3)	189 (91.7)	206
≥ 60	38 (19.3)	159 (80.7)	197
	72 (7.5)	893 (92.5)	965

EEG/ECG METHODOLOGY AND ANALYSIS

The AEEG recording devices currently available have proved themselves to be quite versatile in their ability to record various other physiologic parameters simultaneously, the most common being ECG. This section will deal with the equipment and techniques used in the recording and analysis of ECG via cassette and rapid-replay units, respectively.

Both the Oxford Medilog and the Bio-Log AEEG recorders can easily be adapted to record one or more channels of ECG. The Medilog recorder can be configured either with a hard-wired board and snap lead set dedicated to ECG, or with the newer ECG-adapter module, which can be mated to any one of the preamplifier lead sockets. Bio-Scan's Bio-Log AEEG unit can likewise be fitted with such an adapter, which attaches directly to the input terminals on the Q.P. preamplifier. These newer adapters provide greater flexibility, since they allow one or more EEG channels to be converted easily to ECG recording without internal reconfiguration.

The Holter ECG application, while relatively simple, requires a disciplined technique. It is essential for quality recording that the technician gain the confidence and cooperation of the patient. Although a sophisticated knowledge of the recorder's electrical or mechanical system is not necessary, the technician must be alert to potential difficulties and take corrective actions when they arise. Technical problems inevitably will occur with the modified Holter ECG lead, but many can be detected prior to attaching the patient during a brief precheck of the recording system including the calibrator, the system monitoring unit, and impedance meter. The latter two items are essential to confirming ECG signal integrity.

By convention, the red snap lead is assigned as the positive electrode terminal. At the time of calibration, a standard 1-mV calibration signal is passed through the ECG snap leads. A smooth alternating deflection of the needle across the microamp meter on the interface unit indicates continuity. During this procedure, the ECG lead wire should be jiggled near the recorder clamp, at the adapter, and at the snap leads themselves. A short at any point in the lead will produce either an intermittent signal deflection or none at all. The ECG snap-lead contacts must also be inspected and cleaned with an appropriate solvent.

Adhesive residue on the contacts may produce an intermittent signal. For purposes of scanning ease, the designated ECG channel is best placed in the channel 8 position. A second Holter lead, if desired, should be positioned alongside it in position 7. This configuration places the ECG leads closest to the cursor line on the scanning unit, which is used to calculate heart rate.

The ECG lead set is usually secured to the patient following the application and gelling of the scalp electrodes. Application to the chest is performed using standard Holter techniques. Disposable, hypoallergenic, offset type, silver/silver chloride cardiac electrodes are recommended. The very small, stress-test electrodes and very large hospital monitoring electrodes are inappropriate for long-term ambulatory monitoring. Special pediatric electrodes are needed for neonates and young children.

In a one-lead conventional ECG application, a left precordial view is standard for the detection of ST segment depression of myocardial ischemia. Although cassette EEG/ECG lead is not well suited for such analysis, a left precordial lead placement does afford the opportunity to record a relatively strong R wave signal, which is important in rapid audio analysis of the cardiac channel on playback. A modified bipolar V5 lead is depicted in Fig. 7. A second lead, which demonstrates good P waves and which is perpendicular to the modified V5, is the modified V1. Muscular areas should be avoided, as artifact or baseline wandering will compromise the signal analysis. In the case of patients with cardiac pacemakers, one must further avoid placing electrodes directly on top of the pacemaker, as it may hinder or mask the recording of normal intraventricular conduction.

Following electrode-site preparation, the backing is removed from pregelled electrode's, and the electrolyte is checked for freshness. A dried-out electrode will produce a very poor signal. The electrode pad should then be firmly placed in position. Before proceeding further, the electrode's impedance should be checked to see that it is less than 10 K Ohms. A continuity check should also be performed. This can be accomplished either by noting an appropriate signal deflection for the ECG channel on the system monitoring unit or by examining a printout from an interfaced EEG machine. The electrode snaps are then additionally secured to the electrode pads with a small piece of surgical tape. Excessive taping over the electrodes should be avoided, however, since it promotes artifact. Slack should be left in the ECG wire leading back to the recorder. The patient is then dressed and instructed in the proper use of the recorder's event marker button and the patient diary.

The importance of the recorder precheck, proper electrode placement, and subsequent ECG signal testing cannot be overemphasized. Unfortunately, the ECG leads are exposed to more physical stress than any other component in typical AEEG attachments and thus fail at a disproportionate rate. Patients should be instructed to perform periodic inspection of the electrodes for accidental disconnection. A quick, even if nonexpert, reattachment can cut down considerably on lost signal time.

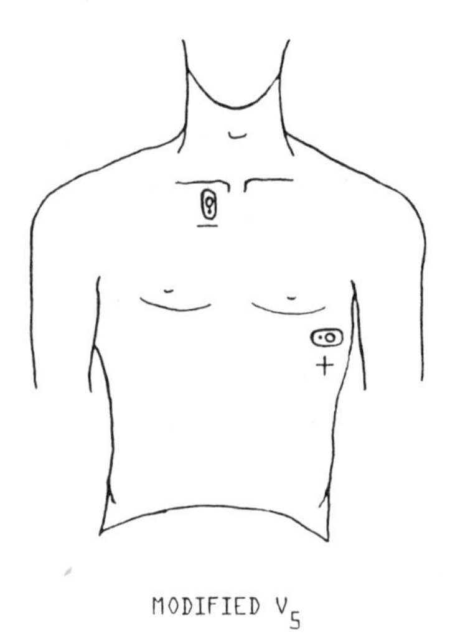

FIG. 7. ECG lead placements for a modified V5 recording.

The manufacturers could do more to reduce the likelihood of cable clamp pressure and patient-induced stress. The "Y" junction along the ECG lead, where the snap lead wires emerge, should also be strengthened. The newer ECG adapter modules have alleviated some of these difficulties, but strain reliefs would be helpful there as well.

Scanning the ECG Channel(s)

In contrast to electrode application, reviewing ECG channels on replay requires significant expertise. The analysis requires not only a knowledge of cardiac electrophysiology and electrocardiography, but also familiarity with Holter ECG scanning technologies from the era prior to microprocessor-assisted arrhythmia detectors, arrhythmiographs, and total beat counters. The Oxford Medilog EEG replay units offer no such mechanisms for automated ECG processing.

Prior to scanning, the technician should review the patient's diary for any relevant entries and later pay particular attention to possible abnormalities during these periods. The review technique employed involves listening to the audio output of the ECG channel played back at rapid speed. The repetitive ECG waveforms, when applied to a speaker or stereo headphones, produce a characteristic "buzzing" sound. The frequency and tonal qualities of the buzz are directly related to the patient's heart rate and the shape of the ECG complexes. As heart rate increases or decreases, so does the pitch of the audio tone. Ectopic beats, as well as other arrhythmias, interrupt the monotonal buzz because they have a different waveform and rhythm, which results in a different sound. Although sound is critical in detection of a possible ECG abnormality, a simultaneous visual analysis is important in confirming an arrhythmia or change in heart rate.

The review speed should be set at the maximum, which, on the Oxford unit, is 60 times real time. Audio perception will suffer dramatically at a lower speed. A 16-sec video page is easier to review in the rapid mode; an 8-sec page is superior for more critical review. In addition, the reviewer may wish to reduce the gains of nearby EEG channels, if they are distracting. If excessive baseline wandering is present, a time-constant adjustment can be made. All filters must, of course, be specified on printout, since they will affect the shape of the complexes. As cardiac pathology is often subtle, the ECG review is best performed in a separate pass from that of the EEG.

While scanning, the technician should stop frequently to ascertain heart rate. The 8-sec page format is best used for P-R interval measurement. Confirmation of a borderline first-degree AV block should be made at printout. Scanning for various forms of second-degree AV block is slightly more difficult. Tapes from patients with pacemakers are difficult to scan even on conventional Holter ECG scanners. Intermittent pacemaker-sensing failures and spike-generator failures can, however, be detected with 1-channel ECG as described above.

PVCs are detected by their distinctive popping sound, although frequency can only be determined by diligent hourly hand counts. While reviewing a particular hour of ECG, sporadic heart-rate measurements and PVC-frequency estimates can be made. High PVC frequency in association with ventricular sequences and/or multiformity is generally considered to be pathologic. Multiformity with respect to PVC configuration should be judged conservatively, especially when only one ECG lead was recorded. PVC couplets and bursts can be picked out easily by their characteristic sounds, as can many supraventricular arrhythmias.

Following ECG replay, the worklog is reviewed, and pertinent ECG rhythm strips are selected for incorporation in the final AEEG/ECG report and printout. The technician's general comments may be added to the report and can include a subjective impression of PVC frequency, the presence of significant bradycardia or tachycardia, multiformity of ventricular ectopia, ventricular sequence, complex arrhythmias, and the presence of AV block. These strips may also be presented to a consultant cardiologist, as long as he is familiar with the unconventional recording technique.

Technical Limitations

Analysis of the ECG portion of simultaneous EEG/ECG cassette recordings is subject to certain limitations. A reviewer must overcome the distortion of waveforms due to a difference in chart speed. ECG is usually printed out at 25 mm/sec versus 30 mm/sec for EEG. This difference will slightly widen the ECG complex and P waves, which are already reduced in this technique. By not using any high-frequency filtering on EEG printer, the complexes may be sharpened to a degree. In general, this type of ECG monitoring is not suitable for proper ST segment evaluation.

Another, more troubling, concern comes from the "bar" artifacts that are peculiar to the Medilog blocked-analog recording system. In this replay error involving transcription back to analog, several channels momentarily appear to have lost their signal. If this affects the ECG lead, the resulting artifact may simulate a cycle of second-degree AV block. A second pass over the same tape segment will usually produce an error-free display.

Artifact and intermittent loss of signal are the major limiting factors in the analysis of ECG monitoring. These tapes must be interpreted most conservatively, since no backup channel is available in case of lead or electrode failure. An alternative view from another lead is not possible to clarify questionable arrhythmias or PVC multiformity. As with EEG, reporting ECG features as abnormal should be based on their repetitive documentation.

If a disciplined technique is employed in attaching patients, and if tapes are scanned by experienced personnel familiar with the limitations of the technique, one channel of ECG is adequate. If these conditions cannot be met, then a conventional Holter ECG may be indicated whenever cardiac monitoring is clinically warranted.

CONCLUSION

The practical, clinical utility of simultaneous EEG/ECG monitoring cannot always be ascertained by literature review. The studies critiqued above, including our own, are not comparable in all spheres. Part of the reason for variability in findings has been the marked differences in patient selection, referral patterns, types of test employed, etc. For example, while one study may include large numbers of patients with syncope (who might be anticipated to have cardiac disease), another may exclude them. Patients with undiagnosed attacks referred to an epilepsy-monitoring center may differ significantly from patients studied in a private-practice setting.

Conclusions drawn from results have also varied greatly. If a patient with unexplained spells has an asymptomatic cardiac arrhythmia detected, does that necessarily "rule in" a cardiogenic etiology for the patient's symptoms and rule out a neurologic cause? In the absence of any epileptiform abnormalities, one may argue that such a finding may take on significance. Similar questions have been faced by cardiologists since the advent of Holter ECG monitoring. Only long-term follow-up studies on large numbers of patients will help resolve these issues. For now, clinical judgment, as applied to each individual case, must be paramount. We hope this will result in proper and judicious use of the modality and appropriate interpretation of the resultant data.

Although no absolute guidelines can be advanced for the use of simultaneous EEG/ECG monitoring, some general recommendations can be made. The relative simplicity of electrode application and the ease with which ECG can be analyzed, when following the guidelines outlined above, are by themselves sufficient criteria for its use in most patients. Regardless of symptoms, older patients who are referred for AEEG, particularly those over 60, should have concurrent ECG monitoring, simply because of the high rate of arrhythmias in this population. The case is less strong for always monitoring the ECG of young patients having AEEG, but there is little to lose by doing so and potentially much to gain. Certainly those patients with attacks not responding to anticonvulsants and those with a family history of sudden death with or without seizures should indeed have combined EEG/ECG recordings.

ACKNOWLEDGMENTS

We wish to thank Dr. Aaron Miller for reviewing the manuscript and Donna Keilson for technical assistance. This work has been supported in part by a grant from the research and development fund of Maimonides Medical Center.

REFERENCES

1. Kapor WN, Karpf M, Wieand S, et al. A prospective evaluation and followup of patients with syncope. *N Engl J Med* 1983;309:197–204.
2. Lipsitz L. Syncope in the elderly. *Ann Int Med* 1983;99:92–105.
3. Radack KL. Syncope—cost effective patient workup. *Postgrad Med* 1986;80:169–178.
4. Gastaut H, Fischer-Williams M. EEG study of syncope. *Lancet* 1957;2:1018–1025.
5. Barlotta F, Grace WJ. Neurologic disorders due to cardiac arrhythmia. *NY State J Med* 1966;66:513–515.
6. Braham J, Hertzeanu H, Yahini JH, et al. Reflex cardiac arrest presenting as epilepsy. *Ann Neurol* 1981;3:277–278.
7. Schott GD, McLeod AA, Jewitt DE. Cardiac arrhythmias that masquerade as epilepsy. *Br Med J* 1977;1:1454–1457.
8. Williams ER. Cardiogenic syncope and epilepsy. *Postgrad Med J* 1967;43:677–679.
9. Woodley D, Chambers W, Starke H, et al. Intermittent complete AV block masquerading as epilepsy in the mitral valve prolapse syndrome. *Chest* 1977;72:369–372.
10. DeBono DP, Warlow CP, Hyman NM. Cardiac rhythm abnormalities in patients presenting with non-focal neurologic symptoms: a diagnostic grey area? *Br Med J* 1982;284:1437–1439.
11. Jonas S, Klein I, Dimant J. Importance of Holter monitoring in patients with periodic cerebral symptoms. *Ann Neurol* 1977;1:470–474.
12. Koudstaal PJ, Van Gun J, Klootwijk APJ, et al. Holter monitoring in patients with transient and focal ischemic attacks of the brain. *Stroke* 1986;17:192–195.
13. Lavy S, Stern S. Transient neurologic manifestations in cardiac arrhythmias. *J Neurol Sci* 1969;9:97–102.
14. Luxon, IM, Crowther A, Harrison MJ, et al. Controlled study of 24-hour ambulatory ECG monitoring in patients with transient neurologic symptoms. *J Neurol Neurosurg Psychiat* 1980;43:37–41.
15. Gastaut H. Syncopes: generalized anoxic cerebral seizures. In: Vinken PJ, Bruyn GW, eds. *Handbook of clinical neurology,* vol 15. Amsterdam: North-Holland; 815–835.
16. Duvoisin RC. Convulsive syncope induced by the weber maneuver. *Arch Neurol* 1962;7:219–226.
17. Kershman J. Syncope and seizures. *J Neurol Neurosurg Psychiat* 1949;12:25–33.
18. Bridgers SL, Ebersole JS. Ambulatory EEG in clinical practice. *Neurology* 1985;35:1767–1768.
19. Callaghan N, McCarthy N. Ambulatory EEG during fainting attacks with normal routine and

sleep EEG records. In: Stefan H, Burr W, eds. *Mobile long-term EEG monitoring.* Stuttgart: Gustav-Fischer, 1982;61–65.
20. Graf M, Brunner G, Weber H, et al. Simultaneous long-term recording of EEG and ECG in "syncope" patients. In: Stefan H, Burr W, eds. *Mobile long-term EEG monitoring.* Stuttgart: Gustav-Fischer, 1982;67–76.
21. Keilson MJ, Magrill JP, Hauser WA. Evaluation of syncope with ambulatory cassette EEG. *Neurology* (suppl.) 1985;35:225.
22. Lai CW, Zeigler DK. Syncope problem solved by continuous ambulatory simultaneous EEG/ECG recording. *Neurology* 1981;31:1152–1154.
23. Haslam RH, Jameson HD. Cardiac standstill simulating repeated epileptic attacks. *JAMA* 1973;224:887–889.
24. Schraeder PL, Pontzer R, Engel TR. A case of being scared to death. *Arch Int Med* 1983;143:1793–1794.
25. Abdon NJ, Malmcrona R. High pacemaker implantation rate following "cardiogenic neurology." *Acta Med Scand* 1975;198:455–461.
26. Editorial. Or in the heart or in the head? *Br Med J* 1976;1:1158.
27. Lin JT, Zeigler DK, Lai DW, et al. Convulsive syncope in blood donors. *Ann Neurol* 1982;11:525–528.
28. Moss AJ, Schwartz PJ. Sudden death and the idiopathic long Q-T syndrome. *Am J Med* 1979;66:6–7.
29. Ballardie RW, Murphy RP, Davis J. Epilepsy: a presentation of the Romano-Ward syndrome. *Br Med J* 1983;287:896–897.
30. Bricker JT, Garson A, Gillette PC. A family history of seizures associated with sudden deaths. *Am J Dis Child* 1984;138:866–868.
31. Pignata C, Farina V, Andria G, et al. Prolonged Q-T interval presenting as idiopathic epilepsy. *Neuroped* 1983;14:235–236.
32. Selby PJ, Driver MV. An unusual cause of apparent epilepsy: ECG and EEG findings in a case of Jervell Lang-Neilson syndrome. *J Neurol Neurosurg Psychiat* 1977;40:1102–1108.
33. Sundaram MB, McMeckin JD, Gulamhussein S. Cardiac tachyarrhythmias in hereditary long Q-T syndromes presenting as a seizure disorder. *Can J Neurol Sci* 1986;13:262–263.
34. Vlay C, Mallis G, Brown J, et al. Documented sudden cardiac death in prolonged Q-T syndrome. *Arch Int Med* 1984;144:833–835.
35. Schwartz GD, Periti M, Malliani A. The long Q-T syndrome. *Am Heart J* 1975;89:378–390.
36. Moss AJ, Schwartz RJ, Crampton RS, et al. The long Q-T syndrome: a prospective international study. *Circulation* 1985;71:17–21.
37. Mauck HP, Hockman DH. Central nervous system mechanisms mediating cardiac rate and rhythm. *Am Heart J* 1967;74:96–109.
38. Blumhardt LD, Smith PEM, Owen L. EEG accompaniments of temporal lobe seizures. *Lancet* 1986;1:1051–1055.
39. Erickson TC. Cardiac activity during epileptic seizures. *Arch Neurol Psychiat* 1939;41:511–518.
40. Katz RI, Tiger M, Harner RN. Epileptic cardiac arrhythmia: sino-atrial arrest in two patients. *Epilepsia* 1983;24:248.
41. Keilson MJ, Hauser WA, MaGrill JP. ECG changes during electrographic seizures. (submitted).
42. Kiok MC, Tennence CF, Fromm GH, et al. Sinus arrest in epilepsy. *Neurology* 1986;36:115–116.
43. Lathers C, Schraeder P. Autonomic dysfunction in epilepsy. *Epilepsia* 1982;23:633–647.
44. Lathers C, Schraeder P. Review of autonomic dysfunction, cardiac arrhythmias and epileptogenic activity. *J Clin Pharm* 1987;27:346–356.
45. Marshall DW, Westmoreland BF, Sharbrough FW. Ictal tachycardia during temporal lobe seizures. *Mayo Clin Proc* 1983;58:443–446.
46. Mathew NT, Taori GM, Mathai KV, et al. Atrial fibrillation associated with seizures in a case of frontal meningioma. *Neurology* 1970;20:725–728.
47. Mosier JM, White P, Grant P, et al. Cerebro-autonomic and myographic changes accompanying induced seizures. *Neurology* 1957;7:204–210.
48. Phizackerly PF, Poole EW, Whiuttey CW. Sino-auricular heart block as an epileptic manifestation. *Epilepsia* 1954;3:89–91.
49. Rossi E, Rossi GF. Heart rate behavior during partial epileptic seizures: an electroclinical

study. In: Strober T, Schimrigk K, Ganten D, et al., eds. *Central nervous system control of the heart.* Boston: Kluwer Academic, 1986;187–201.
50. Rush JL, Everett BAS, Adams AH, et al. Paroxysmal atrial tachycardia and frontal lobe tumor. *Arch Neurol* 1977;34:578–580.
51. Schamroth CL, Davidoff R, Myburgh DP. Grand mal epilepsy as recorded during dynamic electrocardiography. *Heart Lung* 1981;10:696–697.
52. Schraeder PL, Lathers CM. Cardiac neural discharge and epileptogenic activity in the cat: an animal model for unexplained death. *Life Sci* 1983;32:1371–1382.
53. Van Buren JM. Some autonomic concomitants of ictal automatism. *Brain* 1958;81:505–528.
54. Van Buren JM, Ajmone-Marsan C. A correlation of autonomic and EEG components in temporal lobe epilepsy. *Arch Neurol* 1960;3:683–703.
55. Walsh GO, Nasland W, Goldensohn ES. Relationships between PAT and paroxysmal cerebral discharges. *Bull LA Neurol Sci* 1972;37:28–35.
56. White PT, Grant P, Mosier J, et al. Changes in cerebral dynamics associated with seizures. *Neurology* 1961;11:354–361.
57. Carnel SB, Schraeder PL, Lathers CM. Effect of phenobarbital pretreatment on cardiac neural discharges and PTZ induced epileptogenic activity in the cat. *Pharmacology* 1985;30:225–240.
58. Natelson BH. Neurocardiology: an interdisciplinary area for the 80's. *Arch Neurol* 1985;42:178–184.
59. Talman WT. Cardiovascular regulation and lesions of the CNS. *Ann Neurol* 1985;18:1–12.
60. Keilson MJ, Hauser WA, MaGrill JP, et al. ECG abnormalities in patients with epilepsy. *Neurology* 1987;37:1624–1626.
61. Gordan S, Saksena S, Parsonnet V. Latent intrahistian block provoked by a seizure. *Am Heart J* 1987;113:837–839.
62. Pritchett EL, McNamara JO, Gallager JJ. Arrhythmogenic epilepsy: an hypothesis. *Am Heart J* 1980;100:683–688.
63. Hirsch C, Martin D. Unexpected death in young epileptics. *Neurology* 1971;21:682–690.
64. Jay G, Leestma J. Sudden death in epilepsy. *Acta Neurol Scand* 1981;63(suppl 82):1–66.
65. Terrence C, Wisotzkey H, Perper J. Unexpected, unexplained deaths in epileptic patients. *Neurology* 1975;25:594–598.
66. Messenheimer JA, Quint SR, Tennison MB, et al. Changes in heart rate period variability during repeated complex partial seizures. *Epilepsia* 1987;28:635.
67. Quint SR, Messenheimer JA, Tennison MB, et al. A procedure for assessing the autonomic activity related to unexplained deaths in epileptics. *Epilepsia* 1987;28:610.
68. Tennison MB, Quint SR, Messenheimer JA, et al. Autonomic effect of seizures assessed by power spectral analysis of heart period variability. *Epilepsia* 1987;28:610.
69. Blumhardt LD. The diagnostic value of ECG/EEG recording. In: DelPalu C, Pessina A, eds. *Isam: proceedings of the fifth international symposium on ambulatory monitoring.* Padua: Cleup Pub, 1985;675–683.
70. Blumhardt LD, Oozeer R. Simultaneous ambulatory monitoring of the EEG and ECG in patients with unexplained transient disturbances in subconsciousness. In: Stott FD, Raftery EB, Clement DL, et al., eds. *Isam-Gent 1981 proceedings of the fourth international symposium on ambulatory monitoring.* London: Academic Press, 1982;171–192.
71. Cull RE. An assessment of 24-hour ambulatory EEG-ECG monitoring in a neurology clinic. *J Neurol Neurosurg Psychiat* 1985;48:107–110.
72. Nousiaianen U, Mervaala E, Tiihonen P, et al. Cardiac arrhythmias in long-term EEG-ECG recordings. *Epilepsia* 1986;27:633.

Ambulatory EEG Monitoring,
edited by John S. Ebersole.
Raven Press, Ltd., New York © 1989

12

Presurgical Evaluations Using Cassette EEG

John R. Ives, Donald L. Schomer, and Howard W. Blume

Beth Israel Hospital, Harvard University, Boston, Massachusetts 02215

EEG MANDATE

Most patients who are considered candidates for epilepsy surgery have been followed medically for extensive periods of time, and considerable information exists regarding the classification of their clinical seizure pattern. This pattern should suggest a focal area of onset that could possibly be resected. Previous EEG findings, as well as other localizing procedures such as computerized tomography (CT) scan, magnetic resonance imaging (MRI) scan, and neuropsychological testing, are extremely helpful (1,2). The patient's history should include failure of adequate control with conventional anticonvulsant treatment (1,3,4) and a form of seizures that is socially disabling, preventing the patient from experiencing a normal life (1).

The effective monitoring of the patient's EEG during the onset of a seizure is the current standard for determining whether a seizure onset is focal. More than 90% of surveyed surgical centers include ictal EEG as a requirement in their presurgical protocol (3). Conventional routine scalp EEGs are most often nonictal. When a seizure occurs during such a recording session, these centers are not very efficient technically in localizing the spontaneous seizure activity. The long-term monitoring (LTM) of the EEG by telemetric means has the potential to record consistently the physiological markers of the onset and progression of a seizure. This is the technique that is used by approximately 80% of surgical centers (3).

Until the advent of LTM techniques, fewer than 25% of the patients who underwent temporal lobectomies for medically refractory focal epilepsy at Montreal Neurological Institute had their spontaneous seizures recorded, despite extensive recordings with conventional EEG (5–7). Even the seizures that were recorded under these circumstances did not demonstrate the onset well, because of technical considerations that included the effects of movement, muscle artifact, choice of inappropriate montages, and connecting cables. The seizures that were recorded provided a variable contribution to the localization for surgery in this large group of surgical candidates. The major contribution of the EEG was in the lateralization and localization of the patient's interictal epileptiform activity.

During the 1970s, LTM techniques at several institutions (8–15) permitted the majority of patients to have their habitual seizures recorded prior to surgery (3). Currently, at our institution, it is a prerequisite that several seizures be recorded with a consistent focal origin in order for the patient to be considered a surgical candidate for focal corticectomy. This is accomplished by the use of inpatient and outpatient LTM technology tailored to the individual needs of the patient under investigation.

Other parts of the investigation aid in determining that the patient has a focal neurological problem and that the focus of seizure onset is in an operable area of the brain. These investigations include imaging techniques and neuropsychological testing, as well as the routine clinical neurological examination (1,3). However, the localization of an epileptic focus currently is still dependent on a consistent and unequivocal focal onset as determined by EEG criteria. If there is an anatomical lesion such as an arteriovenous malformation, tumor, or cyst, confusing or ambiguous ictal EEG findings should not necessarily affect the neurosurgeon's decision to operate. The localization of the seizure onset may be in an area near or adjacent to the anatomical lesion. More extensive removal that would include this surrounding area may then be considered. However, in some cases, the anatomical lesion appears to be unrelated to the localization of the onset of the patient's seizures, and further EEG evaluation may be required.

Level of Diagnostic Intervention

There are three relative levels of invasiveness of EEG electrode evaluation that may be required for surgical candidates. The first level is standard conventional scalp electrodes routinely placed according to the international electrode placement procedure for direct EEG recordings or telemetry. The placement of either mini (16) or standard chronic sphenoidal electrodes (17–19) constitutes a minor invasive procedure. The third and most invasive form of investigation is the placement of recording electrodes into (20) or over (21) the surface of the brain in order to record electrical activity from structures that are not well recorded with scalp, sphenoidal, or other extracranial electrodes. This is considered only when the less invasive techniques fail to show a discrete focal onset to seizures (22).

At some institutions, a brief investigation with scalp electrodes is performed prior to the use of sphenoidal electrodes. In most situations, sphenoidals are extensively used (23). If a diffuse generalized onset of the seizures is demonstrated under these conditions, a generalized or multifocal epileptic disorder may be suspected, particularly if this correlates with the clinical characteristics. These cases usually cannot be helped through a surgical intervention, and more invasive electroencephalography is unlikely to demonstrate a focal problem. Under these circumstances, the patient is no longer considered a surgical candidate.

However, some focal areas of epilepsy may present with seizures that appear as generalized forms, particularly if the origin is frontal cortex. Awareness of this possibility will guard against premature termination of surgical evaluation in these patients.

If a consistent onset of seizures is found during ictal recordings, and if collaborating localization information is obtained from other independent clinical tests, the patient's presurgical EEG workup is complete and surgery is considered as a therapeutic option (1,2). In our experience, the need to delineate further a focus with more invasive intracranial electrodes is not required (22). If there is ambiguity regarding the lateralization or lobe of the brain involved in the onset of seizures using scalp or sphenoidal techniques or if the other clinical tests are highly inconsistent with the EEG data, there may be a need to proceed with the more-invasive EEG recordings with implanted electrodes. Data from the less-invasive studies may help to determine the location and type of electrode system to be used. With implanted electrodes, the concept of recording and localizing a consistent focal seizure onset is of paramount importance.

Patients with a surgically approachable problem of epilepsy may show any of several findings. In some, a focus has been demonstrated that is consistently associated with the initiation of the onset of the patient's seizures. In these cases, removal of that area usually benefits the control of the patient's spontaneous seizures. In other cases, his seizures may appear to have a multifocal pattern of onset. If the vast majority of seizures or the more socially disabling type of seizures have a consistent focal onset in an area that can be safely removed, excision of that area may significantly help the patient's control of that specific seizure pattern. However, there is a risk that the frequency of seizures from another epileptic area that is not part of the area of excision may increase after surgery and give poor overall long-term control (24). Finally, when the patient's primary seizure focus appears to be in an inoperable functional area that evolves into a disabling seizure by spread into medial temporal gray matter, surgical excision of the mesial temporal structures may be of benefit (25). These latter patients, in whom the primary area of onset is not in a resectable area, cannot be expected to have as promising a prognosis as those who have resection of the primary area of onset. However, the evolution of complex partial seizures may often be reduced to an aura or a simple partial seizure following medial temporal excision with a primary focus remaining.

Hierarchy of Focal Problems

In seizure disorders of focal onset, the focus frequently resides in one of four major anatomical regions: the temporal lobes, the frontal lobes, the parietal lobes, or the occipital lobes. The temporal-limbic type of seizure is the most prevalent, and seizures of frontal-lobe origin are the next most common. Clinical observations and description by the patient or reliable witnesses often provide a good indication of the probable location of the patient's seizure onset.

However, seizures of frontal-lobe origin, particularly of the orbital frontal area, may have the same clinical presentation as seizures of temporal-lobe origin. Similarly, seizures of more posterior cortex may spread to anterior and mesial temporal structures and appear as classic "temporal lobe" attacks. EEG data must be relied on for distinguishing area of origin (25,26).

The next consideration in localization is laterality of onset. Determining the laterality of onset is usually fairly straightforward in temporal-lobe seizures. Occasionally, the presence of a secondary contralateral independent focus or rapid spread from one medial temporal area to the other may confuse the issue and implanted electrodes may be necessary. Truly independent bilateral temporal foci giving rise to seizures cannot be approached surgically. In cases of frontal-lobe onset, the two sides are anatomically close to each other and have very extensive physiological connections that may lead to a rapid spread of epileptic discharges at the onset. In addition, significant areas of the frontal lobes are deep and not easily sampled with surface electrodes. In these cases, implanted electrodes are of great value but, in a few instances, may still not give sufficient information about laterality to permit a surgical decision. Independent bifrontal seizure foci are also not resectable because of the functional deficits that would occur with any bilateral excision. Computer analysis may eventually assist in determining the true site of origin of seizures.

EQUIPMENT PREREQUISITE

General Requirements

The evaluation of patients for excision of epileptogenic tissue mainly requires the localization of the brain area that is initiating and/or sustaining the epileptic discharge. Traditionally, the EEG has been the major source of that crucial information. Long-term EEG monitoring units have brought the capability of recording seizure onset and duration with less artifact. Units with 16-, 24-, or 32-channel capacities or more now permit a high level of accuracy in localization. Ambulatory long-term monitoring with a 16- and 24-channel coverage allows more freedom for the patient and still provides the same degree of sophistication of EEG recordings.

Ambulatory EEG and Its Use with Surgical Candidates

In the past, because of the relatively limited number of EEG recording channels available on ambulatory devices, the outpatient evaluation of a presurgical candidate was not taken seriously. We have been using ambulatory cassette recorders (A1-A2) that have either 16 or 24 channels of simultaneous EEG coverage (27,28). These event-type recorders store up to 2 min of delayed EEG prior to the activation of the seizure/event push button. They emulate PDP-12 and PDP-11 computer-based delay systems described in earlier reports (8,29). These ambulatory cassette recorders may also be programmed to perform frequent nighttime/sleep sampling of the patient's EEG (e.g., a 20-sec sample every 5 min from 2300 hr to 0700 hr the next morning) and thus may emulate the sleep-sampling function previously described (30). The ambulatory recording system and methodology can also accommodate chronic sphenoidal electrodes, which are well tolerated and extensively used in the outpatient environment (17,18,31). Using a surface/sphenoidal bipolar montage, the ambulatory cassette coverage is equal to or exceeds conventional EEG machine capacity. If a 24-channel system is used in conjunction with sphenoidal electrodes, all head regions can be recorded in a bipolar montage array. Both the 16- and 24-channel recording systems are compatible with our depth-electrode arrays. Any individually designed bipolar montage can be selected from the depth electrodes. This can give more freedom to the hospitalized patient with depth electrodes in place.

In addition, a small, portable take-home computer (ELB) (32,33) can extend the capabilities of the ambulatory cassette for outpatients with scalp and sphenoidal electrodes. Figure 1 illustrates the setup in a typical home environment. The ELB has a 40-Mybte hard disk that provides up to 3.5 hr of storage capacity and performs on-line automatic spike and seizure detection on the multiplexed EEG, which is available from the A1-A2. It can be easily interconnected to the ambulatory unit by the patient. Thus, the enhanced ambulatory EEG monitoring system can emulate the large and more-extensive PDP-11/60–based system but has the advantage of home use.

Obviously, the ambulatory system can also be used in a hospital environment. The patient may be free to move around on the ward wearing the 16- or 24-channel system, restricted only by nursing and medical precautions. Alternatively, his ambulatory unit may be interconnected and time-locked with a video system or with the ELB on-line seizure/spike-detection unit. This necessitates patient cooperation in order to connect himself during the night or at other times when ictal events may occur. In other diagnostic situations, he may require continuous video monitoring and/or automatic detection surveillance with only short, necessary breaks. If he is away from the video camera and/or the automatic detection system during those times, the A1-A2 is still operational and capable of recording clinical seizures, should they occur. The ambulatory coverage makes the hospital routine far more amenable to patient compliance,

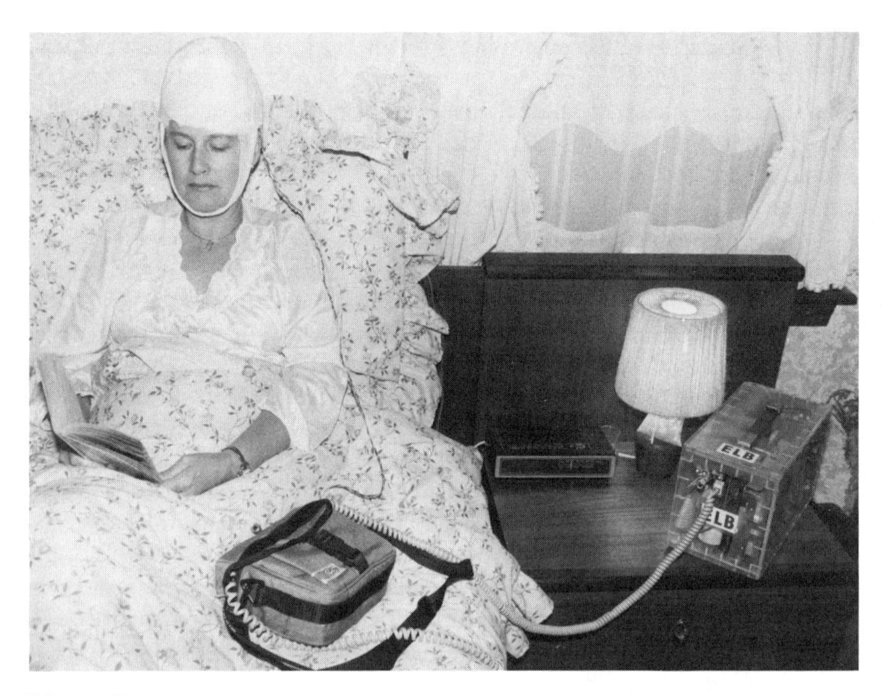

FIG. 1. This subject illustrates the equipment used to monitor the patient in the home environment. The 16- or 24-channel ambulatory cassette, or A1-A2, is contained in the camera bag on the bed. It is connected to the head-mounted electrodes, preamplifiers, and multiplexor via a thin woven cable. This equipment is installed during setup in the lab and is worn by the patient until the end of the recording session. The other unit on the bedside table, labeled ELB, was the first prototype system to be sent home; it contained a 30-Mbyte hard disk. The current unit is about half the size and has a 40-Mbyte hard disk. After being set up on the A1-A2, the ELB is given to the patient to take home and install near the bed. On retiring, the patient interconnects the A1-A2 and the ELB with a 25-ft coiled telephone cable. In the morning, the patient disconnects and returns to the lab with all the equipment.

since it is not dependent on his remaining confined to a room or ward. The universal incorporation of an ambulatory setup on all patients requiring some form of LTM is convenient and efficient.

The bandwidth of the ambulatory EEG is from 0.5 to 70.0 Hz with a digitizing sample rate of 200 samples/sec/channel. It compares favorably to the frequency resolution of the conventional EEG machines. The A1-A2– and the ELB-acquired EEG can be replayed onto any conventional EEG machine or viewed on a high-resolution graphics display screen. Since the EEG is recorded in standard PC-DOS files, it can be stored on bulk-storage media such as cartridges or large disks for future reading or filing.

Off-line analysis of the recorded seizures captured by either the A1-A2 or the ELB is also possible. We have built into the replay demulitplexor a 6-pole switched-capacitor–type high-frequency filter (34). Thus, any events contaminated with high-frequency muscle activity can be selectively and repeatedly filtered at any cutoff frequency between 8 and 70 Hz in an attempt to determine if unequivocal localizing seizure activity is present but masked by overlying muscle activity. Further off-line digital analysis of the EEG may be easily accomplished with a variety of available software techniques.

THE RELATIVE IMPORTANCE OF VIDEO

Ambulatory monitoring in the past meant that the patient was released to his home environment and simultaneous video recording was impractical. However, as discussed in the preceding section, an ambulatory patient can be restricted and interconnected to a video system to permit simultaneous time-locked monitoring. It has not been our experience that *all* surgical candidates benefit for having *all* their seizures simultaneously documented by both EEG and video. In some circumstances, the diagnosis and plan for treatment may benefit significantly as a result of video documentation of these events. This does *not* appear to be the case for the majority of patients. One of the main reasons for our observation is that the majority of the patients considered for surgery have an epileptic focus in one of the temporal lobes. The clinical expressions of those seizures as documented with video do not seem to have consistent lateralizing or localizing features (35). Our use of video is to supplement the EEG recording and localization procedures.

IMPORTANCE OF AUTOMATIC EEG-DETECTION SYSTEMS

Systems that automatically detect, classify, log, and record EEG phenomena have been introduced recently. Presently, their significance appears to be in the area of data reduction rather than data analysis. They permit an efficient use of long-term monitoring on several patients for extended periods of time with fewer personnel. Relevant events are automatically extracted for later confirmation by an experienced electroencephalographer.

Automatic detection *does not* replace the event/seizure push button. This is still the more-important event to document. Automatic detection gleans from a 24-hr EEG morphological events that may be significant. The system is biased on the side of overdetections or false positives. The only events that have been successfully detected on a routine basis are spikes, sharp waves (36), electrographic seizures (37), and spike-and-wave discharges (38). The detection algorithms are not absolute. In our lab, they are used only to scan for morphologically significant events and not as a detection device that competes with the experienced electroencephalographer.

Frequent periodic sampling of the EEG, particularly during sleep, is also an essential part of our 24-hr recordings (30). We take 20- to 30-sec samples every 5 min between 2300 and 0700 hr. This permits us to look at about 7 to 10% of the total sleep EEG in a totally periodic fashion that is independent of seizure/event push buttons and automatic detections.

INPATIENT VERSUS OUTPATIENT

The principal reason for bringing a patient with epilepsy into the hospital is that the equipment necessary for his monitoring is hospital-based. He does not need hospitalization per se. If he is experiencing seizures at a level of one to several per week, it is now as easy and as sophisticated from an EEG point of view to monitor him on an outpatient basis using a 16- or 24-channel ambulatory recorder with surface/sphenoidal electrodes as it is to bring him into the hospital for monitoring. There are advantages to monitoring a patient in the outpatient environment besides the obvious savings in direct medical cost. Hospitalization disrupts his life and is often inconvenient to family members. In addition, there appears to be a significant reduction in spontaneous seizure occurrence on hospitalization in a large percentage of patients (39). This frustrating phenomenon has been observed by many investigators in this field. Additionally, the casual nursing coverage on a standard ward is usually not sufficient for a patient who is unaware of his seizures. Arranging special nursing observation is expensive.

The advantages of ambulatory outpatient monitoring include the observation that, in our experience, the frequency of spontaneously occurring seizures does not usually change. The level of dedication in terms of patient observation and documentation of events is usually better than on an inpatient unit if a family member is asked to participate. Even if the patient must travel long distances, outpatient monitoring can be obtained with relatively simple instructions that include only a tape change to extend coverage for a second day. If the patient comes from a considerable distance, staying at a local hotel or motel is a reasonable alternative to hospitalization.

Exceptions to successful outpatient monitoring include relative infrequent rate of occurrence of spontaneous seizures, i.e., less than one seizure per week. If the reduction of anticonvulsant medication is needed to increase seizure frequency, the patient should be hospitalized. If he is unreliable in terms of his ability to push the event button or if family members are not available, hospitalization may be required. When the preliminary investigation of a patient indicates that simultaneous video/EEG documentation of a spontaneous seizure is necessary, he needs to be hospitalized. If the investigation of a patient requires implanted electrodes, he needs to be hospitalized for close supervision during monitoring while the electrodes are in place.

INTERICTAL VERSUS ICTAL

It has only been in the past 10 to 15 years that documentation of ictal events can consistently be accomplished on a large number of presurgical candidates. The long-term follow-up results of basing a surgical decision on documented ictal recordings rather than interictal findings is limited. Table 1, which has been reorganized from a previous study (7), indicates that a significant and probably important prognostic trend exists. In Table 1, 57 patients with more than 2 years of follow-up after an anterior temporal lobectomy were analyzed. A relevant predictor of long-term outcome may be seen by cross correlating the degree of ictal localization with the degree of interictal localization. In patients whose EEGs demonstrate a focal onset without spread to the contralateral temporal lobe and who have exclusively ipsilateral interictal spiking, the prognosis for a seizure-free long-term outcome approaches 100% after an anterior temporal lobectomy. However, if there is significant spread to the contralateral side, the prognosis for a seizure-free result is less optimistic.

The ability consistently and successfully to document the location of an ictal phenomenon may now permit surgery in some patients who, in the past, would not be candidates on the basis of interictal findings. Additionally, the ictal EEG is, by definition, a recording of the physiological activity of the seizure itself and may be a more-relevant event than the interictal activity, which is a secondary phenomenon (7). The morphology of ictal and interictal activity from the same

TABLE 1. *A combination of ictal and interictal findings versus the results of a >2-year follow-up of 57 temporal lobe epileptic patients who had a spontaneous clinical seizure documented prior to surgical removal of the temporal lobe*

Localization of ictal activity	Localization of interictal activity											
	Unilateral, independent, and generalized				Unilateral and independent				Unilateral only			
Focal, no spread	0	0	0	0	0	0			0	0	0	0
to contralateral					3				0	0	0	
temporal lobe		0							0	0	0	0
Focal with spread						1						
to contralateral					3	3	3					
temporal lobe					4	4	4	4	3			
		4			4	4	4		4	4		
Generalized		3										
or bilateral	4	4	4	4	3	3			3	3	3	3
	4	4	4							1		
Unreadable						3						
		4			4	4	4		4	4	4	

0, Seizure-free; 1,
became seizure-free; 3, marked reduction (< 1–2%); 4, moderate or less reduction (> 1–2%). From Ives (7).

patient is usually not similar, nor does it appear that there is a clear transformation from interictal to ictal event. The only feature that these two phenomena appear to have in common is that they cohabit the same general area. In previous work, it appears that the ictal events seem to increase the frequency of the occurrence of interictal phenomena (40).

The documentation of the ictus itself may contain other information in addition to localization. The seizure morphology or "seizure signature" of individual patients is usually unique, complex, and stereotypic (7). This implies that information may be contained in these wave forms. One such observation based on preliminary analysis of the frequency of the electrical phenomena at the onset of the temporal lobe seizures suggested a correlate with the presence of a space-occupying lesion (7,41). In those cases, if the event started with less than a 1-Hz rhythmic discharge, there was a high correlation with the coexistence of a tumor.

To explain this observation, one theory suggests that the temporal neocortex, which is seen by the surface/sphenoidal electrode array, has an inherent rhythm of electrical activity. When irritated or stimulated during a seizure, the rhythm that this neocortex can generate is a reflection of the state of health of that tissue. If it is significantly damaged, it will not oscillate at its more-typical frequencies. Thus, the frequency of the electrical activity when stimulated by a seizure correlates with the extent of the tissue damage.

Ictal information that is now systematically recorded by advanced LTM techniques has not been extensively studied other than for localization purposes. It is felt that it will contain information that will contribute to the understanding of seizure disorders. One area that may be explored is the distinction between areas of primary epileptogenic tissue and area of recruitment and spread of seizure discharge.

TYPICAL MONITORING SESSIONS

The workup of a surgical candidate is governed by individual requirements and seizure frequency. An initial attempt to record seizures with outpatient monitoring should be made using sphenoidal electrodes and an ambulatory system supplemented with ELB automatic detection. It is logistically easier and more efficient to perform ambulatory outpatient studies rather than inpatient recordings. The results of these studies can serve to triage patients for the more expensive and limited inpatient monitoring resources.

After an outpatient monitoring session, the results segregate into several distinct categories. The most-useful results are seen in those patients whose spontaneous seizures are recorded and have a consistent focal onset with automatically detected events as well as the interictal sampling, all correlating with other clinical lateralizing and localizing tests. Patients whose monitoring results are in this category can be scheduled for the Wada tests of speech and memory lateralization with intracarotid amytal injection and for subsequent surgery. In another group of patients, the seizures may be too infrequent and necessitate the hospitalization of the patient in order to taper anticonvulsant medication. In another category of patients, there may be discrepancies between the actual pushing of the button marking the seizure-event recorder, the EEG onset of the seizure, or the clinical description of the event. Therefore, an in-hospital EEG-monitoring session with simultaneous video recording may be necessary to clarify the problem. In a further patient group, it may be obvious from the ictal and interictal EEG that the localization of the onset escapes the still-limited coverage obtained with sphenoidal and surface electrodes. The patient then requires depth-electrode placement in order to identify a potential focus. If ictal and interictal EEG markers indicate that his seizure disorder is nonfocal or of a primary generalized type, further investigation with more-invasive electrodes is not warranted.

In summary, the outpatient EEG telemetry procedure can be conveniently combined with the battery of other outpatient procedures such as CT scan, MRI, and neuropsychological testing, as well as physician and nurse practitioner visits.

RESULTS

From September 1983 to the end of March 1988, 1209 ambulatory EEG studies were performed in our laboratory on three groups of patients. In the first group, an epilepsy diagnosis was only one of several clinical considerations. There were 702 studies in this group. The second group was comprised of patients with a definite diagnosis of epilepsy, who were having clinical events that needed further study and documentation. There were 167 studies in this group. The third group consisted of 77 patients who had intractable focal epilepsy and were under investigation as surgical candidates. In this group, 340 EEG studies were carried out with specific details noted in Table 2.

Five patients with depth electrodes in place had recordings using the ambulatory EEG event recorder in a hospital setting. All the initial depth recordings on these patients were obtained with our intensive inpatient 16-channel EEG/video/computer system. Near the end of their investigation period, when video was no longer essential, they were switched to the ambulatory unit to test its effectiveness.

In the remaining presurgical group of patients, the ambulatory EEG system appeared to provide a reliable assessment of the patient's interictal and ictal EEG activity. A combination of surface and sphenoidal electrodes was used in a majority of the studies as only 6 of the 77 patients were assessed without chronic sphenoidal electrodes. In some instances (15% of the outpatients studied), the results of the outpatient recording sessions provided enough information that further inpatient monitoring was not necessary. In the remainder, it was obvious

TABLE 2. *Surgical candidates monitored with ambulatory event recorder*

Ambulatory studies	340
Patients	77
Ambulatory outpatient studies	164
Events recorded during outpatient studies	>300
Ambulatory inpatient studies	176
Events recorded during inpatient studies	>400
Patients recorded with sphenoidals	71
Patients with depth electrodes	5
Inpatient ambulatory studies with depth electrodes	26

that hospitalization coupled with withdrawal from anticonvulsants was necessary to document a sufficient number of clinical events.

CASE STUDIES

Of the 77 presurgical candidates studied in our institution by means of ambulatory cassettes, three individual patient situations have been selected to illustrate the versatility of the ambulatory cassette in evaluating them for surgery and in determining which patients required the more-limited resource of intensive inpatient monitoring.

Case 1. A 35-year-old female patient was referred for an outpatient-monitoring session with sphenoidal electrodes. She had a previous history of temporal lobe seizures, which were felt to be under good control. Her major complaint was episodic severe abdominal pain occurring several times each day. She underwent a hysterectomy 10 years earlier in an attempt to alleviate her pain. The initial referral was not for a surgical opinion but rather for a diagnostic evaluation of her episodic complaints. She underwent outpatient monitoring to record the EEG during times of abdominal pain. These occurred several times per day.

A 2-day recording session with the ambulatory unit yielded five such episodes of abdominal pain. Two seemed to be followed by complex partial seizures as witnessed by a friend. All five events demonstrated rhythmic epileptiform activity from the right temporal lobe with phase reversal at SP2 (Figs. 2A and B). The interictal sampling (Fig. 2C) also revealed consistent unilateral interictal spike discharges phase-reversing at SP2 (right sphenoidal lead).

After a 6-month period with additional trials of anticonvulsant medication, this patient was reinvestigated at another EEG facility as an inpatient using sphenoidal electrodes, a 16-channel cable telemetry system, and video. Seven similar clinical events occurred and had the same associated electrographic findings. This patient subsequently had a right temporal lobectomy at our institution and has been seizure-free now for 2 years.

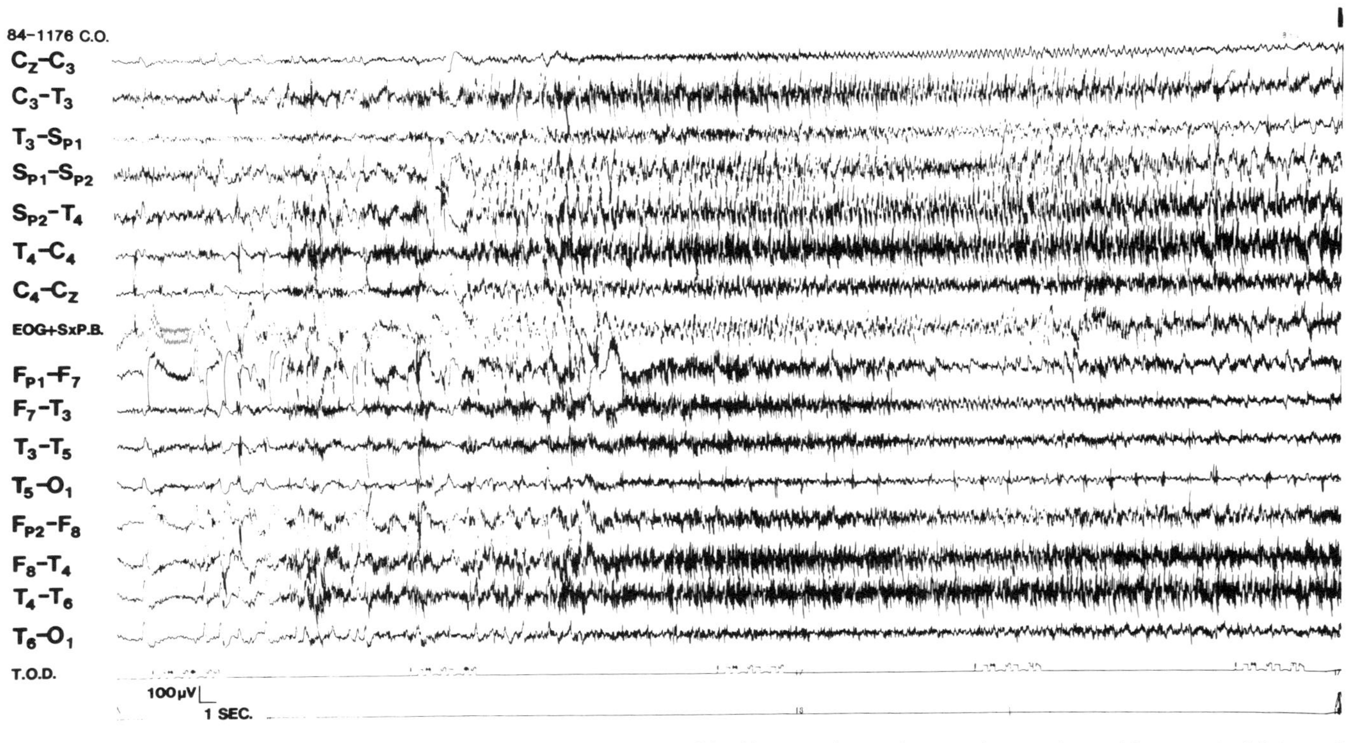

FIG. 2. A: This illustrates one of three spontaneous seizures captured in this outpatient, who experiences the sudden onset of "stomach pain." The event shown occurred on the second day of a 2-day monitoring session at 1851 hr. Her actual activation of the event button can be seen as a high-frequency artifact on channel 8, which is labeled EOG + SxP.B. This replay is done with the 6-pole filters set at 70 Hz. It demonstrates the presence of considerable muscle artifact. Some rhythmic focal activity can be seen over the right temporal lobe area, specifically at the right sphenoidal contact (SP2), where phase reversals are demonstrated between channels 4 and 5. The replay of this seizure with a 6-pole, 15-Hz filter is shown in Fig. 2B. (*Fig. 2 continues on pp. 208–209.*)

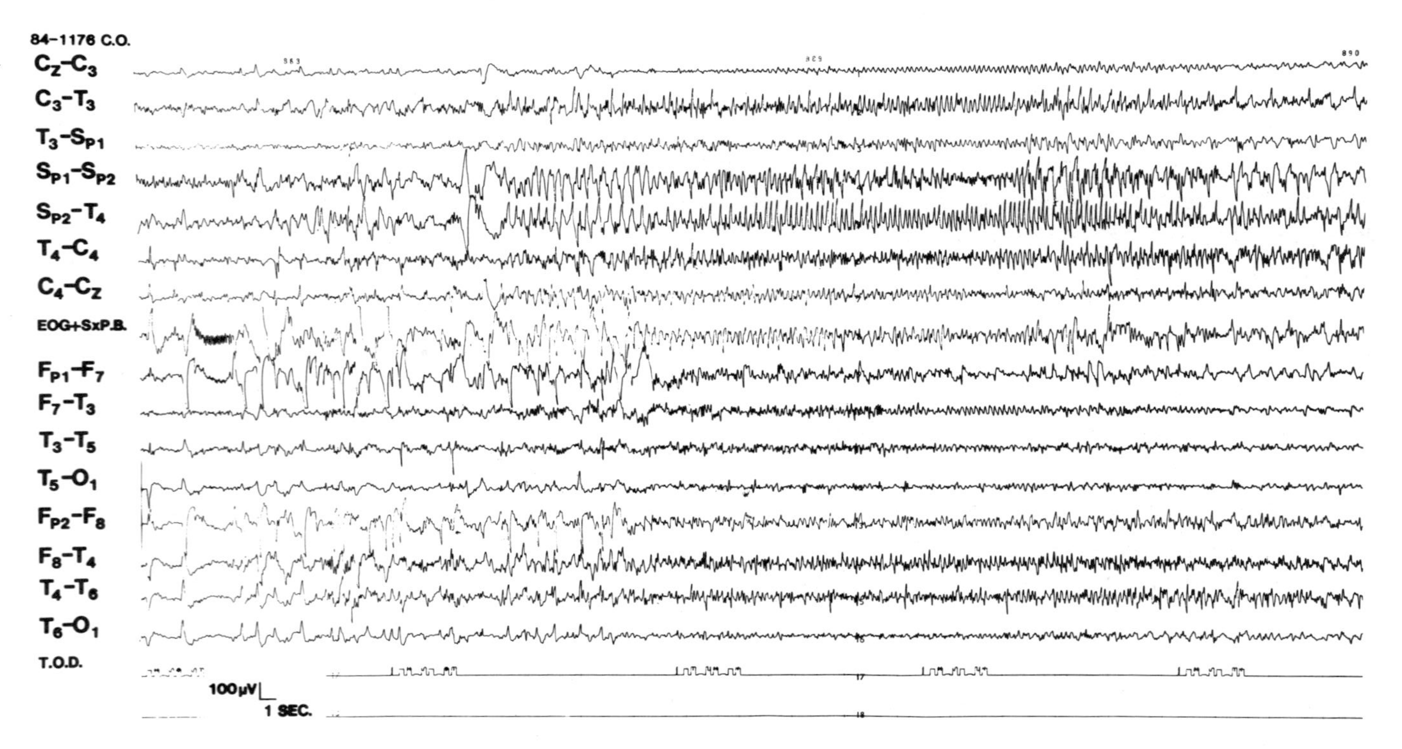

FIG. 2. B: The same event shown in Fig. 2A has been replayed with a 6-pole, 15-Hz filter. The underlying slower frequencies consistent with an epileptic discharge can be more easily seen. (*Fig. 2 continues on p. 209.*)

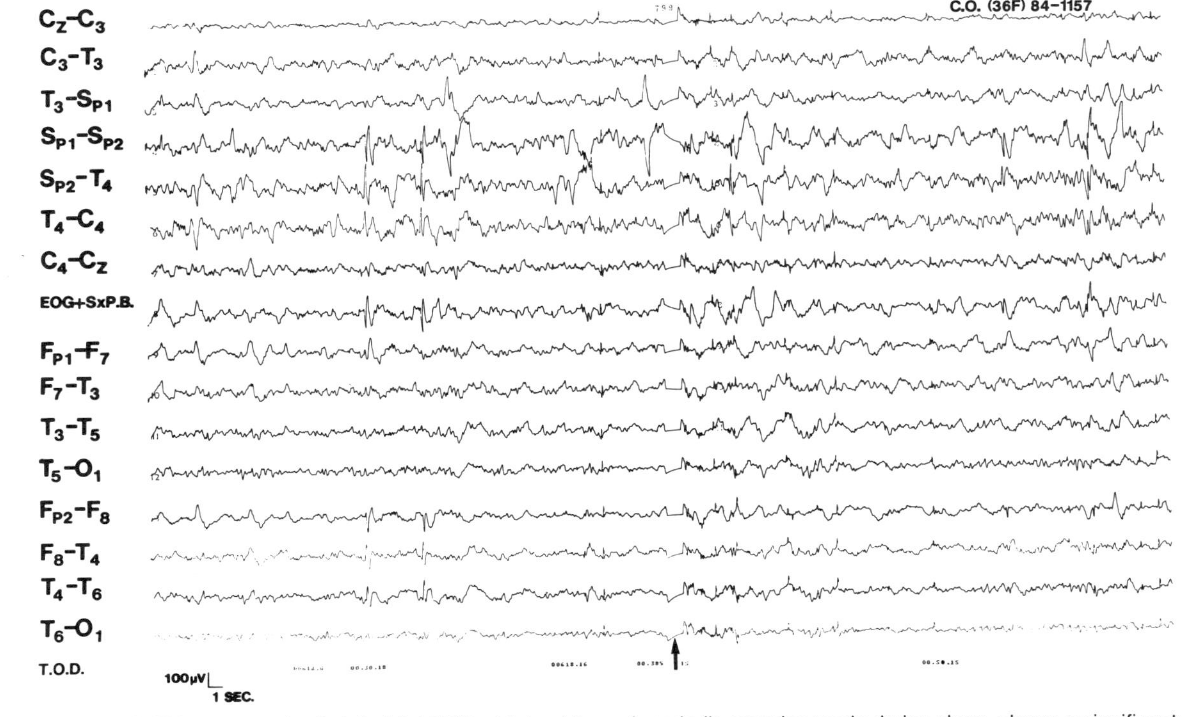

FIG. 2. **C:** This same patient's interictal EEG, obtained through periodic samples made during sleep, shows a significant number of focal interictal discharges in the same region as the patient's seizures. The samples in this case were obtained at 0030 and 0050 hr in the morning. The *arrow* shows the separation between these two samples. The interictal abnormality is confined to the right temporal lobe with distinct phase reversals seen at SP2, channels 4 and 5, and the F8-T4 surface area. The spikes seen on channel 8, EOG, are picked up by the EOG electrodes, which are near the T1 and T2 electrode locations.

Case 2. A 35-year-old male patient was referred for outpatient monitoring with sphenoidal electrodes to evaluate a worsening seizure problem that was intractable to anticonvulsant therapy. A previous CT scan had been read as normal, but the radiologist had commented on a possible asymmetry in the size of the ventricles. A 1-day outpatient recording session using the sphenoidal-temporal montage yielded five push-button events for "a funny feeling in the stomach, associated with strange tastes and smells, and for a feeling in the head." The first three push-button events revealed no changes from baseline activity on the EEG. The fourth and fifth events demonstrated a slow 1-cps rhythmic discharge over the right inferior mesial temporal area followed by a rhythmic 2- to 3-cps discharge from the same location that occurred immediately after the push button (see Fig. 3A). Interictal sampling demonstrated epileptiform spike activity from the same area (see Fig. 3B). The extremely slow frequency at the onset was considered to be suggestive of a possible mass lesion. In this patient's case, the original CT scan was obtained and a new scan performed with contrast enhancement. The original scan was re-read as abnormal. Both CT scans revealed a low-density lesion in the right frontal temporal areas with no enhancement with i.v. contrast infusion. Angiography was performed to rule out an arteriovenous malformation. A brain biopsy was subsequently performed, and an oligodendroglioma was confirmed by this procedure. Removal was not contemplated at that time, and, instead, the patient was started on anticonvulsant therapy. This was associated with a reduction in the number and severity of the seizures.

An interesting note is that the significant EEGs were all obtained through an outpatient-monitoring device. During his hospitalization for the angiography and biopsy, monitoring with the in-hospital EEG-monitoring system with video was repeated for 3 days and no seizures or bursts of focal slowing occurred.

Case 3. A 26-year-old male was referred for a surgical opinion because of a medically intractable seizure disorder. Because he lived alone and was not an entirely reliable observer of himself, he was admitted for inpatient monitoring. During that admission, 4 days of monitoring were performed. Three days used the inpatient-based intensive EEG/video system and 1 day used the 24-channel ambulatory cassette recorder. Many seizures were obtained on the EEG/video system that had consistent focal onset during the ictus, and he had corroborating interictal abnormalities. The video demonstrated that he developed confusional and belligerent states following a seizure. Having documented his behavior with the video, we elected to use the 24-channel ambulatory system more fully to evaluate frontal head regions during a seizure. A typical seizure was documented using the 24-channel system, and the results are seen in Fig. 4. The findings were consistent with a focal seizure in the right temporal lobe without significant involvement or spread to the contralateral hemisphere or within the ipsilateral hemisphere. The patient recently underwent a right temporal lobectomy.

C.J. (35M) 85–0291

C_Z–C_3
C_3–T_3
T_3–S_{P1}
S_{P1}–S_{P2}
S_{P2}–T_4
T_4–C_4
C_4–C_Z
EOG+SxP.B.
F_{P1}–F_7
F_7–T_3
T_3–T_5
T_5–O_1
F_{P2}–F_8
F_8–T_4
T_4–T_6
T_6–O_1
T.O.D.

75µV
1 SEC.

FIG. 3. **A:** This figure illustrates a low-amplitude 2-cps restricted seizure discharge captured in a recording when the patient pushed the event button. The push button was followed by a 1-cps discharge that developed into the electrical discharge seen in this figure. The discharge is very focal, essentially involving only the right sphenoidal contact. Under these circumstances, an event of this type that displayed such a limited field would be conservatively interpreted, but another similar seizure was captured during this 2-day outpatient examination and it had similar morphology. The interictal abnormality also exhibited a similar location. (*Fig. 3 continues on p. 212.*)

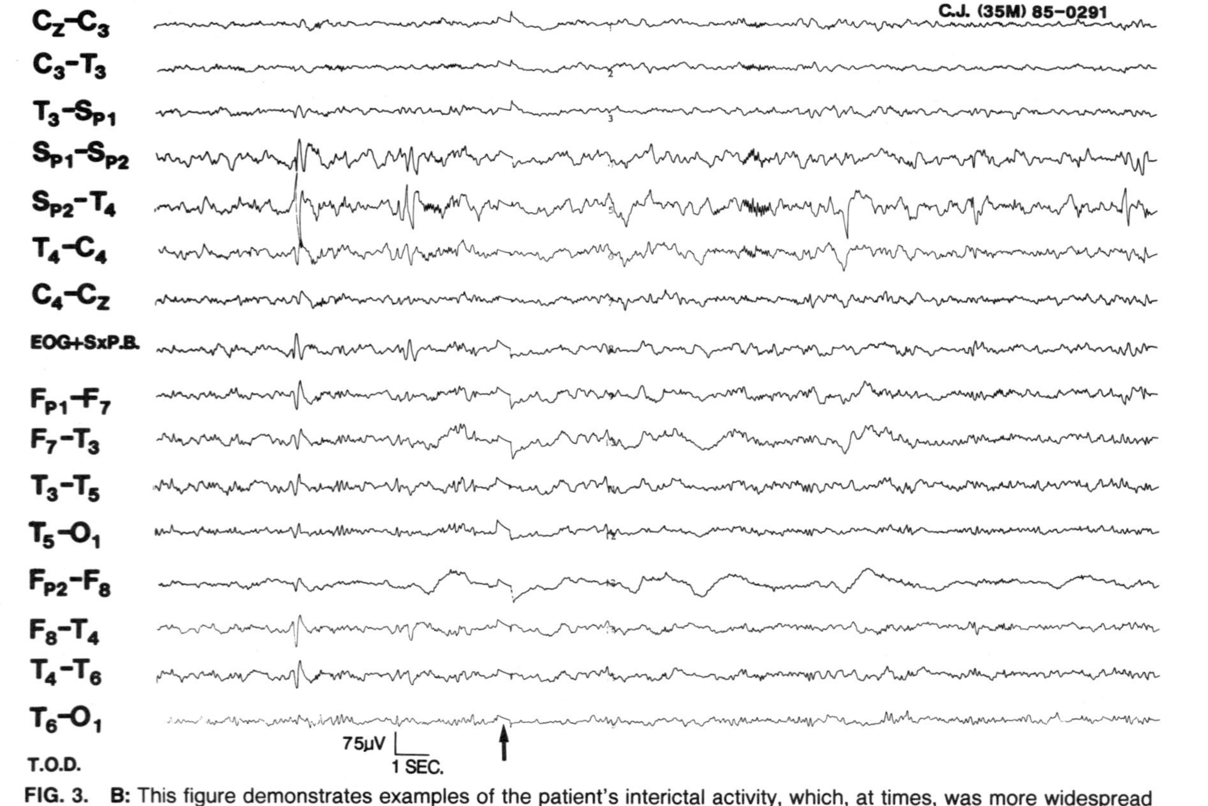

FIG. 3. B: This figure demonstrates examples of the patient's interictal activity, which, at times, was more widespread than the ictal events but still demonstrated phase reversals at the SP2 electrode site and in some examples was uniquely confined to just the SP2 electrode. The *arrow* separates the two samples taken at 0534 and 0539 hr. The automatic sampler was programmed to take samples every 5 min between 2300 and 0700 hr.

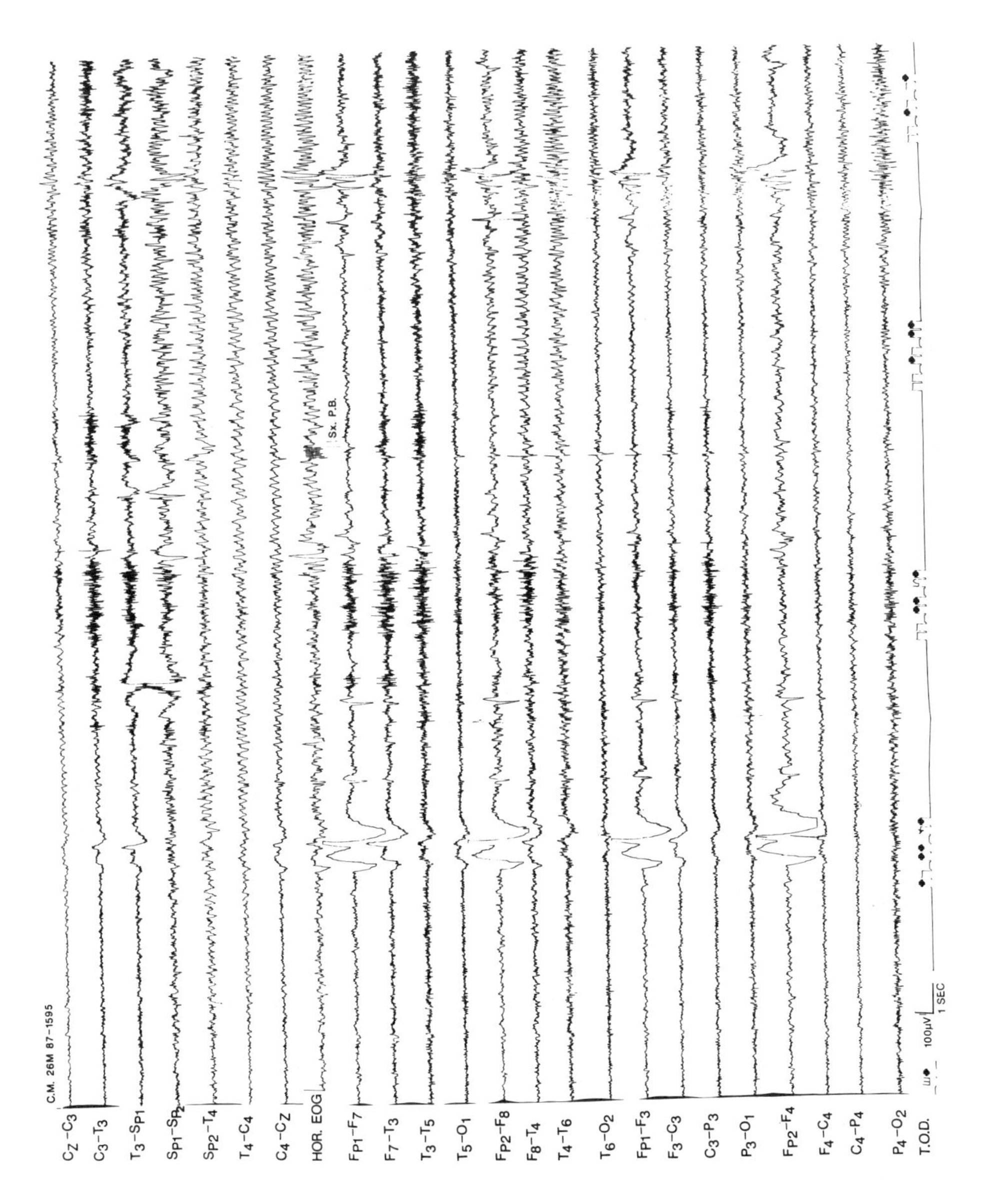

FIG. 4. The 24-channel ambulatory recorder was used to perform this study on an inpatient. The button was pushed because the patient experienced a sudden onset of a feeling of fear associated with a feeling "as if someone was coming up behind me." The artifact of the push button is marked on channel 8. In this right temporal seizure occurring at about 1100 hr, the significant phase reversals can be seen in the right sphenoidal SP2 site. This event slowly spread and ultimately incorporated all the right temporal contacts but did not spread significantly to the contralateral temporal lobe or to the frontal or parasagittal regions.

CONCLUSION

Ambulatory outpatient monitoring in a group of patients who are candidates for surgical intervention appears to contribute significantly and may obviate the need for a major inpatient workup.

Ambulatory outpatient and inpatient monitoring using a 16- or 24-channel event/periodic sample system bridges the gap between routine and prolonged conventional EEG and the more-elaborate, expensive, intensive, inpatient EEG/video monitoring systems and allows for the more efficient use of the inpatient unit.

Ambulatory monitoring increases the chances of efficiently documenting the EEG during major symptoms of the patient's epilepsy and, thus, provides information to further the understanding of the phenomena.

REFERENCES

1. Andermann F. Identification of candidates for surgical treatment of epilepsy. In: Engel Jr J, ed. *Surgical treatment of the epilepsies.* New York: Raven Press, 1987;51–70.
2. Rasmussen T. Surgical treatment of patients with complex partial seizures. In: Penry JK, Daly DD, eds. *Advances in neurology,* vol 11. New York: Raven Press, 1975;415–449.
3. Gumnit RJ. Postscript: who should be referred for surgery? In: Engel Jr J, ed. *Surgical treatment of the epilepsies.* New York: Raven Press, 1987;71–74.
4. Engel Jr J. Approaches to localization of the epileptic lesion. In: Engel Jr J, ed. *Surgical treatment of the epilepsies.* New York: Raven Press, 1987;75–95.
5. Ives JR, Woods JF. The contribution of ambulatory EEG to the management of epileptic patients. In: Littler WA, ed. *Clinical ambulatory monitoring.* London: Chapman and Hall, 1980;122–147.
6. Rasmussen T. Localization aspects of epileptic seizure phenomena. In: Thompson RA, Green JR, eds. *New perspectives in cerebral localization.* New York: Raven Press, 1982;177–203.
7. Ives JR. Long-term monitoring in epileptic patients. In: Buser PA, Cobb WA, Okuma T, eds., *Kyoto symposia* (EEG suppl 36), Amsterdam: Elsevier Biomedical Press, 1982.
8. Gotman J, Ives JR, Gloor P, et al. Monitoring at the Montreal Neurological Institute. In: Gotman J, Ives JR, Gloor P, eds. *Long-term monitoring in epilepsy* (EEG suppl 37). Amsterdam: Elsevier Science Publishers BV, Biomedical Division, 1985;327–340.
9. Binnie CD, Aarts JHP, Van Bentum-De Boer PTE, et al. Monitoring at the Instituut voor Epilepsiebestrijding Meer en Bosch. In: Gotman J, Ives JR, Gloor P, eds. *Long-term monitoring in epilepsy* (EEG suppl 37). Amsterdam: Elsevier Science Publishers BV, Biomedical Division, 1985;341–356.
10. Ebersole JS, Mattson RH, Williamson PD, et al. Monitoring at the West Haven VA/Yale University School of Medicine Epilepsy Center. In: Gotman J, Ives JR, Gloor P, eds. *Long-term monitoring in epilepsy* (EEG suppl 37). Amsterdam: Elsevier Science Publishers BV, Biomedical Division, 1985;357–370.
11. Egli M, O'Kane M, Mothersill I, et al. Monitoring at the Swiss Epilepsy Center. In: Gotman J, Ives JR, Gloor P, eds. *Long-term monitoring in epilepsy* (EEG suppl 37). Amsterdam: Elsevier Science Publishers BV, Biomedical Division, 1985;371–384.
12. Nuwer MR, Engel Jr J, Sutherling WW, et al. Monitoring at the University of California, Los Angeles. In: Gotman J, Ives JR, Gloor P, eds. *Long-term monitoring in epilepsy* (EEG suppl 37). Amsterdam: Elsevier Science Publishers BV, Biomedical Division, 1985;385–402.
13. Kellaway P, Frost Jr JD. Monitoring at the Baylor College of Medicine, Houston. In: Gotman J, Ives JR, Gloor P, eds. *Long-term monitoring in epilepsy* (EEG suppl 37). Amsterdam: Elsevier Science Publishers BV, Biomedical Division, 1985;403–414.
14. Sato S, Long RL, Porter RJ. Monitoring at the National Institute of Neurological

Communicative Disorders and Stroke. In: Gotman J, Ives JR, Gloor P, eds. *Long-term monitoring in epilepsy* (EEG suppl 37). Amsterdam: Elsevier Science Publishers BV, Biomedical Division, 1985;415–422.
15. Roberts R, Fitch P. Monitoring at the National Hospital, Queen Square, London. In: Gotman J, Ives JR, Gloor P, eds. *Long-term monitoring in epilepsy* (EEG suppl 37). Amsterdam: Elsevier Science Publishers BV, Biomedical Division, 1985;423–436.
16. Laxer KD. Mini-sphenoidal electrodes in the investigation of seizures. *Electroencephalogr Clin Neurophysiol* 1977;58:127–129.
17. Ives JR, Gloor P. New sphenoidal electrode assembly to permit long-term monitoring of the patient's ictal and interictal EEG. *Electroencephalogr Clin Neurophysiol* 1977;42:575–580.
18. Ives JR, Gloor P. Update: chronic sphenoidal electrodes. *Electroencephalogr Clin Neurophysiol* 1978;44:789–790.
19. Quesney L. Extracranial EEG evaluation. In: Engel Jr J, ed. *Surgical treatment of the epilepsies.* New York: Raven Press, 1987;129–166.
20. Ojemann GA, Engel Jr J. Acute and chronic intracranial recording and stimulation. In: Engel Jr J, ed. *Surgical treatment of the epilepsies.* New York: Raven Press, 1987;262–288.
21. Luders H, Lesser RP, Dinner DS, et al. In: Engel Jr J, ed. *Surgical treatment of the epilepsies.* New York: Raven Press, 1987;297–321.
22. Gloor P. Commentary: approaches to localization of the epileptogenic lesion. In: Engel Jr J, ed. *Surgical treatment of the epilepsies.* New York: Raven Press, 1987;99–100.
23. Olivier A, Gloor P, Andermann F, et al. Occipito-temporal epilepsy studied with stereotaxically implanted electrodes and successfully treated by temporal resection. *Ann Neurol* 1982;11:428–432.
24. Bloom D, Jasper H, Rasmussen T. Surgical therapy in patients with temporal lobe seizures and bilateral EEG abnormality. *Epilepsia* 1959/60;1:351–365.
25. Quesney LF, Gloor P. Localization of epileptic foci. In: Gotman J, Ives JR, Gloor P, eds. *Long-term monitoring in epilepsy* (EEG suppl 37). Amsterdam: Elsevier Science Publishers BV, Biomedical Division, 1985;165–200.
26. Williamson PD, Wieser H, Delgado-Escueta AV. Clinical characteristics of partial seizures. In: Engel Jr J ed. *Surgical treatment of the epilepsies.* New York: Raven Press, 1987;101–127.
27. Ives JR. A completely ambulatory 16-channel cassette recording system. In: Stefano H, Burr W, eds. *EEG monitoring,* Stuttgart: Gustav Fischer, 1982;205–217.
28. Ives JR, Schomer DL. Recent technical advances in long-term ambulatory outpatient monitoring. *Electroencephalogr Clin Neurophysiol* 1986;64:37p.
29. Ives JR, Thompson CJ, Gloor P. Seizure monitoring: a new tool in electroencephalography. *Electroencephalogr Clin Neurophysiol* 1976;41:422–427.
30. Ives JR, Gloor P. Automatic nocturnal sleep sampling: a useful method in clinical electroencephalography. *Electroencephalogr Clin Neurophysiol* 1977;43:880–884.
31. Ives JR, Schomer DL. The significance of using chronic sphenoidal electrodes during the recording of spontaneous ictal events in patients suspected of having temporal lobe seizures. *Electroencephalogr Clin Neurophysiol* 1986;64:23p.
32. Ives JR, Schomer DL. Preliminary technical experience using a portable computer (PC-AT) for on-line data analysis of epileptic spike activity on 16 channels of telemetric EEG data. *Epilepsia* 1986;27(5):626.
33. Ives JR, Mainwaring NR, Gruber LJ, et al. Home computing: a remote intelligent EEG data acquisition unit for monitoring epileptic patients in the home environment. *Electroencephalogr Clin Neurophysiol* 1988;64:49p.
34. Ives JR, Schomer DL. A 6-pole filter for improving the readability of muscle contaminated EEG. *Electroencephalogr Clin Neurophysiol* 69:486–490.
35. Ochs R, Gloor P, Quesney F, et al. Does head turning during a seizure have lateralizing or localizing significance? *Neurology* 1984;34:884–890.
36. Gotman J, Ives JR, Gloor P. Automatic recognition of interictal epileptic activity in prolonged EEG recordings. *Electroencephalogr Clin Neurophysiol* 1979;46:510–520.
37. Gotman J. Automatic recognition of epileptic seizures in the EEG. *Electroencephalogr Clin Neurophysiol* 1982;54:530–540.
38. Koffler DJ, Gotman J. Automatic detection of spike and wave bursts in ambulatory EEG recording. *Electroencephalogr Clin Neurophysiol* 1982;61:165–180.
39. Riley TL, Porter RJ, White BG, et al. The hospital experience and seizure control. *Neurology*

1981;31:912–915.

40. Gotman J, Koffler D. Temporal distribution of interictal spikes in epileptic patients. *Electroencephalogr Clin Neurophysiol* 1987;67:54p.
41. Ives JR, Gotman J, Rasmussen T. Comparing the EEG seizure onset frequency of temporal lobe epileptic patients with and without space occupying lesions. *Electroencephalogr Clin Neurophysiol* 1980;50:186p.

Ambulatory EEG Monitoring,
edited by John S. Ebersole.
Raven Press, Ltd., New York © 1989

13

Evaluation of Episodes of Altered Awareness or Behavior

Samuel L. Bridgers

Neurology Service, Veterans Administration Medical Center, West Haven, Connecticut 06516; and Department of Neurology, Yale University School of Medicine, New Haven, Connecticut 06510

Cassette electroencephalography (EEG) has been offered as a clinical service through the Clinical Neurophysiology Laboratory at Yale–New Haven Medical Center (YNHMC) since October 1981. Originally, the Oxford 4-24 4-channel recorder and PMD-12 playback system were used, with subsequent transition to the Oxford 9000 system. Provision of cassette EEG as a clinical service followed the performance of comparative studies that established the accuracy and reliability of detection of epileptiform abnormalities and seizures with fixed-montage limited channel recording and rapid review (1,2). Developmental studies have continued, through both the Epilepsy Center at the Veterans Administration Medical Center, West Haven, Connecticut (3–8), and YNHMC (9–11), as clinical experience has accumulated at YNHMC (12–15). Since initiating cassette EEG recording at YNHMC, we also have been called on by physicians and hospitals in our geographic area to provide interpretive services for cassette recordings obtained through their clinical laboratories.

Since clinical information is provided at the time of referral and diaries are routinely maintained by either patients or observers during cassette recording, it has been possible for us to monitor the yield of cassette EEG in the detection of evidence to support a diagnosis of epilepsy, in association with specific circumstances of referral and specific varieties of clinical events during recording. As our experience has grown to include hundreds, and now thousands, of cassette-tape interpretations, recurring relationships between questions asked, events recorded, and abnormalities detected seem worthy of some sort of codification. The purpose of this chapter is to present these variable complaint-related yields of cassette EEG. From the results, it will be evident that some clinical circumstances are very likely to result in productive cassette recording. The farther afield one travels from the generally recognized somatic and behavioral manifestations of seizures, however, the less likely cassette EEG will be systematically useful. Nevertheless, there is no circumstance in which it will not yield occasional surprises.

OVERALL YIELD OF CASSETTE EEG

For this review, results of cassette EEG interpretations were correlated with referral information and diary information for 2097 patients. Cassette recordings performed for research purposes were specifically excluded. Cassette EEG interpretations were provided through the Clinical Neurophysiology Laboratory on all of these patients, although the actual recording acquisition took place through outside institutions for 944 patients. Recording was performed with the Oxford 4-24 recorder in 1345 patients and with the Oxford 9000 recorder in 752. The montages used have been validated (1,2,6) and are described elsewhere in this volume (see Chapter 4).

Cassette tapes were reviewed for evidence to support a diagnosis of epilepsy. The ideal, of course, was recording of actual EEG seizure activity. We have also considered the detection of interictal epileptiform abnormalities as evidence to support a diagnosis of epilepsy, although it is appreciated that such abnormalities do not constitute proof on the same level as correlation of a specific clinical event with EEG seizure activity. Interictal epileptiform abnormalities are found in a small percentage of healthy individuals with no history of epilepsy (16,17), and this phenomenon is encountered most often in children (18,19). Furthermore, such abnormalities sometimes will be seen in patients with medical or psychiatric illness, suggesting a transient increased susceptibility to seizures (20,21). For convenience, interictal epileptiform abnormalities will be referred to as evidence of epilepsy in this chapter. However, the caution necessary for interpretation of the significance of epileptiform abnormalities must not be forgotten.

Epileptiform abnormalities and/or seizures were detected in 328 of 2097 patients, for an overall yield of 15.4% of positive evidence of epilepsy. Epileptiform abnormalities alone were detected in 203 patients, with epileptiform abnormalities and seizures detected in 98 and seizures alone in 23. The yield of 3-channel recording was somewhat higher than that of 8-channel recording, with abnormalities in 17% of the former and 13% of the latter. This was felt to be a reflection of the greater number of children recorded with the Oxford 4-24. Table 1 illustrates the age-related yield of abnormalities in 2091 patients for whom age was known. Pertinent clinical events occurred during cassette recording for 756 patients, and these were documented to be seizures for 87 (11.5%).

TABLE 1. *Age-related yield of cassette EEG*

	Age (years)									
	< 1	1–10	11–20	21–30	31–40	41–50	51–60	61–70	71–80	81–94
Total patients	131	355	471	386	290	136	116	110	79	17
EA[a] only	5	59	40	33	20	13	13	13	11	1
EA and seizures	5	32	25	19	10	2	2	0	1	2
Seizures only	8	2	2	4	2	1	2	1	0	0
Total positive	18	93	67	56	32	16	17	14	12	3
% Positive	13.7	26.2	14.2	14.5	11.0	11.7	14.7	12.7	15.2	17.7
% Seizures	9.9	9.6	5.7	5.9	4.1	2.2	3.4	0.9	1.3	11.8

[a] EA, Epileptiform abnormalities.

SEIZURES

In a previous review of our clinical experience after three years, we found that evidence of epilepsy was more often detected on cassette EEG if the referring physician indicated without equivocation that the episodes in question were seizures, or at least that the patient had experienced clinically definite seizures some time in the past (12). With more extensive experience, this relationship remains. In the current series, a positive indication of this sort accompanied 445 patients, and evidence of epilepsy was detected in 174 or 39%.

A similar relationship exists for clinical events noted during recording. For 74 patients, such events were noted simply to be "seizures," and seizures were exactly what they were documented to be by cassette EEG for 38 patients, or 51%.

No other referral information or event description has been associated with these levels of positive information obtained. The relative yields obtained in different clinical circumstances are illustrated in Figs. 1 and 2, and are discussed in detail below.

INVOLUNTARY MOTOR ACTIVITY

The occurrence of stereotyped episodes of motor activity is obviously one of the cardinal manifestations of seizure activity (22), and it would be anticipated that cassette EEG recording in this circumstance would be of high yield. Nevertheless, not all such episodes are seizures, and improved diagnostic precision makes cassette EEG a worthwhile undertaking.

We have identified 173 patients in our series who underwent cassette EEG recording because of episodes of involuntary motor activity or for whom such episodes were reported during recording (14). Of these, 42 (24%) had cassette EEG evidence to support an epilepsy diagnosis, including 25 (14%) with actual correlation of clinical events with cassette-recorded EEG seizure activity. The latter constituted one-quarter of the patients reporting clinical events during

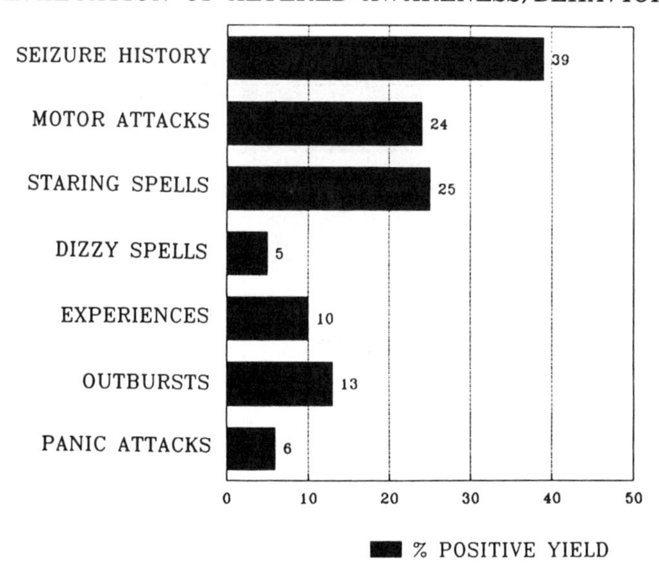

FIG. 1. Yield of cassette EEG in relation to history. The types of episodes reported by history at referral are indicated at **left,** and *bars* indicate the relative yield of epileptiform abnormalities and/or seizures on a percentage scale. The number at the **right end** of each bar indicates the actual percentage. Full explanation of the various categories is included in the text, but it should be noted that the category "dizzy spells" includes patients with syncope as well.

cassette recording. For 33 of these patients, there was a confident indication on the part of the referring physician that the patient had epilepsy, and cassette EEG evidence of epilepsy was discovered in 13 (39%), a somewhat higher yield than in the overall group, as would be expected.

The group can be further divided, on the basis of episodes, into those with bilateral or complex motor activity, those with lateralized motor activity, and those with subtle motor phenomena such as facial twitching or eye deviation. Patients reported to have eyelid fluttering in association with absence episodes were specifically excluded (see below).

Yields in the groups with bilateral or complex motor activity and the group with lateralized motor activity were essentially the same. In the former group, consisting of 102 patients, 26 (25%) had evidence of epilepsy. Clinical events were documented to be seizures in 26%, or 16 of 62. Evidence of epilepsy was obtained in 12 of 48 with episodes of lateralized motor activity, again a yield of 25%. Clinical events were documented as seizures in six of 27 (22%). Among the smaller group of 23 patients with subtle motor activity, only five had evidence of epilepsy, but clinical events were documented as seizures in four. An additional three patients in this group had clinical events not associated with EEG change.

Acceptance of the lack of an EEG correlate to a clinical event as evidence that the clinical event is not a seizure clearly requires qualification, particularly

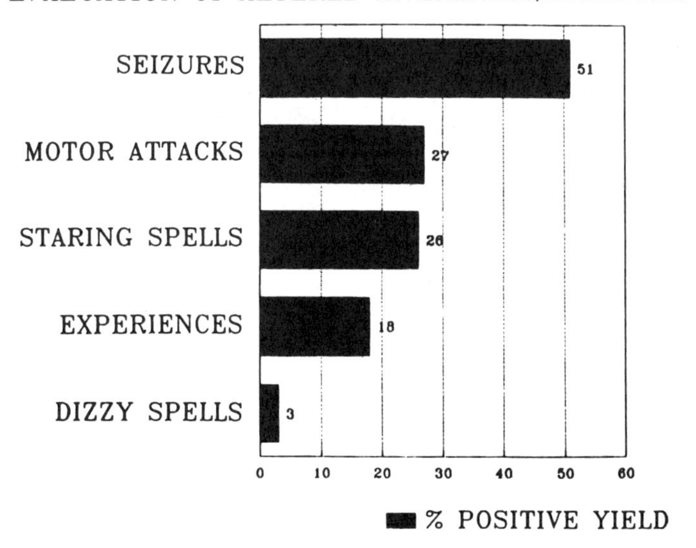

FIG. 2. Yield of cassette EEG in documenting seizures. The types of specific episodes occurring during cassette EEG recording are indicated at **left,** and *bars* indicate the percentage of each type of episode documented as seizures by correlation of the behavior with EEG change. Full explanation of each category is included in the text.

where episodes of focal motor activity are concerned. We know of three specific instances where clinical events that were clearly focal motor seizures were not associated with cassette EEG seizure activity, and we imagine that more such instances may exist. This is not a limitation of the cassette EEG technique as such, but a problem that besets all forms of EEG limited to the scalp (5). However, the need to consider cassette EEG data as part of the entire clinical picture cannot be overemphasized.

A related group of patients, with cassette EEG of lower yield, is those patients with episodic loss of tone. These 20 patients were predominantly infants, and episodes were described as drop attacks or episodes of head bobbing or head dropping. Eleven had episodes during recording, and in only one were episodes documented to be seizures. None of the others had even interictal abnormalities. Only one had a prior diagnosis of seizures, and that child had clinical episodes unaccompanied by EEG change during cassette recording. Interestingly, two of four adolescents with episodes of loss of tone were found to have daytime sleep attacks and early onset of nighttime REM sleep, suggesting a diagnosis of narcolepsy when this had not been suspected clinically.

EPISODES OF LOSS OF CONTACT OR CONFUSION

Another group of patients in whom a high yield of cassette recording could be anticipated consists of those with episodic loss of contact, variously characterized by such terms as staring spells, absence attacks, petit mal attacks, and "spacing out," at least when described by an observer rather than a patient (14). Patients who had both loss of contact and eyelid flutter were included in this group.

In our series, we were able to identify 173 patients with episodes of loss of contact, a number identical to that of patients with episodes of involuntary motor activity. The yield of evidence of epilepsy was also similar, with epileptiform abnormalities and/or seizures detected in 45 patients (25%). Clinical events were documented to be seizures in 18 (10%), and these patients constituted 26% of the 69 for whom episodes of loss of contact were reported during cassette recording.

Not surprisingly, a preponderance of patients undergoing cassette EEG recording because of episodic loss of contact were preadolescent children. There were 104 children age 12 or under in this group, but the yield was actually slightly lower (23%) than in adolescents and adults (30%).

Practically speaking, two important issues in differential diagnosis exist for patients with episodes of staring or apparent loss of contact. First, are these episodes seizures? If they are not, they are unlikely to be diagnosable at all. Staring off into space is a commonly observed phenomenon among children and individuals with all variety of cognitive and emotional disturbances. The second issue is this: If the episodes are seizures, are they manifestations of primary generalized epilepsy or partial epilepsy? Optimal therapy rests on appropriate differentiation, since some agents useful in absence epilepsy are of no benefit in treatment of partial complex seizures (23), and the most effective agents for partial epilepsy may actually exacerbate absence seizures (24–26).

Regarding the first issue in differential diagnosis, it is notable that one-third of these patients with cassette EEG evidence of epilepsy were not receiving any anticonvulsant medication at the time. Furthermore, one-third of the patients with episodes of loss of contact during recording unassociated with EEG change were receiving anticonvulsants. While lack of EEG change does not definitely exclude the possibility that such events are seizures, they certainly could not be typical absence seizures.

Regarding the second issue, it was notable that 23 of the 45 patients with abnormalities had focal epileptiform discharges and/or seizures. Furthermore, seven of the 22 patients with staring spells and generalized spike/wave discharges were being treated with phenytoin or carbamazepine, rather than one of the anticonvulsants more likely to be effective in absence epilepsy.

A related, but smaller, group consisted of patients referred for evaluation of episodes of confusion. We were able to identify 39 such cases, of whom 36 were adults. Epileptiform abnormalities were documented in five (13%), and episodes of confusion were documented as seizures in two (5%) of the total group and 15% of the subgroup of 13 with actual episodes during recording.

DIZZINESS AND SYNCOPE

Early in the evolution of clinical application of ambulatory EEG, the prospect of differentiating loss of consciousness from seizure and loss of consciousness from cardiac arrhythmia promised a specific application of the technique that would be particularly valuable, as anecdotal experience proved that ambulatory EEG could perform reliably in this circumstance (27,28). Our own initial clinical series suggested that the actual yield might prove disappointing (12). Further experience has borne this out. We have found that cassette EEG yields occasional positive evidence of a cerebral or cardiac etiology of episodic dizziness or syncope, but the primary accomplishment of use has been to indicate that episodes of interest do not appear to be either seizures or cardiac-rhythm disturbances (14).

In the current series, a total of 377 patients underwent ambulatory EEG because of episodes of dizziness or syncope or reported such episodes during ambulatory EEG recording. Of this group, 221 underwent simultaneous cardiac monitoring. Only four patients, or less than 2% of the cardiac-monitored group, had cardiac-rhythm disturbances that explained unequivocally the reported clinical problem, and only 11% (26 patients) had evidence of a cardiac-rhythm disturbance potentially responsible for symptoms. These classifications were based on those used in a prior prospective evaluation of syncope (29). We have encouraged the use of simultaneous ambulatory EEG and ambulatory ECG as a means of evaluating troublesome and confusing cases, rather than as a first-line assessment in patients with syncope, anticipating that simple cardiac monitoring or other evaluations aimed at the cardiovascular system are more likely than ambulatory EEG to provide an answer. Our yields of cardiac-rhythm disturbances indicate that our syncope and dizziness population is one skewed away from the cardiogenic etiologies that account for half of patients presenting with syncope.

Despite what would seem like a bias favoring the inclusion in our series of patients likely to benefit from ambulatory EEG, the yield of useful positive information remains unimpressive. Evidence of epilepsy was discovered on ambulatory EEG in only 20 of 377 patients (5%), including five patients in whom EEG seizure activity was recorded, four in association with clinical episodes of dizziness. There were 45 patients identified with a history of epilepsy unrelated to the referral episodes and 12 of these (27%) had evidence of epilepsy on ambulatory EEG. In three of these patients, including one in whom a clinical episode of dizziness was positively identified as a seizure on ambulatory EEG, the history of seizures was remote and anticonvulsants were not being given at the time of ambulatory EEG.

Omission of the patients with a prior history of seizures leaves 332, of whom evidence of epilepsy was discovered in eight, just over 2%. Of these patients, 47 reported episodes of dizziness during recording, but referral information was insufficient to be sure that dizziness and syncope were pertinent clinical issues, and two of these had ambulatory EEG epileptiform abnormalities, one with clinically correlated seizure activity. Thus, of 285 patients clearly referred for the express purpose of evaluating episodes of dizziness or syncope without preexisting clinical evidence of epilepsy, only five (just under 2%) had evidence of epilepsy on ambulatory EEG, and none of these had actual seizures recorded.

A numerically more impressive yield of ambulatory EEG is in the correlation of clinical episodes of dizziness with normal EEG. In this series, a total of 149 patients reported clinical episodes of dizziness, and two reported frank syncope. Four of these episodes of dizziness were documented to be seizures. It is a safe presumption that the vast majority of the remaining episodes were not epileptic.

Thus, our experience to date supports the use of ambulatory EEG in patients with dizziness or syncope, particularly in combination with ambulatory ECG, as a source of occasional dramatic positive diagnostic information, but more frequently as a source of reassurance, to physicians and patients that such events do not appear to represent seizures or cardiac-rhythm disturbances, allowing for watchful waiting rather than a rush to therapy.

APNEIC EPISODES

We have performed cassette EEG recording for the purpose of evaluating apneic episodes in 68 children, all but three under 1 year of age and 55 under 2 months. Recording through documented apneic episodes has been obtained in 43 of these children. We have yet to document EEG seizure activity in association with an apneic episode, although one full-term neonate did manifest three EEG seizures for which no clinical manifestations were observed (9). Since this infant was recorded specifically because of apneic episodes, and these episodes ceased with phenobarbital therapy, the diagnosis of apneic seizures seems highly likely as circumstantial evidence and cassette EEG provided critical supportive information. In general, however, we find cassette EEG recording of neonates with apnea an unproductive pursuit. This is particularly true of recording during the typical episodes of apnea and bradycardia frequently seen in premature neonates. This does not appear to be a limitation of the technique, which has been successfully employed to record neonatal seizures (10,30), but merely a manifestation of the limited role of seizure activity as an etiologic factor in such episodes.

EXPERIENTIAL PHENOMENA

Since the earliest definition of psychomotor epilepsy, it has been recognized that a seizure originating in the temporal lobe may give rise to illusions of experience (31). Frank hallucinations may occur, or more complex internal and sometime indescribable feelings may arise paroxysmally manifesting seizure activity (32). Since perceptions such as deja vu, dreamy detachment, and olfactory or other sensory distortions and illusions may also be encountered in other circumstances, most notably in association with psychiatric disorders, it is not surprising that electroencephalographic techniques will be used to differentiate those patients with epilepsy. With enhanced opportunity for the capture of interictal abnormalities in sleep, and EEG correlation with actual events through extended daytime monitoring, cassette EEG can be particularly useful.

In our series, we have identified 93 patients who underwent cassette EEG recording for evaluation of such experiential phenomena (15). Seizures and/or interictal abnormalities were detected in nine (10%), of whom two had a confident diagnosis of epilepsy at the time of referral. Actual events occurred during cassette recording in 45 (48%) and were documented as seizures in eight.

Abnormalities were not equally distributed among patients reporting different varieties of experiential episodes. Among 51 patients with hallucinations or perceptual distortions, EEG evidence of epilepsy was found in only one, for a 2% positive yield from cassette recording. Among those with more complex experiences such as deja vu, dreamlike states, or inner feelings that defied clear description, such evidence was found in eight (19%), with experience-correlated EEG seizures in seven. Interestingly, none of 14 patients reporting episodes of illusory or hallucinatory olfactory experiences had evidence of epilepsy on cassette EEG, despite the prominent diagnostic significance attached to the olfactory aura (33).

ANXIETY AND PANIC

A sensation of anxiety may characterize the onset of a complex partial seizure, but episodes of anxiety or panic are much more commonly encountered as an independent psychiatric disorder. Because epilepsy is in the differential diagnostic list, though an unlikely explanation for such episodes, referral for extended EEG monitoring can be anticipated when the resource is readily available.

In our series, 32 patients were referred because of episodes of anxiety or panic attacks or reported such episodes during cassette recording. Only two of these patients had a prior diagnosis of epilepsy, and both had normal cassette EEG. Evidence of epilepsy was encountered in only two patients (6%) and in neither in association with such episodes, which did occur during recording for both. One patient had EEG seizure activity in association with a focal motor episode unrelated to her episodes of anxiety, and the other had only interictal abnormalities during sleep. In both, it remains possible that anxiety episodes represented focal seizure activity not transmitted to the scalp. Since neither patient was thought to have a seizure disorder at the time of referral, cassette EEG provided useful information in guiding therapy. Nineteen other patients experienced anxiety or panic episodes unassociated with EEG change during cassette recording.

As in a number of other situations, cassette EEG can play a useful role in ferreting out the small minority of patients with this sort of complaint who may actually be experiencing seizures. Because the yield across-the-board is so low, however, it seems that cassette recording might best be deferred until conventional management has failed, or applied in cases where there is some additional historical or physical information, beyond the occurrence of the attacks themselves, to suggest an etiologic role for seizure activity.

BEHAVIORAL DISTURBANCES

The relationship between epilepsy and explosive or aggressive behavior is controversial (34,35). While some have promoted the concept of episodic dyscontrol as a phenomenon somehow similar to epilepsy (36), demonstration of aggressive behavior as an ictal phenomenon has been difficult (37). Nevertheless, epileptiform abnormalities are more frequently encountered in children and adolescents with explosive behavior than in psychiatric patients in general (21). Furthermore, population screening has revealed an increased incidence of behavioral disturbances in children discovered to have epileptiform abnormalities, but without a history of seizures (19). The difficulties of dealing with these patients may account for the general lack of enthusiasm among inpatient epilepsy monitoring centers for a concerted effort to clarify this purported relationship. Cassette EEG offers the opportunity to evaluate patients with explosive behavior in a more suitable atmosphere, whether at home or within a psychiatric facility.

Thus far, we have had the opportunity to review cassette EEG results on 92 patients with episodic behavioral disturbances, variously characterized as episodic dyscontrol, rage attacks, aggressive outbursts, impulsive outbursts, violent outbursts, or temper tantrums. Of these patients, 65 (71%) were under age 21. Pertinent episodes occurred during recording in 37 (40%). None of these was documented to be seizures. However, cassette EEG evidence of epilepsy was discovered in 12 (13%). All three adults with epileptiform abnormalities had a prior diagnosis of epilepsy. However, this was not the case for five of the nine children and adolescents with abnormalities, three of whom also had EEG seizures unrelated to outbursts. Furthermore, for one of the four younger patients with a prior history of epilepsy, seizures were remote and she was no longer receiving anticonvulsant medication.

Although the significance of these results is not clear, it does seem that cassette EEG can identify a subgroup of younger patients with behavioral disturbances who might at least be more likely to benefit in some way from anticonvulsant therapy.

CONCLUSIONS

The yields of positive information from cassette EEG associated with episodes of involuntary motor activity and with staring spells are substantial. In fact, they compare favorably with the yield of ambulatory ECG monitoring in the evaluation of patients with syncope (29). Considering that few would be willing to forgo the latter, it seems that cassette EEG deserves to be a standard part of the evaluation of any patient with either of these complaints, at least when routine EEG has failed to provide definitive evidence to suggest an epilepsy diagnosis.

In the other circumstances explored above, the yield of positive information drops considerably. It is difficult to justify the routine use of cassette EEG in the evaluation of patients with syncope or episodic dizziness, for example, when viewed simply from the standpoint of cost effectiveness. However, there can also be little doubt that a small percentage of such patients will be having seizures. At this point, cassette EEG is probably the simplest way to identify these patients reliably.

In all the circumstances examined, there was a high yield of clinical events during cassette EEG, even though most such events were not accompanied by EEG seizure activity. We have repeatedly cautioned that failure to detect an EEG correlate does not eliminate the possibility that an event is actually a seizure (5,12,13,38). However, it is not farfetched to suggest that the likelihood that such an event is a seizure is considerably reduced. Such negative events are useful in clinical decision-making, because they force careful reconsideration. Faced with such information, the physician cannot simply presume that the episodes in question are seizures but must carefully marshal all other evidence available to override the evidence against epilepsy provided by cassette EEG.

While it remains difficult to establish firm guidelines showing when cassette EEG should be used in low-yield situations, we consider it prudent neurologic practice to pursue some form of monitoring before affixing a diagnosis of epilepsy, once routine EEG has failed to provide definitive supportive evidence. For many, cassette EEG will be the only form of extended monitoring available. Once attached, a diagnosis of epilepsy may be extremely difficult to dislodge. Furthermore, the social and medical consequences of the diagnosis can be far-reaching, even life-long. It seems less than ideal to settle for a diagnosis on historical grounds alone, when solid supporting evidence may be readily acquired.

REFERENCES

1. Leroy RF, Ebersole JS. An evaluation of ambulatory, cassette EEG monitoring. I. Montage design. *Neurology* 1983;33:1–7.
2. Ebersole JS, Leroy RF. An evaluation of ambulatory, cassette EEG monitoring. II. Detection of interictal abnormalities. *Neurology* 1983;33:8–18.

3. Ebersole JS, Leroy RF. Evaluation of ambulatory, cassette EEG monitoring. III. Diagnostic accuracy compared to intensive inpatient EEG monitoring. *Neurology* 1983;33:853–860.
4. Ebersole JS, Bridgers SL, Silva CG. Differentiation of epileptiform abnormalities from normal transients and artifacts on ambulatory cassette EEG. *Am J EEG Technol* 1983;23:113–125.
5. Bridgers SL, Ebersole JS. The clinical utility of ambulatory cassette EEG. *Neurology* 1985;35:166–173.
6. Ebersole JS, Bridgers SL. Direct comparison of 3 and 8-channel ambulatory cassette EEG with intensive inpatient monitoring. *Neurology* 1985;35:846–854.
7. Bridgers SL, Ebersole JS. Supervision of ambulatory cassette EEG screening: a strategy based on the temporal distribution of epileptiform abnormalities. *Electroencephalogr Clin Neurophysiol* 1987;66:219–224.
8. Bridgers SL, Ebersole JS. EEG outside the hairline: detection of epileptiform abnormalities. *Neurology* 1988;38:146–149.
9. Bridgers SL, Ment LR, Ebersole JS, et al. Cassette EEG recording of neonates with apneic episodes. *Pediatr Neurol* 1985;1:219–222.
10. Bridgers SL, Ebersole JS, Ment LR, et al. Cassette EEG in the evaluation of neonatal seizures. *Arch Neurol* 1986;43:49–51.
11. Ebersole JS, Bridgers SL. Cassette EEG monitoring in the emergency room and intensive care unit. *J Clin Neurophysiol* 1987;4:213.
12. Bridgers SL, Ebersole JS. Ambulatory cassette EEG in clinical practice. *Neurology* 1985;35:1767–1768.
13. Bridgers SL. Ambulatory cassette electroencephalography of psychiatric patients. *Arch Neurol* 1988;45:71–74.
14. Bridgers SL, Ebersole JS. Cassette EEG: defining circumstances of high yield. *J Ambulatory Monitoring* (in press).
15. Bridgers SL, Ebersole JS. Cassette EEG in the evaluation of experiential phenomena. (Submitted).
16. Gibbs FA, Gibbs EL, Lennox WG. Electroencephalographic classification of epileptic patients and control subjects. *Arch Neurol Psychiat* 1943;50:111–128.
17. Bennett DR. Spike-wave complexes in "normal" flying personnel. *Aerospace Med* 1967;38:1276–1282.
18. Eeg-Olofsson O, Petersen I, Sellden U. The development of the electroencephalogram from the age of 1 through 15 years. Paroxysmal activity. *Neuropaediatrie* 1971;2:375–404.
19. Cavazzuti GB, Capella L, Nalin A. Longitudinal study of epileptiform EEG patterns in normal children. *Epilepsia* 1980;21:43–55.
20. Zivin L, Ajmone-Marsan C. Incidence and prognostic significance of epileptiform activity in the EEG of non-epileptic subjects. *Brain* 1968;91:751–777.
21. Bridgers SL. Epileptiform abnormalities discovered on electroencephalographic screening of psychiatric inpatients. *Arch Neurol* 1987;44:312–316.
22. Dreifuss FE. Proposal for revised clinical and electroencephalographic classification of epileptic seizures. *Epilepsia* 1981;22:489–501.
23. Browne TR. Ethosuximide (Zarontin) and other succinimides. In: Browne TR, Feldman RG, eds. *Epilepsy: diagnosis and management.* Boston: Little, Brown and Company, 1983;215–224.
24. Johnsen SD, Tarby TJ, Sidell AD. Carbamazepine-induced seizures. *Ann Neurol* 1984;16:392–393.
25. Horn CS, Ater SB, Hurst DL. Carbamazepine-exacerbated epilepsy in children and adolescents. *Pediat Neurol* 1986;2:340–345.
26. Browne TR, Pincus JH. Phenytoin (Dilantin) and the hydantoins. In: Browne TR, Feldman RG, eds. *Epilepsy: diagnosis and management.* Boston: Little, Brown and Company, 1983;175–189.
27. Lai C, Ziegler DK. Syncope problem solved by continuous ambulatory simultaneous EEG/EKG recording. *Neurology* 1981;31:1152–1154.
28. Blumhardt LD. Ambulatory ECG and EEG monitoring in the differential diagnosis of cardiac and cerebral dysrhythmias. In: Gumnit R, ed. *Advances in Neurology,* vol 46, *Intensive neurodiagnostic monitoring.* New York: Raven Press, 1987;183–202.
29. Kapoor WN, Karpf M, Wieand S, et al. A prospective evaluation and follow-up of patients with syncope. *N Engl J Med* 1983;309:197–204.
30. Eyre JA, Oozeer RC, Wilkinson AR. Diagnosis of neonatal seizures by continuous recording

and rapid analysis of the electroencephalogram. *Arch Dis Child* 1983;58:785–790.
31. Feldman RG. Complex partial seizures (psychomotor or temporal lobe seizures). In: Browne TR, Feldman RG, eds. *Epilepsy: diagnosis and management.* Boston: Little, Brown and Company, 1983;39–50.
32. King DW, Ajmone-Marsan C. Clinical features and ictal patterns in epileptic patients with EEG temporal lobe foci. *Ann Neurol* 1977;2:138–147.
33. Blumer D, Benson DF. Psychiatric manifestations of epilepsy. In: Benson DF, Blumer D, eds. *Psychiatric aspects of neurologic disease, vol II.* New York: Grune & Stratton, 1982;25–47.
34. Ramani V. Intensive monitoring of psychogenic seizures, aggression and dyscontrol syndromes. In: Gumnit R, ed. *Advances in Neurology,* vol 46, *Intensive neurodiagnostic monitoring.* New York: Raven Press, 1987;203–217.
35. Pincus JH. Can violence be a manifestation of epilepsy? *Neurology* 1980;30:304–307.
36. Mark VH, Ervin FR. *Violence and the brain.* Hagerstown: Harper and Row, 1970.
37. Delgado-Escueta AV, Mattson RH, King L, et al. Special report. The nature of aggression during epileptic seizures. *N Engl J Med* 1981;305:711-716.
38. Ebersole JS, Bridgers SL. Ambulatory EEG monitoring. In: Pedley TA, Meldrum BS, eds. *Recent advances in epilepsy,* vol 3. Edinburgh: Churchill Livingstone, 1986;111–135.

Ambulatory EEG Monitoring,
edited by John S. Ebersole.
Raven Press, Ltd., New York © 1989

14

Cassette EEG Monitoring in the Emergency Room and Intensive Care Unit

John S. Ebersole and Samuel L. Bridgers

Department of Neurology, Yale University School of Medicine, New Haven, Connecticut 06510; and Neurology Service, Veterans Administration Medical Center, West Haven, Connecticut 06516

In devising cassette EEG recorders that are suitably portable to be worn by ambulatory subjects, the developers of this technology have accomplished another goal, perhaps not sought but potentially of great value. If a recorder is small enough and light enough to be worn at the waist, even by a child, then it is also compact enough to be brought to the bedside easily and unobtrusive enough to be left there without interfering with ongoing attention to the patient, even in an intensive care unit. It was first evident to us in obtaining cassette EEG in a neonatal intensive care unit (1,2) that the presence of the small device was readily tolerated by staff members attending to the patient, even in cramped quarters. The same could not be said for conventional EEG equipment.

The capacity for unobtrusive, extended, and simplified monitoring at the bedside might have particular utility in emergency situations, where treatment decisions must often be made without benefit of EEG backup. Too often, the acute situation has come and gone, managed pragmatically and without a clear-cut diagnosis, before EEG can be obtained. In retrospect, one can only presume that episodic alterations of behavior or consciousness were seizures when the resolution of such episodes bears a temporal relationship to institution of anticonvulsant therapy. Too often, however, one is presented with an unsatisfactory description of episodes, which may or may not have been seizures, on which a decision for continued and long-term anticonvulsant therapy must be based. In a time of increasing concern over the deleterious effects of such therapy (3), some objective and permanent evidence of the nature of such episodes is clearly desirable. Even when immediate interpretation of such episodes is not feasible, cassette EEG at least offers the prospect of a permanent record that can be reviewed after the fact to assist in long-term management decisions.

Possession of the simplest and smallest of EEG machines sets the stage for practical EEG monitoring in acute situations but is not, in itself, sufficient. The use of cassette EEG for ambulatory monitoring requires all the skills of conventional EEG technology and more. Electrodes are placed in accordance with the 10-20 system and must be anchored securely to assure artifact-free recording in freely mobile patients. Setting up a patient for ambulatory cassette EEG often requires more than an hour, even when performed by an experienced technologist. Since the situations in which emergency cassette EEG might prove useful often arise when no technologist is available, some alternative to the standard ambulatory recording arrangement is necessary.

Our own approach to emergency cassette EEG has borrowed from the experience of inpatient ECG monitoring. Disposable ECG electrodes are quickly applied when patients enter the intensive care unit or coronary care unit to allow ongoing monitoring of heart rhythms. A similar technique using self-adhesive disposable electrodes, which would allow the initiation of EEG monitoring with only a few minutes' effort, seemed the only approach that was likely to be achievable. Available self-adhesive electrodes presented what seemed a tremendous obstacle in that they would not adhere to hairy skin. Most of the electrode positions of the 10-20 system are located in areas of the head that are covered with hair in most people. The logical means of circumventing this problem was placement of the electrodes over parts of the head without hair. From the standpoint of conventional EEG technique, however, this notion represented an apparent disregard of time-honored standards. Knowing the efficacy of anterior temporal electrodes (T1, T2) in detecting epileptiform abnormalities (4) and the nonrandom distribution of epileptiform abnormalities over the scalp (5), we had reason to believe that electrode positions outside the hairline might function quite well. Our thinking in this direction was given a substantial boost by the success of Dyson et al. in performing polysomnography using disposable electrodes placed outside the hairline (6). We devised a system for simplified EEG recording using subhairline electrode positions keyed to obvious anatomic landmarks. It seemed that such an approach would allow ready initiation of EEG monitoring by individuals without extensive EEG training who would be involved in the care of patients to be recorded. We describe below our experimental and clinical experience with this approach and provide a detailed description of the technique so that others who are interested may adopt it.

EXPERIMENTAL STUDIES

The original subhairline montage was a 7-channel circumferential left-to-right chain linkage of eight electrodes. The electrodes were placed in mastoid, preauricular, suprazygomatic, and frontal positions on each side of the head. The initial test was a comparison to simultaneous standard EEG monitoring in the detection of epileptiform abnormalities (7). This study is discussed in detail in Chapter 4 of this volume and the montage is illustrated in Fig. 6 of that chapter. The general result was detection of at least some epileptiform abnormalities on blind analysis in all members of a series of 25 epileptic patients. Acceptable rates of false-positive and false-negative interpretations of individual complexes were encountered. Since false-negative judgments usually involved posterior temporal epileptiform complexes, and since we noted on open analysis that the preauricular-mastoid derivations often failed to demonstrate the posterior dominant rhythm in a satisfactory manner, it was elected to change the montage to a 5-channel circumferential left-to-right arrangement, eliminating the preauricular electrodes. This montage is also illustrated in Fig. 6 of Chapter 4. With the greater interelectrode distance of the suprazygomatic-mastoid derivations, we were able to demonstrate posterior activity, normal or abnormal, more successfully.

In our montage validation study, electrode application was performed by one of us (SLB) with a substantial amount of prior technical experience with both conventional and cassette EEG. Although recordings could be set up within 5 min, our real aim was for equally rapid setup to be accomplished by individuals without that kind of experience. Therefore, we embarked on a project wherein neurology resident physicians, after one or two half-hour training sessions, obtained cassette EEG recordings from patients experiencing seizures at night or on weekends, when standard recording through the clinical neurophysiology laboratory was unavailable.

The goals of this investigation were twofold. First, we hoped to demonstrate that cassette EEG recording obtained in this decidedly unconventional manner could yield interpretable EEG monitoring data. Second, presuming that interpretable recordings were obtained, we wanted to compare their yield to that of the realistic existing alternative—routine EEG obtained as soon as possible after the event, usually on the following morning.

The residents were generally capable of performing skin preparation, electrode attachment, and initiation of cassette EEG recording within 10 min. The results of interpretation of cassette EEG tapes thus obtained were compared to the yield of conventional EEG obtained through our clinical neurophysiology laboratory in a series of 25 patients (8). Of these patients, 14 were admitted to Yale–New Haven Medical Center with apparent seizures, while the other 11 experienced events thought to be seizures while already in the hospital. Two-thirds of the patients had no history of seizures prior to the events that led to acquisition of emergency cassette EEG. All the cassette EEG recordings obtained by residents were interpretable, although 10 were marred by the loss of at least one recording channel. Loss of mastoid electrodes was a particular problem.

Some sort of abnormality was detected on both cassette EEG and routine EEG in 20 of the 25 patients, but the abnormalities detected on routine EEG were usually limited to lateralized or generalized slowing. Two additional patients had abnormalities only on cassette EEG. Twelve of the cassette EEGs

(48%) had epileptiform features, meaning seizures, interictal epileptiform abnormalities, or both. This was true for only six of the routine EEGs (24%). Most important, actual seizure recording was obtained on cassette EEG for six patients (24%), and this did not occur in a single routine EEG in this patient group. More than 90 clearly identifiable seizures were detected in those six recordings.

By involving acutely ill adult inpatients in cassette EEG recording for the first time, we encountered some patterns of abnormality not seen in our usual experience with ambulatory recording, although we did encounter a number of fairly typical examples of interictal epileptiform abnormalities. Abnormalities of

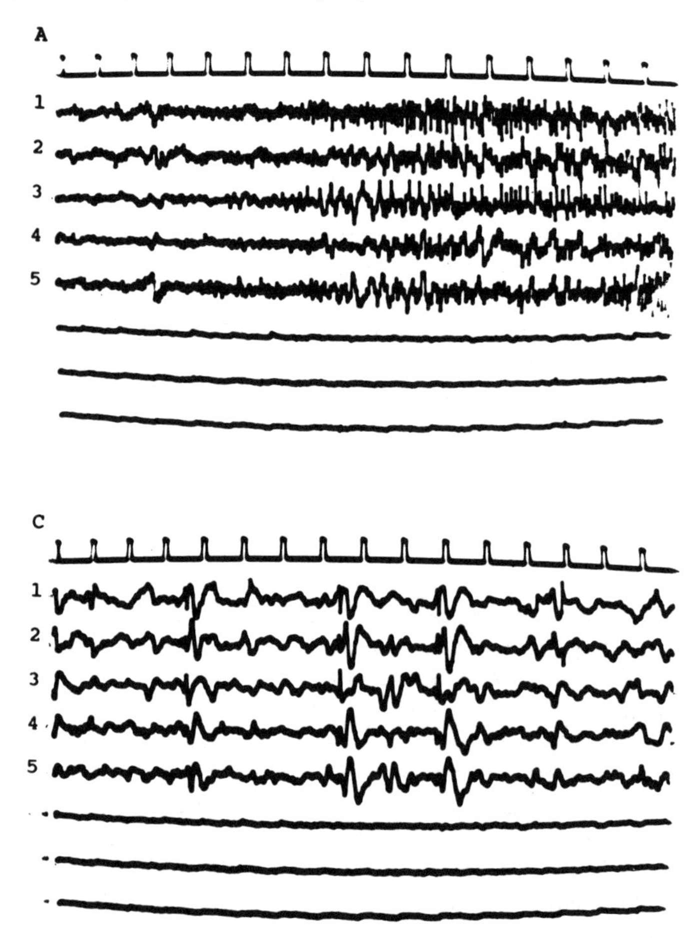

FIG. 1. Photos of 16-sec epochs from an 8-channel cassette EEG playback unit illustrating the onset of a generalized convulsive seizure **(A),** a right hemisphere partial seizure **(B),** bilateral isolated spike-wave discharges **(C),** and a left hemisphere isolated sharp and slow-wave complex **(D).** All examples show five channels of data derived from the subhairline montage depicted in Fig. 6 of Chapter 4.

the sort seen with both emergency and elective cassette EEG are illustrated in Fig. 1, while some examples of novel patterns seen with emergency recording are illustrated in Fig. 2.

Findings we had not encountered previously included periodic lateralized epileptiform abnormalities (PLEDs) and intermittent rhythmic delta activity (IRDA), although these were readily identified, because of their similarity to such abnormalities recorded with conventional EEG. PLEDs were particularly interesting, when examined over several hours, because of their tendency to exhibit varying and migratory morphology and variation in frequency, often building up over extended periods to culminate in overt EEG seizure activity, followed by a diminution and gradual return. In our experience, this comprehensive picture of PLED phenomenology will rarely be grasped from conventional 20- to 30-min recordings, even when obtained serially.

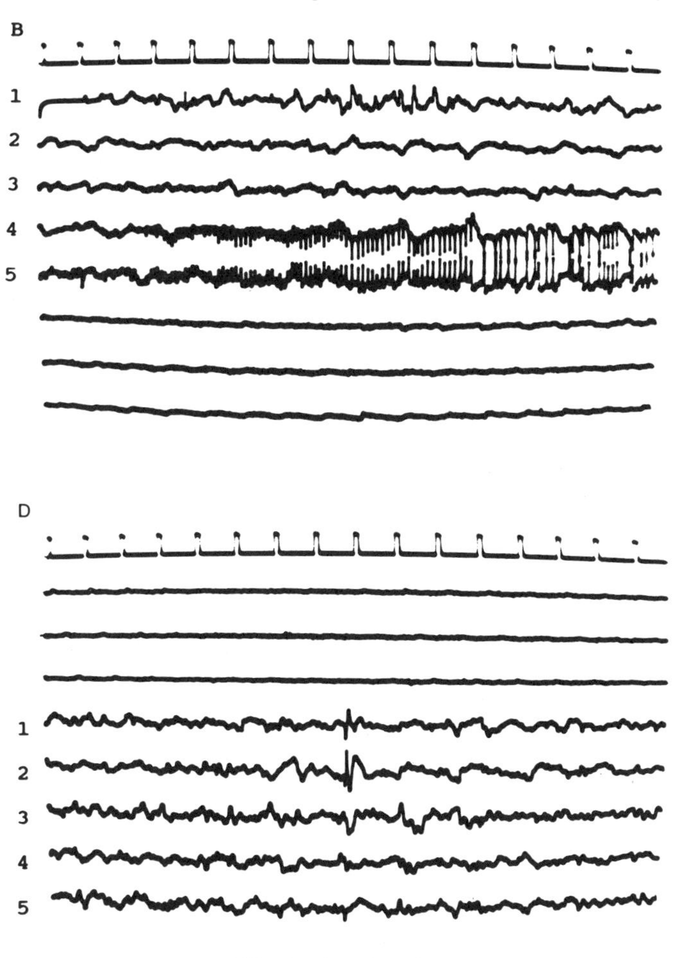

FIG. 1. (*continued*).

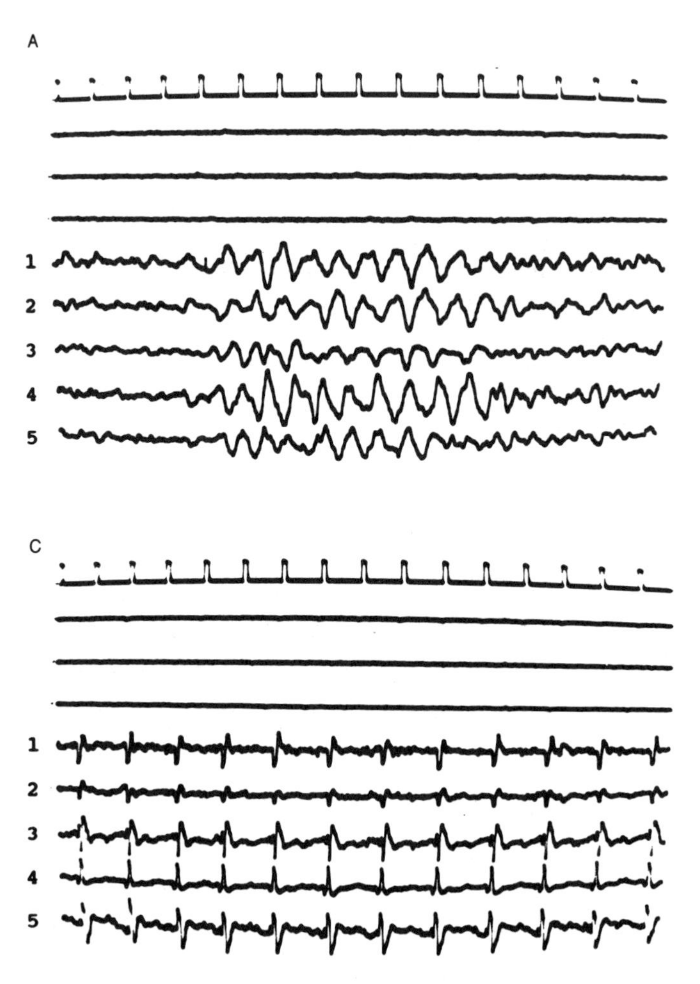

FIG. 2. Photos of 16-sec epochs from an 8-channel cassette EEG playback unit illustrating intermittent rhythmic delta activity (IRDA) **(A),** rhythmic bilateral sharp waves in the midportion of an electrographic seizure **(B),** predominantly right hemispheric, periodic lateralized epileptiform discharges (PLEDs) **(C),** and independent bilateral periodic epileptiform discharges (BiPLEDs) **(D).** All examples show five channels of data derived from the subhairline montage in Fig. 6 of Chapter 4.

The overall results of this study offered convincing evidence that emergency cassette EEG, even with the subhairline montage, offered a distinct advantage over conventional EEG obtained at the earliest practical opportunity. Of course, we have no way of knowing what findings we might have missed with the restricted spatial coverage, since simultaneous cassette and conventional EEG was just not feasible. However, the emergency cassette recordings did not fail to reveal any of the significant abnormalities, epileptiform or nonepileptiform, obtained with subsequent routine recording. This is not an indication that

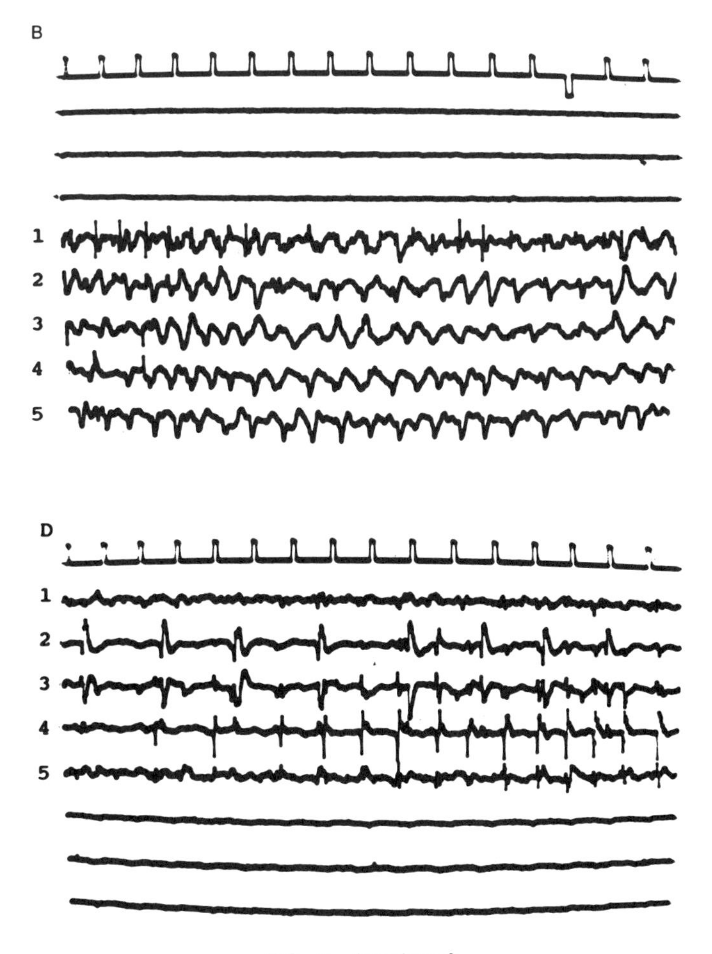

FIG. 2. (*continued*).

conventional EEG need not be performed, but the results clearly supported the continued use and development of emergency cassette EEG as an adjunct to standard techniques.

The limitations of the subhairline montage and the lack of technical expertise were outweighed by the gain of a prolonged temporal sample obtained in an extremely timely manner. There was only one patient in whom a 30-min EEG sample, obtained at any point in the first several hours after presentation, would have offered even a 50-50 chance of capturing a seizure. In our hospitals, such a recording, performed in off hours by a technologist, is not even an option, except in the most unusual circumstances. We suspect that most electroencephalographers operate under similar constraints. Considering that the yield of actual seizures in this sample was more than twice that we have obtained with elective ambulatory cassette EEG in patients with a clinical diagnosis of epilepsy, we

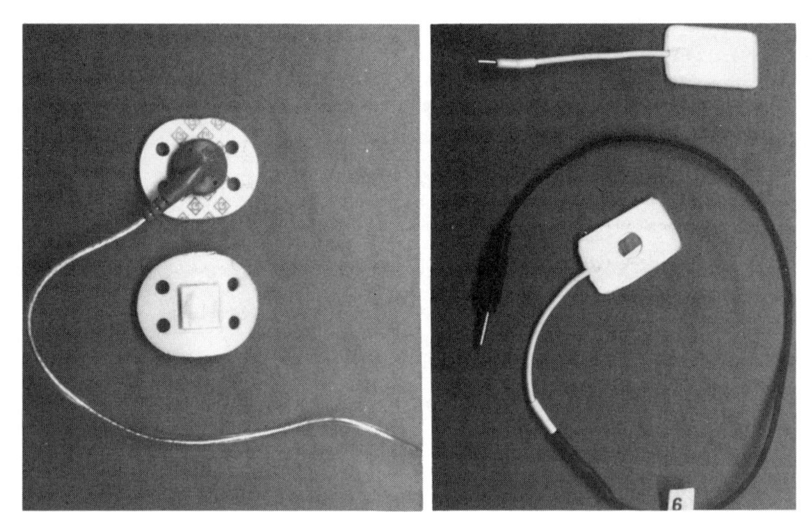

FIG. 3. Self-adhering disposable electrodes used in subhairline montages for emergency cassette EEG recording. At **left** are front and back views of MediTrace pellet electrodes and connections; at **right,** front and back views of Dantec 13L20 electrodes and connections.

cannot escape the conclusion that the timing as well as the duration of the recording is crucial.

CLINICAL APPLICATION

With the technique adequately validated, we have moved forward to offer emergency cassette EEG as a service of the Clinical Neurophysiology Laboratory at Yale–New Haven Medical Center. During normal working hours, applications are performed by EEG technologists, but we rely on neurology residents at other times. Although, at present, the clinical experience is limited, it coincides reasonably with the results of our initial study. Thus far, our series includes an additional 27 patients. This is a heterogeneous population, ranging in age from 2 days to 87 years. Eight of the patients have had a prior diagnosis of seizure disorder. Three were recorded specifically because of a suspicion of pseudoseizures. The others were recorded not only for apparent seizures, but also when encephalopathy or confusional state led to a suspicion of subclinical or atypical seizure activity. Thus, the nature of the problems evaluated might have predicted a lower overall yield than in our initial experience, where patients were recorded only after experiencing episodes thought to be seizures.

Among these patients, the yield of epileptiform features with cassette EEG was 11 of 27 recordings (41%). Actual seizure recording was achieved in four patients (15%). Although somewhat lower than in the pilot study, these yields still represented a substantial gain over subsequent conventional EEG, which yielded epileptiform features in six (22%) and actual seizures in one (4%). Thus,

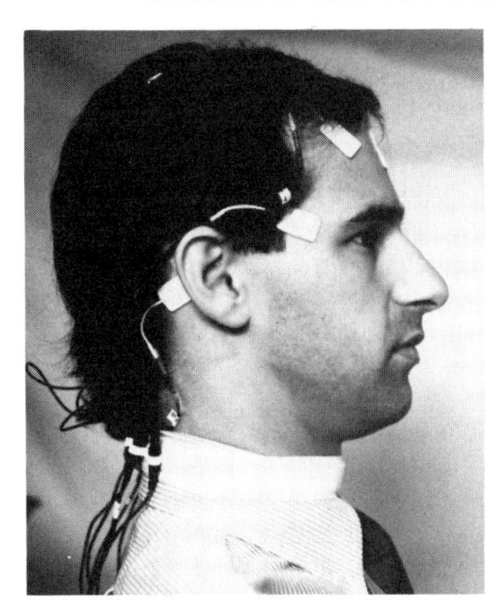
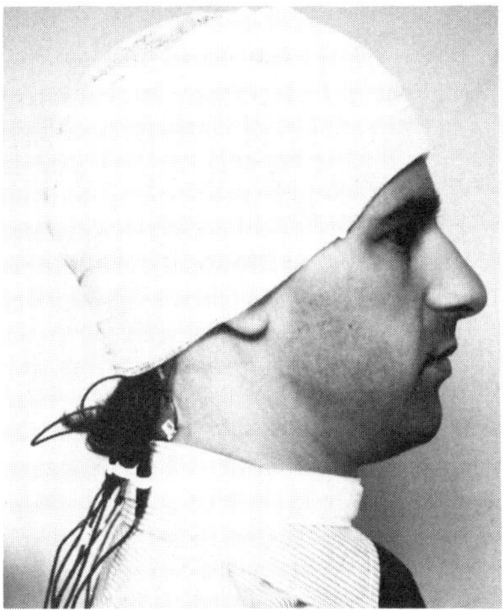

FIG. 4. Subject with subhairline electrodes in place. A midforehead electrode(s) serves as ground. Mesh gauze is routinely wrapped around the head in a turban to help secure the electrodes, connections, and leads.

emergency recording nearly doubled the yield of epileptiform features and resulted in a fourfold increase in seizure detection over routine EEGs obtained afterward. Nonepileptiform abnormal features such as lateralized or generalized slowing and intermittent rhythmic delta activity were equally detected by the two techniques, although such abnormalities were clearly better defined with standard EEG. Channel wastage was still encountered, as in the pilot study, but all the emergency recordings contained at least several hours of readily interpretable EEG data.

Two of the three patients with suspected pseudoseizures experienced clinical episodes during emergency recording, which were unaccompanied by EEG change, and none of them had similar episodes during conventional recording sessions lasting 20 to 30 min. As we have emphasized elsewhere in this volume, such findings do not absolutely eliminate the possibility that such episodes are seizures, but they certainly raise the odds against that possibility.

TECHNICAL ASPECTS

In this section, we shall present our methods for obtaining rapid cassette EEG monitoring. Since this technique has worked, we have not felt much pressure to modify it. Nevertheless, it can be assumed that there are a number of alternative pathways to the goal of successful recording. Therefore, this guide can be taken literally by those who wish to get involved as quickly as possible in emergency recording, or it can serve as a framework for considering technical problems that will be encountered, which may stimulate others to devise their own, perhaps even better, systems.

We have had experience with two varieties of disposable electrode—the MediTrace pellet electrode manufactured by Graphic Controls, Ltd., and the Dantec 13L20 surface electrode. Both are illustrated in Fig. 3. The pellet electrode offers the advantage of an inset polymer gel electrolyte pellet, which obviates the need for any electrolyte paste or gel application. The pellet is a solid square and also eliminates the attendant messiness of most electrolyte preparations. However, with dimensions of 32 × 25 mm, the self-adhesive backing must often be trimmed to assure placement with no hair contact in the mastoid and preauricular positions. If there is any hair contact, the electrodes are very much prone to come loose. With a clean connection, though, attachment is very secure. The pellet will provide a good, low-resistance skin-electrode interface for at least 24 hr. We have not attempted recording for longer periods. The pellet electrode connects to typical ECG monitoring lead wires and snap-on connections for the electrode and typical 0.08-in. phone pins. Since the Oxford 9000 recorder requires a lead for each input of each channel, and the frontal and zygomatic electrodes are each included in two channels, one must fashion a connection of two lead wires to a single snap-on connector for each of these four electrodes. To our knowledge, such lead wires cannot be purchased. An alternative is to place side-by-side electrodes, which is not difficult in adolescents or adults. This approach offers a potential advantage in the more straightforward identification of electrode artifacts. A more secure connection to the recorder can be obtained by replacing the phone pin of the ECG-type lead wire with the locking pin from an Oxford ambulatory EEG electrode, although pin disconnection has not been a problem in our experience. At the microvolt sensitivities of EEG recording, the snap-on electrode connections are prone to artifact with even slight movement, particularly if the lead has been in long use, which makes the snap-on connections somewhat looser.

The Dantec 13L20 electrode was originally designed for surface recording in EMG and nerve conduction studies. It is a silver chloride electrode with vinyl adhesive backing and a 0.7-mm pin for connection to the lead wire, rather than a snap. Its principal advantage is the smaller size of the adhesive backing, which measures 15 × 25 mm. We have not had a need to trim the backing of these electrodes to avoid hair contact. Electrolyte paste or gel must be applied at attachment, and this must be done carefully to avoid smearing the electrolyte preparation over the adhesive surface, which can prevent secure attachment. Obviously, the lead wire that connects this electrode to the 9000 recorder must have a phone pin at one end and a 0.7-mm pin receptacle at the other. Since such leads are not, to our knowledge, commercially available, we have made our own by replacing the electrodes on Oxford ambulatory EEG electrode leads with appropriate pin receptacles. At the time of setup, this connection is taped for secure connection. Again, disconnections at the pin-plug interface have not been a problem. The electrode-lead interface does not present the same sorts of difficulties with artifact as encountered with the snap-on attachment, as would be expected.

With either type of electrode, skin preparation is straightforward. A few vigorous wipes with a cotton ball or gauze square soaked in a standard alcohol-acetone mixture work quite well. Typical individually packaged alcohol prep pads, which have the advantage of being readily available on hospital wards, can also be used, but fairly aggressive rubbing is advisable. We have checked electrode resistances and find them to be in the 20 to 40 kΩ range. Although these resistances are somewhat higher than the standards of the American EEG Society (9), we find the results satisfactory when viewing the tapes on rapid playback.

Figure 4 illustrates a subject with electrodes in place. The mastoid electrodes are placed just above the mastoid eminence behind the ear. The suprazygomatic electrodes are placed in the shallow indentation just above the zygomatic arch. We place the frontal electrodes directly above the midline of each eye just below the hair's margin. When seven channels are used, the preauricular electrodes are placed anterior to and slightly above the tragus. This position is one where hair is often very difficult to avoid, especially in males. Because of the relatively unstable nature of our quick connections, the application of a turban to hold everything in place is particularly important. With either 5- or 7-channel recording, the employment of an additional channel for ECG monitoring is advisable.

When recording is complete, the Dantec 13L20 electrodes are easily peeled off. The MediTrace pellet electrodes are more prone to continued tight adhesion, but application of acetone, which soaks under the electrode through the four small holes in the adhesive backing, quickly loosens the attachment.

Because recordings are usually initiated by neurology residents, who often have other pressing concerns when on call at night, the entire process of setting up emergency cassette EEG must be made as easy and hassle-free as possible. To this end, we maintain a tackle box with all the necessities, including a recorder with fresh batteries and a calibrated tape in place, in an easily accessible place. The lead wires are pre-plugged in a configuration appropriate for the subhairline montage and labeled to assure proper order of attachment of the electrodes. Once the electrodes are attached to skin and lead wires, the resident need only turn on the recorder. Following each use, the box is restocked by a technologist. Included in the box is a checklist for the process, which assures that the responsible individual will not forget some crucial step such as turning on the recorder.

CAVEATS AND CONCLUSIONS

Emergency cassette EEG recording as described is not without problems. Although all the recordings we have obtained have been interpretable, channel loss will be commonly encountered. Fortunately, the three most anterior channels, which are most crucial to interpretation, are also the most secure, and our previous investigations using the Oxford 4-24 recorder have demonstrated how much useful information can be obtained from 3-channel recording (10–12). It is unlikely that even these channels could withstand the rigors of unrestrained ambulatory recording, and we have not attempted using this arrangement of disposable electrodes in a subhairline montage. It is crucial that the emergency recording system be viewed as what it is—a compromise that has clear advantages over the alternative of no EEG data at all. It should not be looked on as a "quick and dirty" approach to ambulatory recording in outpatients that will obviate the need for careful technique, nor should it be pursued, even in emergency situations, without the backup of eventual conventional EEG. As long as these limitations are respected, however, emergency cassette recording offers a range of new opportunities in studying seizures and improving diagnosis at the bedside.

REFERENCES

1. Bridgers SL, Ment LR, Ebersole JS, et al. Cassette EEG recordings of neonates with apneic episodes. *Ped Neurol* 1985;1:219–222.
2. Bridgers SL, Ebersole JS, Ment LR, et al. Cassette EEG in the evaluation of neonatal seizures. *Arch Neurol* 1986;43:49–51.
3. Pedley TA. Discontinuing antiepileptic drugs. *N Eng J Med* 1988;318:982–984.
4. Sperling MR, Engel J. Electroencephalographic recording from the temporal lobes: a comparison of ear, anterior temporal and nasopharyngeal electrodes. *Ann Neurol* 1985;17:510–512.
5. Leroy RF, Ebersole JS. An evaluation of ambulatory, cassette EEG monitoring. I. Montage design. *Neruology (Cleve)* 1983;33:1–7.
6. Dyson RJ, Thornton C, Dore CJ. EEG electrode positions outside the hairline to monitor sleep in man. *Sleep* 1984;7:180–188.
7. Bridgers SL, Ebersole JS. EEG outside the hairline: detection of epileptiform abnormalities. *Neurology (Cleve)* 1988;38:146–149.
8. Ebersole JS, Bridgers SL. Cassette EEG monitoring in the emergency room and intensive care unit. *J Clin Neurophysiol* 1987;4:213.
9. American Electroencephalographic Society. Guidelines in EEG and evoked potentials. Guideline 1: Minimal technical standards for performing electroencephalography. *J Clin Neurophysiol* 1986;3:1–6.
10. Ebersole JS, Leroy RF. Evaluation of ambulatory cassette EEG monitoring. III. Diagnostic accuracy compared to intensive inpatient EEG monitoring. *Neurology (Cleve)* 1983;33:853–860.
11. Bridgers SL, Ebersole JS. The clinical utility of ambulatory cassette EEG. *Neurology (Cleve)* 1985;35:166–173.
12. Ebersole JS, Bridgers SL. Direct comparison of 3 and 8-channel ambulatory cassette EEG with intensive inpatient monitoring. *Neurology (Cleve)* 1985;35:846–854.

Ambulatory EEG Monitoring,
edited by John S. Ebersole.
Raven Press, Ltd., New York © 1989

15

Techniques of Cassette Polysomnography

Moshe Reitman

University Sleep Center, Department of Medicine, New York Medical College, Valhalla, New York 10595

Many feel that proper sleep-disorder evaluations require a complete polysomnogram (PSG) in which brain waves (EEG), eye movements (EOM), and chin-muscle EMG are monitored to determine the stages of sleep (1,2). Other parameters, such as air flow from the nose and mouth, respiratory effort from the chest and abdomen, blood oxygen saturation levels, and an electrocardiogram (EKG), are routinely monitored to evaluate disordered breathing during sleep. For the most part, these evaluations have required the use of equipment that is bulky and stationary. In consequence, studies have been limited to sleep centers.

For many reasons, including patient comfort and costs, a more portable system that would allow evaluation outside centers is desirable. Until recently, portable monitoring systems have been able to record only a limited number of parameters, making accurate sleep staging and complete evaluation difficult, if not impossible.

Using a portable recorder to perform the evaluation in a residence other than the sleep center has several advantages. There are many patients who are appropriate candidates for a nocturnal polysomnogram (NPSG), who cannot, or are unwilling to, be evaluated in a sleep-disorder center. Some patients do not have a sleep center available in their locality. There are patients for whom travel problems or cost makes home studies more desirable. This latter consideration argues that the expense of a clinical-center evaluation might well be reserved for research or for those studies that require a more controlled environment and not simply for diagnostic screening studies.

In recent years, portable polysomnography, in which all essential parameters are recorded, has been used to evaluate patients in critical-care units of hospitals, at chronic-care centers, and at home. In each instance, the feasibility of this approach has been demonstrated and a significant clinical utility demonstrated. It is the purpose of this chapter to discuss the equipment and techniques of cassette polysomnography.

RECORDING TECHNIQUES

We have performed several hundred studies using an 8-channel cassette recorder (Oxford Medilog 9000). It is currently the preferred method for obtaining portable recordings of sleep data from patients. The most frequent evaluation requested in our experience is that of respiration during sleep; the most infrequent, that of periodic movements in sleep (PMS). The evaluation of parasomnias and especially nocturnal seizures is not in the scope of this discussion.

There are many different protocols available for nocturnal polysomnography, each consisting of one or more physiologic measures, depending on the clinical problem. We favor a recorder configured with four electroencephalograph (EEG) amplifiers, one DC amplifier for thermistry, two DC amplifiers to interface with the Respitrace module, which measures chest and abdominal excursions, and one EKG amplifier (see Fig. 1). Channels with EEG amplifiers are used to record the three parameters necessary to identify sleep stages, according to the accepted method of Rechtshaften and Kales (1). These are EEG C3 or C4 referred to the contralateral ear or mastoid, right and left EOG, and submentalis EMG. Some automatic sleep stagers also require this traditional configuration in order to process the data.

EOG is recorded from electrodes placed at the outer canthi of each eye referred separately to the contralateral mastoid or ear (e.g., ROC-A1, LOC-A2). Either the right or left outer canthus electrode is placed about 1 cm higher than that of the other eye. This results in a recording plane that is not perfectly

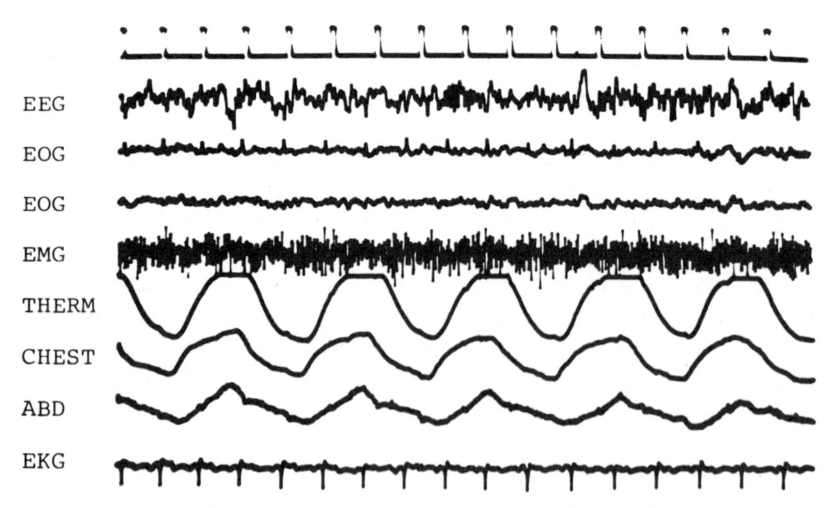

FIG. 1. A 16-sec video display of polysomnographic measures during normal respiration during Stage 2 sleep. Note sleep spindles in EEG, absence of eye movements in EOG, tonic muscle activity in EMG, rhythmic airflow on thermistry, rhythmic in-phase chest and abdomen excursions via Respitrace, and regular EKG rhythm.

horizontal so that vertical eye movements are also detected. Two channels are used to record eye movements so that high-amplitude frontal delta waves can be differentiated from the eye movements seen during dreaming or rapid eye movement sleep (REM). The former appear as in-phase deflections, while REM are seen as out-of-phase deflections.

EOG can be recorded in a single channel. Right outer canthus (ROC) referenced directly to the left outer canthus (LOC) provides a very adequate eye-movement detection channel. This configuration frees an extra channel, which can be used to monitor another parameter, for example, the EMG from the anterior tibialis muscles when evaluating periodic movements. However, EEG background activity, which is usually seen on the eye-movement channels, is less evident when referring the eyes together on a single channel. If, as happens on occasion, the EEG channel is lost or is obscured by artifact, one does not have the backup of monitoring the state of sleep by looking at the EEG present in the eye channels.

The fourth and last signal that is required in traditional sleep staging is the submentalis EMG recorded from the chin. Monitoring this parameter identifies the atonia of the skeletal muscles, which occurs during REM sleep. It is said that this muscle atonia protects us from physically acting out our dreams, which may involve physical activities that would be dangerous if attempted even while awake.

All head electrodes, other then C3 or C4, are off-scalp placements. Great care should be taken in preparing all the electrode sites. We recommend Omniprep (D.O. Weaver, Aurora, CO) as a skin preparation. Pellet electrodes (Graphic Controls Corp.) are extremely versatile and are applied quickly and easily. In order to ensure that the electrodes remain properly affixed throughout the recording period, collodion can be applied around the perimeter of each electrode and inside the four small holes on its surface. A careful collodion application cannot be overemphasized. Every site must be scrutinized prior to securing the electrode to ensure enough room to apply the collodion in a safe manner. This is especially true around the eyes.

The chin and mastoid electrodes are the most likely to come loose during the night and must be affixed very securely. The C3 and C4 electrode is applied via collodion technique exactly as in other ambulatory cassette recordings. Sufficient hair should be woven over the electrode so that it will remain secure (see Chapter 2). On can anticipate difficulty with children between 1 and 4 years old, who are likely to pull at the electrodes. All-night supervision by a trained technician, rather than the general nursing staff, is preferable in these instances. An exceptional patient may not need collodion-applied electrodes. This is limited to those who are known to move very little and who will be recorded with an attendant who can replace them should they come loose.

Respiratory effort is monitored by means of lightweight cloth belts (Respibands, AMI, Ardsley, NY) placed around the trunk, on both the abdomen and thoracic regions. A mesh vest is worn as a retainer over the entire trunk in order to keep the belts from shifting position. These belts detect increase in circumference of both the chest and abdomen by means of inductance measures from a single wire that spirals through each one. This technique is far superior to a strain gauge, which merely indicates the increase in circumference of a very limited area.

The Oxford Medical air flow probe is a combined oral/nasal thermistor constructed from a small triangular piece of silicon in which three thermistry sensors and a small flexible circuit board are embedded. The device, which is available for both adults and infants, has been designed to withstand physical abuse, such as from inadvertent biting. The thermistor, which is fitted between the nose and mouth, is usually worn on a lariat-type nasal cannula that has had the two nasal prongs removed. The cannula and thermistor combination is routinely secured to the cheek on each side with tape (Johnson & Johnson, Dermiform). We also include a single EKG channel in all evaluations. These leads from the chest are usually taped close to the clavicle as a strain relief. Figure 2 shows a patient with all the polysomnographic sensors attached and the typical recording setup.

After the electrodes have been applied, their impedance must be checked to be certain that it is less than 5 kΩ. The thermistor is then positioned between the nose and mouth, and all the wires are connected to the recorder. A monitor box is used to confirm that all channels are working. If one is in doubt about any channel, either because of high impedance or inappropriate deflections of the needle in the monitor dial, the problem must be investigated and corrected. An unresolved question most likely will cause a problem later.

Probably the most crucial step in assuring quality signals during the duration of a study is in organizing and stabilizing all the lead-in wires. They should be gathered together from various parts of the body to run along the back of the neck, strain-relieved at this point, and then continued upward to join all head electrodes at the vertex behind CZ. When this is accomplished, all the leads will be directed in the same direction so they can all eminate from the vertex.

All the leads are gathered together at the top of the head and surrounded by a band formed of tape. One inch of a 4-in. length is folded over onto itself. The folded part of the tape is wrapped around the wires first, so the wires do not stick to it. This allows one to draw the wires through the band to eliminate excess slack. All the wires are snugged tightly, including head electrodes, EKG, thermistor, and respiration leads. The input cables from the recorder are also kept together using tape. The goal is to have all the wires between the scalp and the recorder connectors together in a single bundle. There will be equal tension on all the wires, which will minimize the chances of pulling off single wires during the night.

The vertex location was chosen as the final tethering position, rather than a neck collar, as is used routinely in cassette EEG recordings, so that the patient can turn completely around in bed—front, back, or either side—without placing stress on the leads. Although this technique results in a turbanlike headdress for

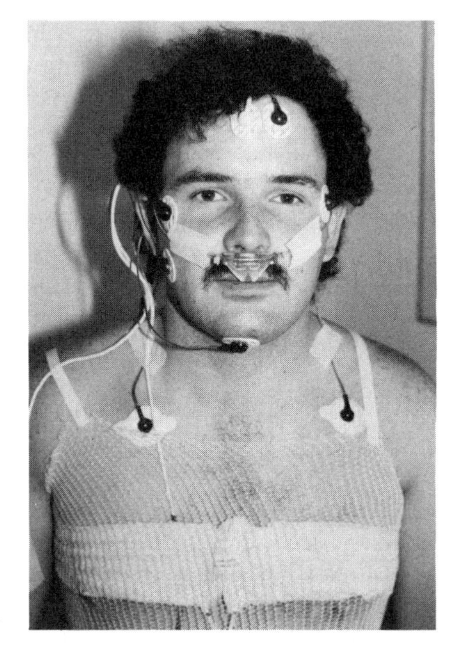

A

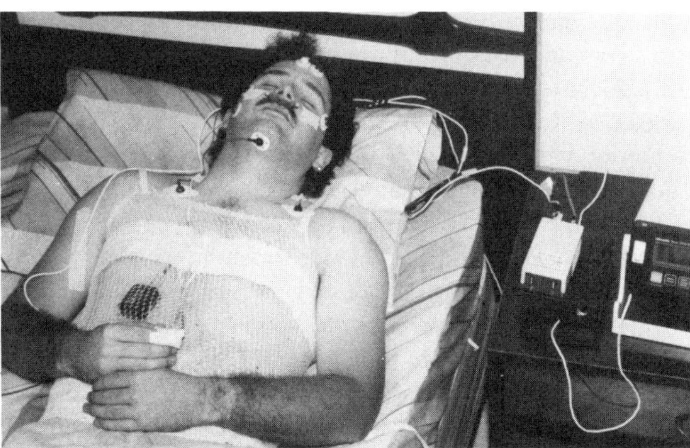

B

FIG. 2. A: Subject with polysomnographic sensors in place as described in the test. **B:** Monitoring setup with cassette recorder, respiration module, and oximeter at bedside. Note oximeter sensor on the subject's index finger.

the patient, there is usually less concern about a cosmetic appearance, since the patient will not be out in public.

EEG, EOG, EMG, EKG, thermistry, and respiratory-movement data use the entire complement of eight cassette channels. Oximeter data are acquired separately from, but synchronized to, the cassette recording, which allows later off-line analysis. We have been using the Ohmeda Biox 3700 Pulse Oximeter, which is very reliable and has the ability to store 8 hr of data internally in computer memory. The sensor probe is affixed on a finger for an adult or on the foot for an infant or child. We have had good success in obtaining long-term oximetry values by this technique. The data can be downloaded easily after the recording session into any IBM-compatible microcomputer through an asynchronous communications port using standard communication programs.

A deficiency in this technique is that the oximeter stores only a single data point for each 12-sec period. Its value corresponds to the lowest saturation level achieved during that period. The data capacity is limited to 8 hr of monitoring, i.e., 2400 points. Points recorded prior to the most recent 8 hr are pushed out of memory as the new ones are stored. The pulse rate associated with that lowest saturation level is also stored. These data are not as valuable as having the actual EKG on the recording, because the tachi-bradi heart-rate irregularities associated with apnea do not occur in either case exactly at the point of lowest saturation.

We have developed a simple computer program that takes the saturation information and organizes it according to total number of data points within each 5% decrease in saturation, starting with 96% saturation through 100%, then 91 through 95%, etc. The program classifies 10% steps or desaturation below 70% and finally totals all points below 49%. Time of day for each data point can also be printed out. This latter feature allows a close temporal correlation between an episode of apnea recorded on cassette tape at a particular time and the associated saturation level. Synchronization is achieved by turning off the oximeter as the cassette recorder's internal clock advances from one minute to the next. With the time of this final oximetry data point identified, all others can be retrospectively calculated. Accurate correlations require that great care be taken in this synchronization procedure.

We are currently evaluating a new oximeter, the Invivo 4500 (Invivo Research, Inc., Broken Arrow, OK), which has overcome the limitations mentioned above. This device collects data points every 2.5 sec. At this faster rate of accumulation, the oximetry trend output provides a greater resolution for both highs and lows of saturation. Several sources have developed software that both manages the data in tabular form and can present them graphically, which makes identification of desaturations easier.

Polysomnographic recordings in the home or other locations where there is no nursing staff may be done with or without a technician in attendance throughout the night, depending on the clinical situation. When equipment is left unattended, the technician tries to have the patient in bed and ready for sleep before he leaves. We advise that a chaperone stay with the patient. Both are instructed how to disconnect and reconnect the oximeter cable if the patient wishes to get out of bed during the night. The technician should also explain how to place the recorder on the bed in such a way that the patient will not accidently go to sleep on it. We have found it important to reassure the patient that there is a technician available and on call to answer even the most trivial questions, regardless of the time. I have rarely been called back to a residence, though many calls have resolved easily correctable problems that would otherwise have ruined the study.

DATA ANALYSIS

After the recording session, the data from the memory of the oximeter are transferred into the computer, freeing it for the next recording. The cassette tape from the recorder is next analyzed using an Oxford Medilog replay unit. It is useful to rewind the tape only a short distance to examine the quality of the recording at the end of the session. It can be determined from this whether that particular recording is of sufficient quality to attempt automated sleep staging. If the data of all four sleep parameters are of high quality, several more points are reviewed as the tape is rewound to confirm that the quality is consistent throughout.

Once assured of the quality, automated staging can be performed by the Oxford Medilog sleep stager at 20 times real time. At the same time, the first video/audio review of the entire tape can be accomplished by the technologist. During this first pass, a general impression concerning the sleep period can be obtained, and any unusual breathing patterns can be identified. If the automated sleep staging appears accurate on first run-through, manual scoring may be unnecessary, and the results of the stager can be added unedited to the final report.

It must be stressed that any recording that is scored by any automated method must also be completely reviewed by a registered polysomnographic technologist. In many cases, editing may be needed to produce an accurate polysomnogram. Although a more reliable automated sleep stager may be available soon, including programs that will quantitate sleep data and prepare a summary report, at present, the data are best prepared by a qualified polysomnographic technologist. It is a major mistake to purchase expensive and sophisticated equipment without giving proper consideration to who will operate it, analyze the data, and, in general, supervise the clinical service.

At present, analyses of apnea, PMS, and EKG anomalies must be visually and/or aurally performed from the replay. However, not having to turn as many as 800 pages of polygraph printout can make it easier for the reviewer to focus on the task. These data are not easily obtained at the same time that sleep is scored. Separate reviews are suggested. Data reduction is best performed in the above sequence, because the sleep architecture must be known before analyzing other phenomena.

Staging sleep from cassette tape is done in nearly the same way as it is from paper, except that, instead of using page numbers to index stage entries, real time from the scanner is used. We have developed a PC program that allows keyboard entry of time, stage, and events. This program produces a comprehensive report, which includes patient information, parametric analysis of sleep, an analysis of oximeter data and apnea, a description of the evaluation, technician's observations, and a technical assessment of the study.

When scoring sleep manually by video/audio review of the tape, the following patterns are usually observed in the evolution of the sleep cycle. The initial transition from wake to sleep, so-called Stage 1, is usually seen as a slowing of the EEG from posterior-dominant alpha activity to mixed theta frequencies and loss of muscle artifact. Alpha breaks up and gradually drops out; slow, rolling eye movements and, especially in young people, high-amplitude vertex waves are seen. Sleep spindles and K-complexes appear when Stage 2 sleep is entered. Synchronized delta, defined as waves greater than 75 μv in amplitude and slower than 0.5 Hz in frequency, further slow the EEG. When delta waves constitute more than 20% of the activity, Stage 3 has been reached. In Stage 4 sleep, more than 50% of the background activity is delta.

After 60 to 90 min of sleep, the EEG becomes low voltage and mixed in frequency like that observed during the onset of sleep. A diminished chin EMG identifies the onset of REM sleep. In some individuals, sawtooth waves are also seen in the EEG during this stage. This full cycle takes about 90 to 100 min. As many as five sleep cycles make up the normal night sleep. The cycles recur every 90 to 100 min, but the amount of slow-wave sleep diminishes during each subsequent sleep cycle, while the REM periods become longer. At first, they occupy 10 min or so in the first cycle, but they increase to as much as an hour in the last cycle of sleep. During the last half of the night, there may be little or no delta sleep observed.

Listening to an audio output from the EEG channel, which is a unique feature of the Medilog 9000 replay, adds a special dimension to reviewing the PSG. Events such as arousals, spindles, and K-complexes are easily identified by their particular audio signature. These can be quickly learned by the scorer. The background activity, whether delta waves or beta, also has a characteristic sound. Listening to the audio of the EKG can also detect subtle EKG rate changes. The data are displayed on the video screen about a second after they are heard, which allows easy identification of each event, because the audio signal alerts the scorer to an upcoming change in state. EEG sounds can also help the scorer identify arousals and cardiac rate or rhythm changes associated with apneic episodes.

Sleep architecture forms a background against which most sleep disorders should be evaluated, even though it may not be considered of primary importance in some clinics. In this regard, it is essential that the EEG is monitored to ensure that negative findings during an all-night recording session are not due to the absence of sleep. Individual disorders are identified by a variety of measures other than those used to stage sleep. Evaluation of disordered breathing during sleep requires the analysis of several phenomena. The two primary ones are respiratory effort, by monitoring thoracic and abdominal-wall movement, and air flow, by measuring temperature changes accompanying exhalation from the nostrils and mouth. We prefer to use Respitrace thoracic and abdominal bands and dual oral/nasal thermistors, respectively, for these purposes. EKG is also routinely recorded in these patients. Figure 1 illustrates the replay display of these various parameters.

An absence of thoracic and abdominal-wall movement lasting more than 10 sec during sleep is considered evidence of a central apnea. If thoracic and abdominal effort continues, accompanied by no air flow at either the nose or mouth that lasts longer than 10 sec, the apnea is considered to be obstructive in type (Fig. 3). Thus, depending on the patterns observed, obstructive, central, or mixed sleep apnea can be identified. Hypopneas, which are periods longer than 10 sec of regular breathing with diminution of respiratory effort greater than 50%, can also be detected by cassette polysomnography. Other breathing anomalies, which can be identified by this method, include Cheyne-Stokes respiration and periodic breathing. The clinical significance of apneas or irregular breathing can be assessed by oximetry, which measures blood oxygen saturation continuously during the recording period. During disordered breathing, oxygen saturation may drop rapidly to dangerous levels.

With the advent and now expansion of serial cassette studies, we are documenting that there is significant night-to-night variability in apnea severity and prevalence. This is especially true of patients with sleep apnea of only moderate severity. Medications, alcohol, and position can greatly affect the results of one night's recording. In these patients, serial studies can be useful and may be necessary for proper diagnosis and documentation. This is not as necessary in those patients with very severe apnea, since they do not have much night-to-night variability in our experience of recording several hundred such cases. False-negative evaluations are unlikely in this group. It used to be thought that, as long as a patient slept on his back for a part of the night and had some REM sleep, one could determine the extent of the apnea. Given the variability we have observed, this may not be true.

As noted above, some patients have apnea that is very position-sensitive. Data about body position are important in their evaluation. Video monitoring is useful in this regard, and it can be accomplished in the home as well as in the laboratory. Although several new devices have been developed recently that offer position data throughout the night, none interfaces easily with our cassette configuration due to the limited number of available channels. Optimal studies in these patients require the presence of a technician who can attempt to get the patient into different positions. This type of intervention can be done in the home as well as in the lab. In these situations, the presence of a well-trained technologist, not necessarily the location, will make the difference.

Excessive or paroxysmal daytime sleepiness is a major complaint of patients seen in sleep centers. The multiple sleep latency test (MSLT) measures this tendency. It is the study of choice in the evaluation of narcolepsy. In this test, the patient is requested to take three to five short naps every 2 hr starting at

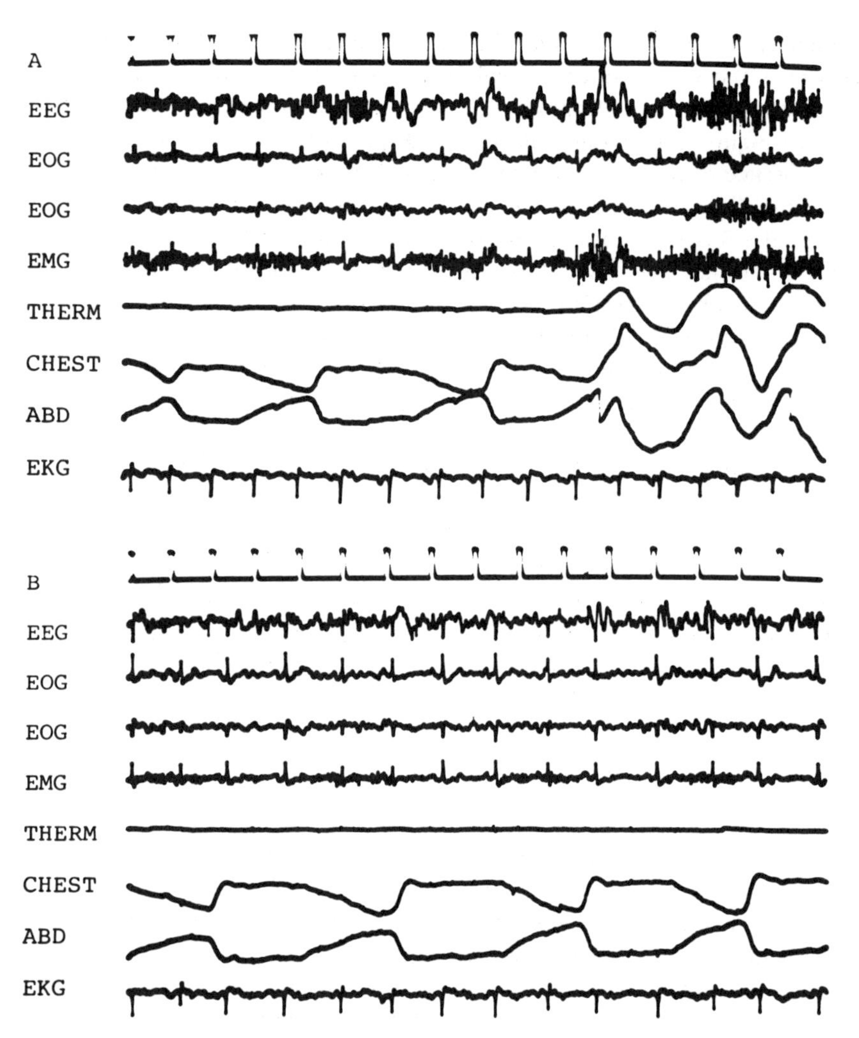

FIG. 3. A: A 16-sec video display of polysomnographic measures during another period of Stage 2 sleep in the same patient as in Fig. 1. Note similar EEG and EOG findings, but EMG tonic activity is reduced during the first 10 sec, and there is no airflow detected by thermistry despite chest and abdomen movements, which are out of phase. Increased EMG activity and artifact on EEG and EOG indicative of an arousal during the latter portion of the traces are accompanied by airflow and increased respiratory movements. This pattern is typical of obstructive apnea. **B:** A video display of data from the same patient during a period of REM sleep. Note attenuated EMG activity and lack of airflow during the entire period despite respiratory efforts marked by out-of-phase chest and abdomen excursions. Obstructive apneas are commonly prolonged during REM sleep.

10:00 a.m. If performed in a sleep laboratory, a patient is allowed to sleep for no longer than 10 min, provided that sleep onset occurs prior to the 20th min.

When using cassette recorders to perform the MSLT in the home setting, we advise that a chaperone, who is usually a family member, friend, or a nurse/technician, be present to allow the patient to nap only for 25 min with each attempt. He is instructed not to allow any sleep between naps. A mean latency to sleep of less than 5 min over all naps, with the presence of more than one REM period, supports the diagnosis of narcolepsy. Patients with moderate to severe sleep apnea, who also complain of excessive sleepiness, also usually have short sleep latencies between 5 and 10 min. In either case, follow-up cassette MSLTs can be of great help in evaluating the efficacy of treatment. (See Chapter 18 for further discussion of the hypersomnias.)

Evaluations of PMS are appropriate for the cassette technique. In order to evaluate PMS, electrodes are routinely placed on the anterior tibialis muscles of both legs. PMS are defined as episodes of five or more leg jerks, each jerk lasting 3 to 5 sec and occurring at a rate of two to three per min. The leg jerks usually involve dorsiflexion of the feet with variable spread into the upper leg in severe cases. Movements may be present in either or both legs. (See Chapter 20 for a more detailed discussion.)

We have had to reevaluate a small percentage of our patients due to technical errors. On rare occasions, tapes have failed to advance properly, resulting in corrupted or no data. For the most part, these failures have been due to inserting the tape improperly and failing to verify tape transport. Also, if the tape is not taut between the cassette spools, it may pull away from the recording head. The recording should not be placed under the patient's pillow, since it is possible that his weight could interfere with tape transport. Oximeter failure has caused several studies to be repeated. A power failure lasting several hours and not securing the oximeter probe properly were the underlying reasons. We have learned from these experiences and have been able to eliminate almost all such failures subsequently. Table 1 summarizes the results of our evaluations to date.

DISCUSSION

Sleep disorder centers have the advantage of a laboratory polygraph with multiple channels. For the present, portable cassette recorders only have eight channels and a time/marker channel. This is a major limitation of the ambulatory polysomnogram. However, leaving aside the question of how many channels are minimally necessary to evaluate a PSG properly, requiring a patient to come to a laboratory for evaluation can also be a limitation. The fact is that many patients do not want to come to the sleep center. This may sound like a weak justification for portable PSGs, but, at a major sleep center during a 2-year period, a follow-up to inquiries that did not result in an appointment revealed that many patients preferred not to be admitted to a hospital laboratory, especially when the sleep center was part of a psychiatric facility.

In reality, many, if not most, PSGs can be performed in the home and eight well-chosen channels plus a free-standing oximeter are usually sufficient. The

TABLE 1. *Cassette polysomnographic evaluations*

Age (yr)	*N*	Sex		Results		Type of Evaluation		Location	
		M	F	Pos[a]	Neg	Apnea	Other	Home	Hosp
1–4	27	18	9	10	17	23	4	4	23
5–19	27	15	12	14	13	22	5	12	15
20–85	175	131	44	110[b]	65	131[b]	44[c]	130	55

[a]Positive results—specific abnormal polysomnographic findings, e.g., apnea index greater than 5, oxygen desaturations below 70%.
[b]Includes 16 studies of CPAP trials, regardless of success, which were second evaluations of patients with initially positive sleep-apnea studies.
[c]Other evaluations—includes 35 multiple sleep latency tests.

capability of doing these evaluations outside the sleep lab is a major advance in the sleep-disorders field. Certainly we have found this to be true at our center, which is part of a pulmonary medicine division, where we perform mostly apnea evaluations. When breathing is to be evaluated during sleep, the appropriate parameters must be recorded. This has little to do with the environment. If one records sleep, air flow, respiratory effort, EKG, and oxygen saturation properly, and the patient sleeps, he will get useful data. There are those few patients who will not sleep enough throughout the night to provide enough data to analyze, regardless of whether in the lab or home. These patients require multiple nights of recording.

Unquestionably, there is a population of patients whose problems are complex and who need to be evaluated in the laboratory. This number is relatively small in our experience. Many more patients have the opportunity of being evaluated in an ambulatory setting, not only those who refuse to be studied in the lab, but also those who simply cannot be studied there, such as institutionalized or hospitalized patients, especially those in critical-care units. For many patients who need PSG evaluation, it may be easier for the "laboratory" to go to them, rather than the other way around. There seems to be little reason for every small hospital or clinic to establish rooms for sleep studies and then have them performed by unqualified, untrained personnel, when there exists the alternative of having quality diagnostic services of credentialed specialists provided via portable polysomnography.

A major motivating factor in the development of a portable sleep study program was the thought that it would be a more cost-effective method of providing evaluations than the traditional hospital-based sleep lab. When considering the tremendous cost of hospital space, followed by that of instrumenting multiple rooms, cassette polysomnography seemed to make eminent sense. Thus far, we and others attempting this service have met with partial success. Disappointments, however, have not come from the technique, which has proved satisfactory, but from other quarters. These include the insurance industry and government-administrated health-care agencies, such as Medicare and Medicaid, all of whom have not shown much interest in or understanding of the field of sleep-disorders medicine, particularly when applied to new innovations in diagnosis such as cassette polysomnography.

We have successfully shown in more than 200 studies that portable polysomnography, which can be performed in a patient's residence, is a reliable alternative to the traditional sleep-center evaluation, especially in sleep apneas. There is every reason to think that the future will bring with it even better portable equipment capable of storing more and different data for more detailed analyses. Then and now, regardless of instrumentation, the essential elements remain the same, however—skilled polysomnographic technologists to perform the evaluation and reduce the data, trained clinical polysomnographers to interpret the findings.

REFERENCES

1. Rechtschaffen A, Kales A, eds. *A manual of standardized terminology, techniques, and scoring system for sleep stages in human subjects.* Los Angeles: Brain Information Service/Brain Research Institute, UCLA, 1968. (Also available as NIH Publ 204, US Govt Printing Office, Washington DC, 1968.)
2. Guilleminaut C, Dement WC. Sleep apnea syndrome and related sleep disorders. In: Williams RL, Karacan I, eds. *Sleep disorders: diagnosis and treatment.* New York: John Wiley and Sons, 1978.

Ambulatory EEG Monitoring,
edited by John S. Ebersole.
Raven Press, Ltd., New York © 1989

16

Data Reduction of Cassette-Recorded Polysomnographic Measures

C. William Erwin* and John S. Ebersole**

**Ambulatory Sleep Laboratory, Duke University Medical Center, Durham, North Carolina 27710; and **Department of Neurology, Yale University School of Medicine, New Haven, Connecticut 06510*

The process of data reduction, when applied to ambulatory cassette recordings, has various meanings determined by the clinical or research interests of the individual doing the task. Widely disparate diseases such as epilepsy, dysomnia, or psychiatric illness require quite different approaches. The epileptologist may be primarily concerned with the presence or absence of epileptiform events (either interictal discharges or electrographic seizures), proper lateralization if not focality of an abnormality, and correlation of behavioral events with EEG activity. The sleep specialist is likely concerned with interruptions of respiratory activity (apnea), whether the apnea is obstructive or central in type, the degree of oxygen desaturation, the patient's position, and sleep stage when the majority or most severe apneas occur. The psychiatrist or psychologist may have primary interest in the general aspects of sleep architecture, the latency from sleep onset to the initial REM period, the abundance (density) of eye movements during REM, and measures of slow-wave activity. In some instances, the presence of paroxysmal myogenic activity (usually leg) associated with EEG arousal, penile tumescence, core temperature, or a host of other measures are required to address the clinical/research questions.

This chapter will discuss the principal methods of reducing polysomnographic data collected by ambulatory cassette recorders and examine the relative advantages and disadvantages of each.

TECHNICAL CONSIDERATIONS

It is not possible to recover directly recorded analog activity below 20 Hz from tape when the transport speed is the same for both recording and playback.

Although the magnetic fields created by slow activity are recorded on analog tape, field changes are so slow during playback that the strength of the signal is reduced below recoverable levels. Frequency modulation is the usual method of recording slow biologic activity, such as EEG, on analog tape. Unfortunately, bulky electronics initially required for this type of recording prevented its use in ambulatory cassette recording.

Another solution to the problem of recovering sub–20-Hz biologic waveforms is to record the signal at one tape transport speed, but play it back at a much faster speed. The ratio between the record speed and playback speed determines the increase in frequency of the biologic signals. Replayed 20 times faster, even 1-Hz delta activity can be reproduced from an analog recording.

Before low-cost computers became available, taped EEG data replayed in this manner were often printed on an ink writing system capable of very fast paper transport speeds. One system has paper speeds to 600 mm/sec so that the typical appearance of EEG at 30 mm/sec can be maintained. The high-frequency signals produced by rapid replay can be written onto paper, if the inertia caused by the mass of a pen stylus is avoided and instead an ink writing system in which varying magnetic fields control the position of the ink-jet nozzles is used.

A major breakthrough in the analysis of ambulatory cassette tape recordings was to replace the high-speed, ink-jet writeout with a digital computer, which could hold large amounts of data in core memory for either display on a video screen or real-time paper printout. It is still necessary to move the tape over the playback head faster than the record speed, but there is a serendipitous value in accelerating EEG signals into the auditory-frequency range. Connecting EEG or other signals from the tape output to an audio amplifier/speaker allows one to hear the activity. For instance, 10-Hz alpha becomes a 200-, 400-, or 600-Hz tone depending on whether the playback is 20, 40, or 60 times real time.

The evolution of EEG patterns that accompany sleep involves mostly alterations in the frequency and amplitude of ongoing activity and the appearance of transient complexes. The sense of hearing is very well adapted to frequency analysis, amplitude or loudness analysis, and random-event detection. Visual perception, on the other hand, is better adapted to spatial-pattern analysis. Since the scoring of sleep by EEG criteria depends principally on the identification of background rhythms and their relative abundance, and very little on the spatial distribution of these features, it would seem logical that sleep staging should be more easily performed by sound, rather than by sight, if only EEG rhythms were audible. As noted above, rapid cassette replay produces this very effect.

An analogy would be attempting to determine when the clarinets began to play in a particular measure of music by scrutinizing the oscilloscopic display of the frequencies produced by the entire symphony orchestra versus doing the same task by listening to the resultant sound. Few would disagree that the former task would be very difficult, while the latter would be relatively easy, once a person learned what a clarinet sounds like. The same is true for the analysis of sleep rhythms, once the characteristic sounds of alpha, theta, delta, and beta are learned.

METHODS OF DATA REDUCTION

In a clinical setting, data reduction of polysomnographic recordings has an interpretative report as the final output. However, several discrete steps must be accomplished before the clinical report can be written. These are event *identification, registration,* and *compilation.* The term "event" is used here in a very general sense and could refer to a spike, an apneic episode, or a period of increased delta activity.

Initially, the entire record is scanned to identify events. After the interpreter recognizes the event, it is registered. This may be simply a note registered on paper or an entry into a variety of computational devices. Usually, it is necessary to register not only that the event has occurred, but also the time the event has occurred and often its correlation with other events. For instance, it is important to know not only that an apneic event has occurred, but also to classify it as obstructive or central, to note the duration of the apneic event, the position of the sleeper, and the degree of oxygen desaturation.

After all events are registered with associated data, there must be a compilation of the various events and their correlations. Compilation includes such features as the total amount of REM as a percentage of the night's sleep, the latency from sleep onset to the first REM period, the average duration of apneic events (both prone and supine), the maxima and minima of various events, etc. Armed with this array of information, the clinician is now ready to make decisions about the degree of normalcy of a study as compared with normal control groups and to interpret the findings in context with the clinical problem.

Cassette data can be presented to the reviewer in a variety of formats. Each requires a different technique for event identification. Regardless of the method, considerable training and skill are necessary on the part of the reviewer. However, much of the review effort, as well as opportunity for error, occurs in event registration and event compilation. Discussed below are the major methods for reducing polysomnographic data.

Paper

Sleep data recorded on cassette tapes can be transferred to standard polygraphic paper either by high-speed, ink-jet write-out, as discussed above, or by real-time printout, using the continuous print function of the replay unit. Obviously, the former technique makes more efficient use of time. The major impetus to do this laborious task is to have data in a format that is still considered the "gold standard." Once on paper, sleep staging and other forms of data analysis can proceed manually in a traditional fashion on a page-by-page basis. Most of the published literature on polysomnographic data reduction and validation, including inter-rater reliability, is based on paper technology. (See Chapter 18 for further discussion.)

Direct Scoring from Video Screen

Polysomnographic data can be directly scored from the screen with event identification based entirely on visual presentation. Currently, ambulatory cassette replay units hold sufficient data in memory so that they can be presented on the screen as discrete epochs or video "pages." These advance screen by screen, although limited scrolling is also available. For example, the Oxford 9000 displays a screen containing 16 sec of data. This instrument provides playback speed options of 20, 40, or 60 times real time. Each screen persists for 0.80, 0.40, and 0.27 sec, respectively, before the next screen appears at these speeds. The slowest playback rate of 20× is quite comparable to data scanning speeds employed with paper records. For example, 2 sec spent examining two pages of traditional polysomnographic data transcribed at 15 mm/sec would be the same as reviewing directly from video at 20 times real time. Of course, with both paper and video data reduction, one can stop "turning pages" to scrutinize some feature more intensely or to go back in time and review certain data.

The effective scanning speed or rate of data evaluation is ultimately dependent on several factors—the complexity of the record, the type of data reduction being done, the amount of artifact present, interindividual differences in data-reduction style, and the time needed for data registration. This latter function is often the most time-consuming.

Hoelscher et al. (1) made comparisons of (a) screen-by-screen video scoring, (b) times-20 video scoring, and (c) traditional paper scoring. Sixteen polysomnograms were analyzed and compared. Eight were from normal subjects and eight from patients with various dysomnias. The *r* correlation coefficients of the clinical descriptors generated from these types of analyses were high, usually exceeding 0.9. The recognition of sleep-stage changes was highly comparable by all techniques. The faster video-scanning techniques suffered in comparison with page-by-page video scoring and paper scoring in the detection of brief events such as short arousals (WASO <2 min) or brief transition stage I periods. (See Table 1.)

Rapid Audio-Video Analysis of Sleep Stages

The review of cassette records for epileptiform events in a large clinical series of suspected epileptic patients provided ample opportunity for both seeing and hearing the EEG of sleep (2–4). It quickly became apparent, as the skills of

TABLE 1. *Correlation coefficients (r) of various sleep statistics for 16 polysomnograms*[a]

Sleep statistic	Screen by screen	Times 20 scanning
Total sleep time	.998	.995
Sleep efficiency	.995	.998
Latency to stage I	.997	.996
Latency to stage II	.991	.991
Latency to REM onset	.996	.991
Total WASO	.995	.995
WASO >2 min	.985	.982
WASO <2 min	.690	.662
Movement time	.927	
Percent stage I	.905	.753
Percent stage II	.979	.889
Percent stage SWS	.976	.831
Percent stage REM	.978	.947

[a] Scored from paper and compared with (a) 16-sec slow screen-by-screen analysis and (b) continuous scanning speed of times 20. No attempt was made to score movement time during the times 20 scanning analysis.

auditory analysis for seizure detection were being learned, that the identification of sleep rhythms and stage changes by sound was relatively simple. Background rhythms were, in fact, far easier to identify than seizures or interictal discharges, because they are nearly continuous. It proved to be easier to discriminate aurally both seizures and sleep-state fluctuations at the higher playback speed of times 60 than at the slower speed of times 20. The temporal compression afforded by rapid data replay helped to resolve more slowly evolving changes of sleep stage, much the same way that a slow paper speed assists traditional polysomnographic analysis.

Active wakefulness, as recorded on cassette EEG, is characterized by an abundance of muscle and movement artifacts superimposed on a background rhythm of mixed frequencies. The resultant combination sounds like white noise and has little tonal quality. The approach of sleep is signaled first by a decrease in this artifact and thus by a quieting of the record. In a nonlaboratory setting, alpha activity appears only briefly during short periods of relaxed wakefulness with eyes closed just before sleep onset, during intermittent nighttime arousals from sleep, and with morning awakening. It is characterized by a pure-tone sound that stands in contrast to the white noise of active wakefulness. It has been likened to a long owl hoot or mourning-dove call. Breakup of this continuous tone into short tone bursts heralds the transition into sleep. Stage I sleep with its theta and mixed beta frequencies is notable to the listener more as an absence of other features, namely alpha or sleep spindles, than for a presence of a particular sound. The lower pitched whir of theta activity can be appreciated in some people. Higher-amplitude paroxysmal theta, such as hypnagogic hypersynchrony in children, is very distinctive, sounding like pure-tone bursts similar to alpha, but of lower frequency. The most distinctive feature of stage I is the onset of intermittent low-pitched thuds, which are the sonic representations of vertex sharp waves. The addition of sleep spindles to this frequency mixture marks the transition into stage II sleep. These spindles, which sound like bird chirps, more specifically turkey gobbles, are the most distinctive auditory marker of stage II sleep and one that will play an important role in defining critical stage changes into and out of that state relative to stage I and REM sleep. Accurate temporal correlations can be made of these latter transitions based on the appearance or loss of sleep spindles.

The transition from stage II into slow-wave sleep, stages III and IV, is a gradual one. It is signaled by the progressive buildup of delta frequencies. These sound on audio review like the distant rumble of thunder or of an approaching train. Because of its low frequency, even at 60 times real time, delta activity is more often felt as a vibration than heard as a tone. Sleep spindles are not lost in this transition, but they become progressively overshadowed by the rumbling delta background. Precise temporal correlations are difficult to make by auditory staging, since the transition into deeper sleep is gradual. It is not simply a matter of presence or absence of a frequency or event, but of a relative contribution to the background. For this same reason, the distinction between stage III and IV is usually not attempted by rapid auditory analysis. Fortunately, these transitions into deeper sleep are usually not as clinically pertinent as those involving stage I, II, or REM. On the other hand, transitions upward from stage III or IV into II or REM are rather abrupt and can be easily and accurately appreciated by sonic features, namely the loss of delta rumble with or without, respectively, a reemergence of a prominent sleep-spindle chirp.

The transition from either stage II or III into REM sleep is also very characteristic in aural terms. As with stage I, the most striking feature is a lack of significant sound. There is a quieting of the record in which movement artifact, sleep spindles, vertex sharp waves, delta, or alpha is, for the most part, not present. Seldom commented on in the classic sleep literature, but often quite distinctive during this relatively quiet time, is the high-pitched hiss of 18- to 24-Hz low-voltage beta activity. This sound has been likened to wind blowing through trees. Its presence and the absence of the other features are a clear indicator of REM sleep. Rapid eye movements themselves are also heard as intermittent thuds, but they often do not begin until well after the REM period has begun by EEG criteria.

The other non-EEG parameters that are traditionally used by polysomnographers to stage sleep provide supportive or confirmatory information in the rapid auditory technique to that which is primarily obtained from the EEG. It is always reassuring to see or hear the rapid eye movements in the EOG channels during periods thought by EEG criteria to be REM, but, as noted above, the correlation is not tight, particularly in regard to exact time of onset or offset of REM versus eye movements. In equivocal situations, EMG diminution associated with the atonia of REM sleep may be more helpful in substantiating a REM period.

The sleep scorer who uses video, audio, or combined techniques to stage from the cassette replay typically also uses context to help maintain accuracy at high rates of review. Anticipation of what change is likely is clearly useful. This is one distinct advantage that the human scorer has over automated staging systems. In the computerized record-keeping and epoch-recording system of Erwin and Hartwell (5), which is discussed in more detail below, entries into a microcomputer signifying stage changes are made by the reviewer by pressing the appropriate function key. By anticipating what the next likely change will be, the reviewer can be ready to enter this transition by positioning his fingers over the one or two keys most likely to be pressed. This will lessen the reviewer's reaction time and make the transition times more accurate. For example, if the patient is in stage I sleep, it is likely that he will either go into stage II or return to wakefulness; it is unlikely that he will go directly into slow-wave sleep and less likely that he will go into a REM period. Precision is important when reviewing rapidly, since, at 60 times real time, a 30-sec staging epoch lasts only 500 msec.

Bursts of myogenic activity associated with movements during sleep are also an aid to predicting that a stage change is about to happen. Many transitions upward from slow-wave sleep into stage II or stage II into REM are heralded by muscle artifact. A burst of white noise that is the resultant sound should alert the reviewer to a potential upward change in state.

Since staging sleep at 60 times real time can be accomplished quickly, it is reasonable to perform at least two passes to improve accuracy. The audio characteristics of sleep stages and transitions particular to that patient can be learned the first time through a record. Periods of multiple or difficult transitions can also be anticipated and thus analyzed better on repeat scoring.

A brief study was undertaken to evaluate the reproducibility of sleep staging ambulatory cassette-recorded data using combined auditory and visual clues at 60 times real time (6). The scoring criteria for stage identification were those of Rechtschaffen and Kales (7), modified as discussed above. One of the authors scored each of the taped polysomnograms from six patients on three occasions in succession. Staging was performed in one continuous run, without interruptions. Thus, a 7-hr polysomnogram was scored in 7 min.

Scoring at this speed was made possible by using a personal computer (PC) for stage registration. Two-sec miniepochs are registered by pressing a specified function key on the keyboard of the PC. The data are stored to disk for later comparison. Because the data are formatted in 2-sec miniepochs, they can be reformatted to longer epochs, up to 120 sec, using a simple plurality rule. Compilation of the registered data produces a hypnogram and numerous sleep statistics, which include sleep-stage percents, latencies from sleep onset to different sleep stages, interstage latencies, sleep efficiency, and several derived ratios of REM and slow waves.

A second computer program was created whose function was to compare the sleep-data files made at different times by the same scorer or files made by

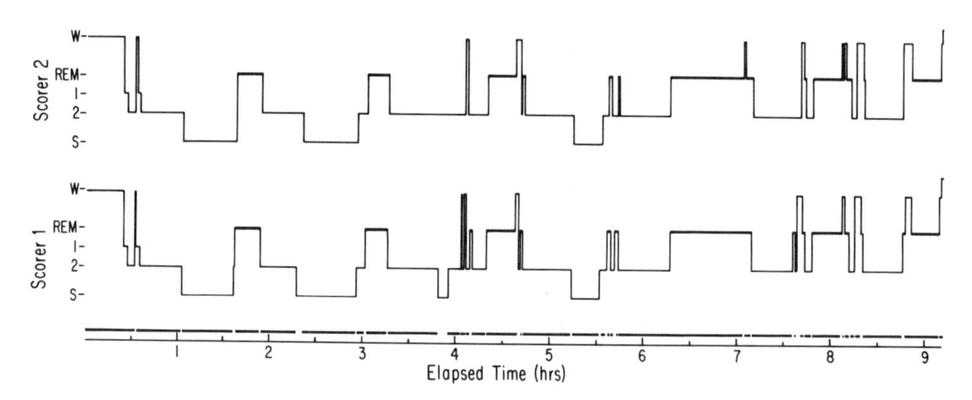

FIG. 1. The results of two consecutive scorings of 9-hr polysomnograms by one of the authors (JSE) using combined auditory and visual clues. The taped record contained the standard polygraphic variables of left and right EOG, chin EMG, and the EEG channel C_3M_2. An additional EEG channel of Oz-Cz was also used. The hypnogram labeled "Scorer 1" was the second scoring of three and "Scorer 2" was the third scoring. Stage N is indeterminate stage and S is combined 3 and 4. The *solid bar* at the bottom, just above the time marker, indicates agreement between the hypnograms, while a *gap* in the bar indicates disagreement.

different scorers. The output of this program produces hypnograms plotted one above the other, with a bar indicator to show areas of agreement and disagreement. In addition, epoch-by-epoch agreement between various stages is tabulated in two formats. In this study, the first sleep analysis was compared to the second analysis for each of the six recordings, and the second analysis was compared to the third analysis.

The mean epoch-by-epoch agreement, comparing first to second analysis, was 90.9% (SD=2.1; range, 87.6–93.7%). Agreement between the second and third analyses was a higher 92.7% (SD=1.6%; range, 90.7–93.8%), which resulted in a difference in means of 1.9% and a difference in SDs of 1.6%. This difference was significant, as determined by a paired *t*-test ($t=2.84$; df= 5; $p=0.03$). Although the difference was small, statistical significance was achieved, because improvement in percent agreement of similar magnitude was found in all six records.

These findings were in keeping with the subjective opinion of the interpreter, who felt his accuracy improved on the second and third interpretive attempts as compared with the first. The data indicate that combined auditory-visual analysis of polysomnograms at 60 times real time can yield highly reproducible anlayses, which compare favorably to comparisons between paper-recorded data and machine-interpreted data. This high level of agreement is, in part, related to the reduced number of stage changes detected by this technique, as compared with other techniques. There is a greater opportunity for error in epoch-by-epoch analysis when there are more stage changes detected. An average of 35 stage changes per night's sleep was seen in this study.

TABLE 2. *Sleep-stage comparison statistics*

A:

File No. Sleep stage	Scorer 1 042-85A.E2 Epochs (*N*)[a]	Scorer 2 042-85A.E3 Epochs (*N*)[a]	Percent agreement
Wake	322	298	92.5
1	41	24	58.5
2	571	528	92.5
R	274	253	92.3
S	112	103	92.0
Total	1320	1206	91.4

B:

	Scorer 1					
S	Wake	REM	1	2	S,3,4	Total
c Wake	6.6	1.2	0.2	0.5	0.0	8.4
o REM	0.3	25.4	0.0	1.2	0.0	26.9
r 1	0.0	0.0	0.7	0.0	0.0	0.7
e 2	0.8	1.5	0.0	43.2	2.2	47.8
r S,3,4	0.0	0.2	0.0	0.5	15.5	16.2
2 Total	7.7	28.3	0.9	45.3	17.7	91.6

[a]Epoch length, 30 sec.

Table 2A presents an epoch-by-epoch comparison of the same files graphed in Fig. 1. Although the format of the comparison seen in **A** is simpler to read than **B,** it makes the implicit assumption that "Scorer 1" is correct. Quite different values are obtained if Scorer 1 and Scorer 2 are interchanged.

Table 2B makes no assumption as to which is the correct scoring and is further able to indicate how epochs were scored differently on the two scorings. For both **A** and **B,** the total agreement is 91.6%, which was less than the average agreement for second versus third scorings (see text).

CONCLUSIONS

Data reduction attempts to make sense of a complex, otherwise unintelligible mass of data. In the process, by definition, information is lost. Which data are important and thus should be retained depends entirely on the clinical or research question being asked. Our experience suggests that rapid, audio-visual scoring of cassette polysomnograms is reproducible and accurate, if the question is confined to identification of traditional sleep stages. At present, there is not a more efficient way to analyze sleep, either manually or by computer, for obtaining basic sleep architecture and certain specific information, such as REM onset latency. Analysis of more microscopic and brief events, such as occur in fragmented sleep with short arousals or periodic nocturnal movements, cannot be accomplished by a technique of an uninterrupted analysis. They are better done at slow scanning speeds with frequent stops for visual inspection of stationary data.

Ultimately, all forms of electrophysiologic data reduction will be by automated, electronic means. A number of early attempts have been met with varying degrees of success. A major problem of the early attempts has been the "black box" approach. Physiologic data go in, and a printed report comes out. Only minimal validation is possible, as the criteria for event identification versus artifact recognition are obscured by the hardware and software.

Undoubtedly, future methods will include artificial intelligence, raw-data screens for visual validation of correct event identification, and calibration techniques to ensure proper functioning of the entire system. This latter includes not only the usual amplitude and analog filter characteristics, but also analog-to-digital conversion, and the algorithms for data reduction. Fortunately, current ambulatory techniques allow data from studies of normal subjects and patients with sleep disorders to be stored on the cassette medium, which is inexpensive and available for later processing as better analytic techniques become available. For the time being, manual analysis, by any of the techniques discussed, must be considered more dependable and the standard for comparison.

REFERENCES

1. Hoelscher TJ, McCall WV, Powell J, et al. Sleep scoring with the Oxford Medilog 9000: comparison to conventional paper scoring. *Sleep* 1988. (In press.)
2. Ebersole JS. Ambulatory cassette EEG. *J Clin Neurophysiol* 1985;2:397–418.
3. Ebersole JS. Ambulatory EEG monitoring. In: Aminoff MJ, ed. *Electrodiagnosis in clinical neurology.* New York: Churchill Livingstone 1986;125–148.
4. Ebersole JS, Bridgers SL. Ambulatory EEG monitoring. In: Pedley TA, and Meldrum BS, eds. *Recent advances in epilepsy,* vol 3. Edinburgh: Churchill Livingstone, 1986;111–135.
5. Erwin CW, Hartwell JW. Sleep staging of ambulatory tape-recorded polysomnographic data: what a difference an epoch makes. *J Clin Neurophysiol* 1987;4:215.
6. Erwin CW, Ebersole JS, Marsh GR. Combined auditory-visual scoring of polysomnographic data at 60 times real time. *J Clin Neurophysiol* 1987;4:214.
7. Rechtschaffen A, Kales A, eds. *A manual of standardized terminology, techniques, and scoring system for sleep stages in human subjects.* Los Angeles: Brain Information Service/Brain Research Institute, UCLA, 1968. (Also available as NIH Publ 204, US Govt Printing Office, Washington DC, 1968.)

Ambulatory EEG Monitoring,
edited by John S. Ebersole.
Raven Press, Ltd., New York © 1989

17

Clinical Utility of Cassette Polysomnography in Sleep and Sleep-Related Disorders

W. Vaughn McCall, Jack D. Edinger, and C. William Erwin

Ambulatory Sleep Laboratory, Duke University Medical Center, Durham, North Carolina 27710

Sleep-related disorders have been recognized and described for centuries but received little more than passing interest by organized medicine until the late 1960s, when investigations of the disorder now known as sleep apnea syndrome began (1). Various investigations of this and other sleep disorders resulted in 1975 in the formation of the Association of Sleep Disorders Centers (ASDC) and publication of an ASDC diagnostic classification of some 80 sleep disorders (2).

Recognition and diagnosis of these disorders were made possible to a large extent by development of polysomnography. Hans Berger's discovery of electroencephalographic (EEG) differences between sleeping and waking was followed by the Loomis et al. classification of EEG sleep stages (3). Aserinsky's (4) finding of rapid eye movements (REM) during discrete sleep periods and the subsequent description of tonic decrease in chin electromyogram (EMG) during REM sleep complete the minimal number of three parameters required for contemporary sleep-stage scoring (5). The discovery of the wide variety of physiologic changes that may occur during sleep has necessitated an expansion of polysomnographic monitoring. In addition to EEG, electrooculogram (EOG), and chin EMG, other parameters are often necessary including measures of respiratory airflow, thoracic expansion, abdominal expansion, esophageal pressure as an indicator of respiratory effort, oximetry, EKG, esophageal pH, anterior tibialis EMG, penile tumescence, multiple EEG derivations, temperature, and others. Various EEG montages may be required, depending on the question being asked, necessitating the use of a minimum of four to, at times, 20 or more channels of polygraphy.

Ambulatory polysomnography has developed closely behind the growth in the corresponding technology. Ambulatory polysomnography implies the recording of physiologic data during sleep from a subject who is free from attachment to stationary physiologic recording devices. Data are either transmitted and stored remotely or recorded on a device attached to the patient. The earliest methods of ambulatory monitoring employed the transmission of data to a remote display and/or recording device. Data transmission was accomplished using radio frequencies and telephone. These methods were employed as early as 1921 for EKG and 1949 for the recording of EEG.

Although these methods were technically feasible, both are encumbered with numerous disadvantages. Radio transmission from an on-the-body transmitter had a short range due to both legal and physical limitations on the range of the transmitter; usually, this was in the range of several hundred feet. With this method, the patient must remain "in range" of the receiver and is not free to be truly ambulatory. In contrast, telephone transmission allows the patient/subject to be a much greater distance from the laboratory. However, the technologist must go to the home of the patient/subject at the beginning and end of the study to attach electrodes, set up equipment, establish the telephone connection, and reverse the process at the end of the study. The patient is no more ambulatory than if the recording were in a typical laboratory and all "trips" away from the bed require a disconnection from the transmission equipment. Nonetheless, telephone equipment has been used for home sleep recordings (6).

More recently developed ambulatory monitoring systems allow for the recording of data on a tape recorder directly attached to the patient/subject. These devices currently record in an analog mode and can store large amounts of data on an inexpensive medium (audiotape). The development of these cassette monitoring systems coincidentally paralleled the establishment of sleep-disorders medicine. Although the "Holter Electrocardiographic Monitor" was first designed in 1961, a multichannel recorder suitable for polysomnographic application did not become available until 1971 (7). Wilkinson was the first to report polysomnographic cassette monitoring of acceptable technical quality in 1973 (8).

AMBULATORY VERSUS LABORATORY POLYSOMNOGRAPHY

Currently, there are several manufacturers offering telephone and radio telemetry and cassette ambulatory polysomnographic monitoring systems. These ambulatory systems have important advantages and disadvantages in comparison with traditional in-laboratory overnight sleep studies. Among the principal disadvantages for sleep recordings is the limited number of channels if continuous recordings are made (6) and compromise of both high and low (DC) response characteristics on some systems. Other limitations of ambulatory techniques relate to the difficulty in making necessary behavioral correlates to polysomnographic events. Examples of this problem include the lack of observation of snoring and grunting respirations in obstructive sleep apnea, leg movements in nocturnal myoclonus, and the complex nocturnal behaviors accompanying the parasomnias and the REM–motor disinhibition syndromes. This lack may be partially compensated by the addition of video monitoring (see Chapter 10, this volume), but currently, the difficulties of sending the technologist to the patient's home or instructing the patient to set up such equipment as well as the problems of synchronizing the physiologic and video data are sufficiently great to make the effort expensive and tedious.

The presence of a technologist at the recording site, as in standard in-laboratory studies, facilitates the reattachment of lost polygraphic leads and repositioning of the sleeper. The technologist is particularly valuable during studies on the sleep-apnea patient. The hundreds of brief arousals that are typical of the sleep-apnea patient often result in dislodging of an electrode or oximetry monitor. Furthermore, many cases of sleep apnea will not manifest their full severity until the patient is supine. In these instances, a technician is needed to monitor and sometimes change the position of the patient.

The Multiple Sleep Latency Test (MSLT) is a standardized assessment of excessive sleepiness. Current recommendations for the MSLT specify that the subject be given a minimum of four opportunities to sleep throughout the testing day while undergoing polysomnographic monitoring. The MSLT is conducted in the laboratory, and, on each sleep opportunity, the patient is connected to the polygraph, given specific instructions to sleep, and disconnected at the end of each test session. The ritual of connecting the patient and giving instructions is an important aspect of the test standardization. Using continuous ambulatory monitoring in lieu of the laboratory polygraph seems intuitively acceptable, but, as yet, this substitution of technique has not been validated (9). In our institution, on occasion, we use ambulatory monitoring on the night prior to the MSLT to assess the quality and duration of sleep. A sleep-deprived patient will obviously have excessive daytime sleepiness and also an increased likelihood of short REM latencies.

Three important advantages counterbalance the disadvantages of ambulatory monitoring. It has long been recognized that testing a normal subject in the novel laboratory setting may introduce disruptions of sleep not seen in the home and, hence, lead to erroneous conclusions. This so-called first-night effect has been best studied in normal volunteers with consistent findings in children (10) and adults (11). The first night of in-laboratory recording is distinguished by a prolonged sleep latency, excessive nocturnal awakenings, poor sleep efficiency, prolonged REM latency, and decreased REM percent and activity. The degree to which this phenomenon is seen in disorders of initiating and maintaining sleep (DIMS) patients is open to some debate. Some depressive disorders may have a lessened first-night effect, and some psychophysiologic disorders may, in fact, have better sleep in the laboratory than at home. It seems likely that ambulatory polysomnography provides a more "natural" sample of the patient's sleep with a lesser degree of first-night effects and, thereby, reduces the need to do multiple overnight studies. Preliminary reports indicate that ambulatory cassette recording is associated with some first-night decrement in slow-wave sleep but not with the other more clinically significant first-night effects of in-laboratory testing (12). Early findings from one of our studies of ambulatory polysomnography show a decrement in total sleep time on the first night of recording as compared with two subsequent nights of recording. Clearly, this work needs replication and extension, even though the results are not unexpected. Not only is the patient left untethered by cassette monitoring, but the electrodes are applied many hours before retiring for the night, thus providing a prolonged period for adaptation to occur.

Naturalistic recording in the patient's home may well be superior to traditional laboratory methods in assessing the severity of those sleep disorders aggravated by interaction with the environment. Persistent psychophysiologic insomnia may be linked to arousal cues associated with the patient's own bedroom. Certain environmental factors such as noise and heat may exacerbate insomnia (2).

An unequivocal advantage of ambulatory monitoring is the extended recording capability. Although the patient's complaint may be limited to either excessive daytime somnolence (EDS) or nocturnal insomnia, in many instances the underlying disturbance affects the entire 24-hr period. Indeed, it is more likely than not that the patient with significant DIMS will have an associated excessive daytime sleepiness and those with disorders of excessive somnolence (DOES) will have an associated nocturnal sleep disturbance. Full 24-hr continuous monitoring is possible on several brands of cassette recorders. An extended recording may reveal excessive daytime napping in an elderly patient complaining of insomnia or the fragmented nocturnal sleep of the narcoleptic patient with daytime sleep attacks.

There is little evidence as yet to show that polysomnographic data obtained by ambulatory monitoring are or are not comparable to the "gold standard" of the traditional in-laboratory paper recording, in terms of intrarater reproducibility or interrater reliability. Good interrater reliability (13) and intrarater reproducibility (14) can be achieved when ambulatory cassette recordings are interpreted directly from a scanner. A recently completed investigation evaluated interrater reliability between ambulatory cassette sleep records scored from the display screen (one screen at a time), from the screen (at 20 times real time), and from traditional paper printout (15). Results show that, for eight normal sleepers and eight DIMS patients, the interrater reliability of three scorers ranged between 85 and 88% (epoch-by-epoch comparisons) for the three techniques, with a greater interrater agreement for paper-scored records than for the other two techniques. Direct epoch-by-epoch comparisons of cassette-recorded data reduction by high-speed screen, slow-speed screen, and paper recordings offer special technical problems related to synchronization of the different formats (16). However, standard sleep parameters computed for the three techniques showed significant correlation coefficients ($p < 0.01$) for the three techniques, indicating that such data can be scored directly on the screen at multiples of real time.

With today's technology, the quality of the raw electrophysiologic data is not as good from the cassette recorders of some manufacturers as that obtained in the laboratory. Although the reduced high-frequency response of some cassette recorders (> 40 Hz) is often given as primary technical difference, we find the lack of a qualified technologist to monitor the study throughout the night to be equally important. Recording of behavioral observation, as well as the correction of defective electrode contacts, makes the average laboratory study more visually appealing. This is obviously a double-edged sword, because the absence of the technologist provides at least two advantages. First, costs of the study are reduced, and, more important, the patient is able to sleep in more familiar home or hospital surroundings, which should lead to a reduced first-night effect.

A study from our laboratory (17) reveals that, despite the increased level of artifact and lack of detailed notation, the majority of ambulatory polysomnographic studies (90.0%; 305/399) were judged to be of good technical quality, and, with the exception of some decrement in the quality of the EMG recordings, were of a quality comparable to polygraphic records. An additional 22 studies (6.5%) were interpretable but had one or more channels compromised; 12 studies (3.5%) were uninterpretable. A critical electrode(s) was lost in four of the 12 uninterpretable studies, the recorder malfunctioned in three cases, three patients prematurely terminated the study by removing the electrodes, and the tape wound around the capstan in two studies. Further, of the 12 inadequate diagnostic studies, 10 occurred in the first 50 patients studied.

Our impression is that patient acceptance of the procedure is high. In an ongoing study, the acceptance factor is being assessed in a formal fashion comparing responses to questionnaires completed the morning after ambulatory polysomnography to various clinical diagnostic and sleep parameters. An issue related to acceptance is the degree of first-night effect as compared to traditional hardwire techniques. Subjects who have experienced both stationary and ambulatory studies report better first-night sleep with the ambulatory apparatus. This is being evaluated in an ongoing study.

In some instances, an ambulatory technique may be preferable for the diagnosis of a particular sleep disorder, while in-laboratory recording may be preferable for a different disorder. The technique selected should be based on the suspected disorder. In general, we find the ambulatory approach best for DIMS patients and in-laboratory studies best for DOES patients. At many centers, the choice is made on the basis of equipment on hand.

Ambulatory monitoring is useful not only in disorders of sleep but also in investigations of the sleep of normal subjects in circumstances not allowing for in-laboratory recordings. Finnegan et al. reported on ambulatory sleep recordings in high-altitude mountaineers (18). A reduction in slow-wave sleep was seen at high altitudes compared against baseline sea-level recordings. The author finds this result consistent with mountain climbers' complaint of poor sleep while climbing.

CLINICAL APPLICATIONS

The remaining chapters in this book focus on a select number of important sleep-related disorders. The following, however, is a discussion of the utility of ambulatory monitoring in sleep disorders, which illustrates the broad applicability of these techniques. The ASDC nosology divides the sleep disorders into four large groups: (a) DIMS, (b) DOES, (c) disorders of the sleep-wake schedule, and (d) the dysfunctions associated with sleep, sleep stages, or partial arousals (parasomnias) (2).

A diagnostic classification of DIMS lists nine major categories and 21 subcategories (2). Historically, physicians have been willing to take the patient's complaint (insomnia) as the correct diagnosis (insomnia) and offer specific medications for its treatment without physical or laboratory findings to corroborate the diagnosis. As a result, there have been few reports on ambulatory monitoring in DIMS. The lack of publication in this area is unfortunate, because of the inherent suitability of DIMS to ambulatory monitoring. Less than 10% of patients with DIMS are diagnosed as having sleep apnea; therefore, the multiple channels often required for sleep-apnea evaluation may be omitted, allowing for 8-channel monitoring (19).

Although the opinion persists that most DIMS sufferers can be accurately diagnosed by history alone (20), our preliminary findings from the study of 85 DIMS outpatients suggest otherwise (21). The EMG bursts and associated EEG arousals of periodic leg movements (PLM) can only be detected by polysomnography. PLM was revealed by ambulatory monitoring in 23.5% of the 85 patients. On clinical grounds, the diagnosis was suspected in 19 patients but confirmed in only 11, and, thus, 42% of the suspected PLM patients would have been inappropriately treated had the clinical diagnosis been accepted. In addition, nine cases were confirmed as having significant PLM in the subgroup of 66 in whom the disorder was not suspected, and, thus, 14% of this group would not have received beneficial treatment had the clinical diagnosis been accepted as final.

Mild apnea was suspected in six patients, but for none was the condition confirmed by polysomnography. Seventy-nine gave no indication of apnea, but apnea, revealed by later laboratory studies to be significant obstructive apnea, was initially discovered in two (3%) of the patients by ambulatory recordings. Five patients were found to have no DIMS abnormality. Their polysomnographic data were markedly discrepant from their sleep diaries for the night of the recording, which did not differ from their chronic complaints.

Of the remainder, 42.3% were diagnosed clinically as "psychiatric," 7.1% as "substance dependence," and 15.3% as "psychophysiologic disorder." With the exceptions noted above, the polysomnographic findings were confirmatory or consistent with the suspected clinical diagnosis.

Sleep apnea, narcolepsy, and periodic movements during sleep account for more than 70% of the final diagnoses of patients with DOES (19). Successful application of ambulatory technique has been reported for all three diagnoses. Peter et al. studied the incidence of sleep apnea in 20 patients with congestive heart failure (CHF), 100 patients with uncomplicated angina, 72 outpatients in a general medical clinic, and 68 healthy young controls (22). The study was performed using a 4-channel ambulatory cassette system measuring abdominal respiratory effort, thoracic respiratory effort, EKG, and transcutaneous Po_2. A higher incidence of sleep apnea was found in patients with CHF (55%) than in healthy controls (10%). This study illustrates the large number of patients who can be screened with this simple technique.

Ambulatory cassette polysomnography in patients with narcolepsy has demonstrated multiple brief spontaneous naps, many with sleep-onset REM periods, and disrupted nocturnal sleep (23). The longest naps were often occurring in the afternoon, reflecting perhaps an exaggeration of the increased tendency of normal subjects to sleep in the afternoon (24). Ambulant recordings of the narcoleptic patient in his home environment indicate that usual activity levels showed a generally successful suppression of daytime microsleep; only 11% of the daytime recording time was spent asleep (25). The authors concluded, however, that ambulatory monitoring does not substitute for MSLT in the evaluation of narcolepsy (see Chapter 18).

One laboratory has reported using ambulatory cassette monitoring routinely and with success in patients with DOES (26). For purposes of diagnosing periodic movements of sleep, this laboratory recommends listening to the anterior tibialis EMG channel played back at 60 times real time for detection of movements, with visual scanning of the EEG for identification of which movements produced arousals.

Sleep apnea is an important cause of "near miss" sudden infant death syndrome (SIDS). Ambulatory cassette monitoring is reported to provide a technically acceptable means of performing at-home evaluations of infants at risk for SIDS (27). For many cases of infantile sleep apnea, no treatable cause can be identified; in these instances, an ambulatory home warning system may alert the parents to recurrent episodes of severe apnea (28).

Extended monitoring may be most directly applicable to disorders of the sleep-wake schedule. These disorders are characterized by the patient's inability to wake at the desired times despite achieving normal overall amounts of unimpaired sleep or to sleep at the desired time despite a normal preceding period of wakefulness (2). These disorders are truly circadian in nature and demand extended monitoring for thorough evaluation.

Among the more common of the disorders of the sleep-wake schedule is that occurring with changing shift work. Ambulatory cassette recording of 25 male paper-mill workers with a continuous three-shift system has demonstrated disrupted sleep periods and involuntary dozing while at work (29). The implications of this study for worker safety and productivity are enormous. Long-term ambulatory temperature monitoring has been useful in understanding delayed sleep phase syndrome (30).

Reports concerning the use of ambulatory monitoring for parasomnias are yet forthcoming. Although limited in scope, our laboratory has found the combination of ambulatory monitoring and videotape monitoring helpful in the diagnosis of sleep-related childhood headbanging. We anticipate that, for certain parasomnias (e.g., sleepwalking), ambulatory monitoring could be particularly revealing. With ambulatory technology, an untethered sleepwalker would be free to engage in walking episodes and have these episodes monitored continuously. This approach should enable clinicians and researchers better to understand the nature of sleep during such episodes. This knowledge, in turn, may lead to a better understanding of the pathology underlying such behaviors.

In addition to these applications, ambulatory monitoring has begun to uncover the relationship between sleep and various medical disorders. The peak time of day for sudden cardiac death occurs at the REM-sleep–rich period of 5 to 6 a.m. (2). Ambulatory monitoring has been employed to study the relationship of ventricular ectopy to sleep stages (31). The investigators concluded that ventricular ectopy diminished during all sleep stages as compared with awake periods.

Ambulatory monitoring has been applied to other systemic dysfunctions associated with sleep, including esophageal reflux and impotence. Ambulatory monitoring of esophageal pH suggests that sleep-related gastroesophageal reflux may be the critical factor in the development of esophagitis (32). Ambulatory monitoring of penile erections during sleep as a basis for investigating the problem of erectile impotence has been reported to be technically acceptable and does not suffer from the "first night" decrease in REM sleep seen in in-laboratory recordings (33). Erections during sleep are REM-linked; first-night-effect loss of REM sleep not uncommonly results in invalid studies.

This brief overview shows the breadth of applications of ambulatory monitoring in sleep and sleep-related disorders. No doubt other applications are yet untapped.

REFERENCES

1. Guilleminault C. Obstructive sleep apnea. *Med Clin NA* 1985;69:1187–1203.
2. Association of Sleep Disorders Centers. *Diagnostic classification of sleep and arousal disorders.* First edition, prepared by the Sleep Disorders Classification Committee, HP Roffwarg, Chairman. *Sleep* 1979;2:1–137.
3. Loomis AL, Harvey EN, Hobart GA. Further observations on potential rhythms of cerebral cortex during sleep. *Science* 1935;82:188–200.
4. Aserinsky E, Kleitman N. Regularly occurring periods of eye motility and concomitant phenomena during sleep. *Science* 1953;118:273–274.
5. Rechtschaffen A, Kales A, eds. *A manual of standardized terminology, techniques, and scoring system for sleep stages in human subjects.* Los Angeles: Brain Information Service/Brain

Research Institute, UCLA, 1968. (Also available as NIH Publ 204, US Govt Printing Office, Washington DC, 1968.)
6. Sewitch DE, Kupfer DJ. A comparison of the telediagnostic and Medilog systems for recording normal sleep in the home environment. *Psychophysiology* 1985;22:718–726.
7. Stott FD. Introductory remarks. *Postgrad Med J* 1976;52(suppl 7):11–13.
8. Wilkinson RT, Mullaney D. Electroencephalogram recording of sleep in the home. *Postgrad Med J* 1976;52(suppl 7):92–96.
9. Carskadon MA. Guidelines for the multiple sleep latency test. *Sleep* 1986;9:519–524.
10. Coble PA, Kupfer DJ, Renolds CF, et al. EEG sleep of healthy children 6 to 12 years of age. In: Guilleminault L, ed. *Sleep and its disorders in children.* New York: Raven Press, 1987.
11. Hauri P. *The sleep disorder.* Kalamazoo: Scope Publications, 1982.
12. Sharpley AL, Solomon R, Cowen P. First night effect on sleep using ambulatory cassette recording. *Sleep Res* 1987;16:579.
13. Patterson N, Ball S, Cohen SA, et al. Medilog 9000: recording quality. *Sleep Res* 1986;15:252.
14. Erwin CW, Ebersole JS, Marsh GR. Combined auditory-visual scoring of polysomnographic data at 60 times real time. *J Clin Neurophysiol* 1987;4:214.
15. Hoelscher TJ, McCall MW, Powell J, et al. Sleep scoring with the Oxford Medilog 9000: comparison to conventional paper scoring. *Sleep* (in press).
16. Erwin CW, Hartwell JW. Sleep staging of ambulatory tape-recorded polysomnographic data: what a difference an epoch makes. *J Clin Neurophysiol* 1987;4:215.
17. Hoelscher TJ, Erwin CW, Marsh GR, et al. Ambulatory sleep monitoring with the Oxford-Medilog 9000: technical acceptability, patient acceptance and clinical indications. *Sleep* 1987;10:606–607.
18. Finnegan TP, Abraham P, Docherty TB. Ambulatory monitoring of the electroencephalogram in high altitude mountaineers. *Electroencephalogr Clin Neurophysiol* 1985;60:220–224.
19. Coleman RM, Roffwarg HP, Kennedy SJ, et al. Sleep-wake disorders based on a polysomnographic diagnosis. *JAMA* 1982;247:997–1003.
20. Tan T, Kales JD, Kales A, et al. Inpatient multidimensional management of treatment-resistant insomnia. *Psychosomatics* 1987;28:266–272.
21. Edinger JD, Hoelscher TJ, Marsh GR, et al. Polysomnographic assessment of DIMS: empirical evaluation of diagnostic value. *Sleep* (in press).
22. Peter JH, Fuchs E, Kohler U, et al. Studies in the prevalence of sleep apnea activity. *Eur J Resp Dis* 1986;69(suppl 146):451–458.
23. deGroen J, Koper M, Bergs PPE, et al. Ambulatory sleep-wake polygraphy in narcolepsy. *Electroencephalogr Clin Neurophysiol* 1985;60:420–422.
24. Broughton R, Dunham W, Suwalski W, et al. Ambulant 24-hour sleep/wake recordings in narcolepsy-catalepsy. *Sleep Res* 1986;15:109.
25. Broughton R, Dunham W, Suwalski W, et al. Can ambulant home monitoring of sleep-wake patterns diagnose narcolepsy? *Sleep Res* 1987;16:318.
26. Kayed K, Wilson J. Ambulatory recording of periodic movements during sleep in patients complaining of excessive daytime sleepiness. *Sleep Res* 1987;16:558.
27. Cornwell AC, Weitzman ED, Marmaron A. Ambulatory and in-hospital continuous recording of sleep state and cardiorespiratory parameters in "near-miss" for the sudden infant death syndrome. *Biotelemetry* 1978;5:113–122.
28. Guilleminault C. Obstructive sleep apnea syndrome in children. In: Guilleminault C, ed. *Sleep and its disorders in children.* New York: Raven Press, 1987.
29. Torsvall L, Akerstedt T, Gillander K, et al. 24 H ambulatory EEG recordings of sleep/wakefulness in shift work. *Sleep Res* 1987;16:256.
30. Kokkoris CP, Weitzman ED, Pollak CP, et al. Long-term ambulatory temperature monitoring in a subject with a hypernychthemeral sleep-wake cycle disturbance. *Sleep* 1978;1:177–180.
31. Pickering TG, Johnston J, Honour AJ. Comparison of the effects of sleep, exercise and autonomic drugs on ventricular extrasystoles, using ambulatory monitoring of electrocardiogram and electroencephalogram. *Am J Med* 1978;65:575–583.
32. Orr WC, Robinson MG. Esophageal reflux during waking and sleeping documented with ambulatory pH recording. *Sleep Res* 1986;15:151.
33. Bennett T, Evans DF, Hosking DJ. A technique for monitoring penile erections during sleep as a basis for investigating the problem of erectile impotence. In: Stott FD, ed. *Proceeding of the second international symposium on ambulatory monitoring.* London: Academic Press, 1978.

Ambulatory EEG Monitoring,
edited by John S. Ebersole.
Raven Press, Ltd., New York © 1989

18

Ambulatory Sleep-Wake Monitoring in the Hypersomnias

Roger J. Broughton

Division of Neurology, University of Ottawa, Ottawa, Ontario K1H 816 Canada

Sleep disorders have been classified (1) into four main groups: the hypersomnias [disorders of excessive sleepiness (DOES), usually associated with increased duration and depth of sleep], insomnias [disorders of initiating and/or maintaining sleep (DIMS)], the sleep-wake schedule disorders (circadian rhythm sleep disorders), and the parasomnias (episodic disorders within sleep).

The hypersomnia group, of interest to us here, includes a large number of individual conditions: narcolepsy-cataplexy syndrome, idiopathic hypersomnia, the many symptomatic hypersomnias (posttraumatic, infectious, demyelinating, tumoral), the non-CNS symptomatic hypersomnias (from fever, metabolic disease, toxic conditions), the recurrent hypersomnias (Kleine-Levin syndrome, menstrual hypersomnia, bipolar affective illness), substance-related forms (CNS depressants, tolerance or withdrawal from stimulants), movement-related disorders (especially periodic movements in sleep and fragmentary myoclonus), and those related to respiratory disorders in sleep (especially obstructive and mixed sleep apnea, and nocturnal hypoventilation). It is, indeed, a heterogeneous group.

Ambulatory monitoring of sleep-wake patterns can be of great assistance in the assessment of the hypersomnias. This important group, moreover, is quite common and represents over 40% of all patients referred to sleep-disorder centers (2). Sleep apnea and periodic movements in sleep are covered by other volume chapters. This chapter will deal with the more traditional neurological hypersomnias, in particular, with narcolepsy, idiopathic hypersomnia, the recurrent hypersomnias, and the assessment of the excessive daytime sleepiness (EDS) present between sleep episodes in all these conditions.

The hypersomnias are of clinical importance for several reasons. The first is their high incidence. The overall group high frequency of presentation for investigation has already been mentioned. Narcolepsy is much more common than previously believed, with current prevalence figures being 40 to 70 per

100,000 (3,4). It is, therefore, about one-half as common as Parkinson's disease and more common than multiple sclerosis or Huntington's chorea. Idiopathic hypersomnia, a genetic condition, appears to be relatively rare in North America; but in some countries, such as Czechoslovakia, is more frequently seen than narcolepsy (5). The symptomatic hypersomnias are very common; unfortunately, no reliable prevalence figures are available. A second reason concerns their marked socioeconomic effects. These are well documented in controlled studies for both narcolepsy (6) and idiopathic hypersomnia (7) and are as great as in major forms of epilepsy (8). A third reason is their typical chronicity, and a fourth their usual poor response to treatment, especially of the EDS (9,10), which is the main cause of the marked socioeconomic effects. Finally, fuller understanding of these conditions has suffered, because of the technical difficulties and high costs in investigating them fully by traditional means.

The usual means of investigating the sleep-wake features of hypersomniac patients have consisted of in-laboratory overnight (or occasionally 24-hr) polysomnography and the Multiple Sleep Latency Test (MSLT) (11) or its variants. Such 24-hr recordings are extremely time-consuming and expensive, requiring three shifts of support staff with attendant overnight work and tie up an entire laboratory room for a prolonged period. Overnight polysomnography will detect respiratory, movement, or other possible EDS causes, but it will not document the nature of either the daytime sleep or the overall sleep-wake disturbances. The MSLT and its variants are very useful to quantify EDS, and, when two or more sleep-onset REM periods (SOREMPs) are recorded, the MSLT assists in the diagnosis of narcolepsy (12). Yet, these tests tie up an EEG room for some 10 hr for a single, if important and reliable, EDS measure; and they give no information concerning daytime sleep in the real-life home or work situation.

Ambulatory monitoring has a number of advantages over these other procedures in the investigation of the hypersomnias. (a) They can readily determine the amount, type, and timing of sleep around the 24 hr. This is of particular importance in the daytime period, when maximum alertness is desired. (b) They can indicate to what extent underlying once-a-day circadian (13,14), twice-a-day circasemidian (15,16), and more rapid ultradian (17,18) biological rhythms of sleep tendency are altered or preserved. Changes in the chronobiological aspects add to our understanding of their physiopathogenesis and, in selected cases, can have actual localizing value for CNS lesions. (c) Such studies can be combined with sleep logs or use of an event marker to explore the frequency and timing of ancillary symptoms like catalexy and sleep paralysis in narcolepsy, or the sleep drunkenness (19) and amnesic automatisms (20) that may be seen in various forms of hypersomnia. (d) Ambulant monitoring is particularly useful in objectifying the response of nocturnal and diurnal sleep to medication. (e) Technologist costs and laboratory overhead are greatly reduced. (f) Representative sleep patterns are documented in the normal environment without unnatural patient restraint by plug-in electrodes. (g) Finally, such unrestrained home studies provide conditions of greater convenience to patients, who need not stay in a hospital setting and can return to their everyday household or work activities.

Our laboratories have been investigating hypersomnia patients using the 24-hr ambulatory recording technique since 1974 (21). These investigations have only been possible by the greatly appreciated assistance of numerous colleagues (see Acknowledgments). The studies have involved several hundred hypersomnia patients and have been performed with a number of objectives in mind. These include patient assessment and diagnosis; controlled research comparisons of sleep between a patient group and matched normals; documentation of effects of treatment; study, in combination with wrist actographs, of rest-activity cycles related to sleep-wake patterns and attempts to define actographic predictors of sleep or wake state; introduction of ambulatory home MSLT tests; development of automatic sleep-wake analysis from the cassette recordings; and efforts (to date unsuccessful) to perform reliable spectral analysis on ambulant data. Examples of most of these will be provided later. We have found that, with due care, entirely satisfactory recordings may be obtained in this group of patients for all these purposes.

As for any procedure, there are, of course, a number of disadvantages as well as advantages. (a) No documentation of behavior is available equivalent to videotape or film studies or even to the notes of technologists written directly on in-laboratory paper-writeout studies. (b) The number of channels is restricted, eight being the maximum in currently available commercial systems. (c) Technical problems (such as electrodes losing firm contact or battery failure) almost always go unnoticed until playback of the data and may require a repeat study. (d) The cassette motor drive causes some degree of noise and may bother the sleep of certain patients.

This chapter will consider the methodology and the results we have had in this group of patients. To our knowledge, there are no publications on ambulatory monitoring in the hypersomnias from other centers so that comparisons can only be made with traditional in-laboratory studies.

METHODOLOGY

Our experience involves the use of both the 4-channel and, since 1982, the 8-channel Medilog apparatuses (Oxford Medical Systems, Abingdon, U.K., and Clearwater, Florida). Because nocturnal sleep in both normals and patients is a main determinant of alertness/sleepiness the next day, and considering convenience for both laboratory personnel and the patient, we have almost always begun 24-hr (or at times 48-hr) recordings in the late afternoon, normally at 1730 hr. The 24-hr recording, therefore, covers the evening, overnight, and following morning and afternoon periods. Essentially all patients have received a prior traditional overnight polysomnogram to rule out clinically significant amounts of sleep apnea or periodic movements in sleep.

The derivations used for 4-channel recorders have generally included a central lead referred to the contralateral earlobe, right outer canthus electrooculogram (EOG) referred to contralateral mastoid, left outer canthus EOG referred to the contralateral mastoid, and submental electromyogram (EMG). Bilateral EOGs are preferable in order to see out-of-phase potentials with lateral eye movements, although, in some studies, a referential occipital lead and a single-channel right-to-left outer canthus EOG (22) have been substituted. The usual montage for the 8-channel recorders has been: C4-A1, O2-A2, RE-M1, LE-M2, submental EMG, precordial EKG, with the remaining two channels as desired (e.g., central body temperature, respiratory rate). All EEG electrode position locations are those of the international 10/20 system (23).

Dissatisfaction with results using ambulatory monitoring in a number of centers has been attributable to transferring the same level of technical care used in overnight polysomnography. Ambulatory monitoring unquestionably requires a higher order of care to ensure the quality of (unseen) tape recordings. The EEG electrodes must be very solidly anchored with gauze and collodion. EOG electrodes are attached using a high-quality sticky tape such as Micropore. (Collodion and gauze should *never* be used for EOG, because facial movements will lift the electrodes off the skin surface, and removal with acetone or alcohol poses risks to the cornea.) The sticky tape covering the EOG electrode wire is carefully anchored with a piece at right angles over its exit end. Submental EMG and precordial EKG are similarly placed with sticky tape using appropriate anchoring crosspieces.

Other technical details can greatly increase the likelihood of acceptable high-quality recordings. Electrode impedances should, of course, be checked carefully and be less than 5000 Ω. A calibration signal should be recorded on the tape through the apparatus' preamplifiers prior to recording physiological data and is used to ensure precise calibration of the paper playback record. (We routinely place a 100-μV sinusoidal signal for 1 to 2 min at the start of the tape.) It is essential to use batteries of known shelf life. If a local supplier cannot supply this information, it is best to order batteries directly from the manufacturer. In subjects bothered by tape motor noise, the recorder may be taken off the belt and placed under the pillow. Such patients, however, if getting up to go to the bathroom in the night and on morning awakening, must first replace the recorder on the belt to ensure that electrode wire stain or pulloff does not occur. In patients with sleep drunkenness, this compliance, of course, cannot reasonably be expected.

In all recordings, it is highly desirable to have the subject keep a sleep-wake log. Our center's log is quite simple and consists of 24 vertical rows each divided into halves and representing 0000 to 0030, 0030 to 0100, 0100 to 0130, 0130 to 0200 hr, etc. The patient is instructed to note in each half-hour square whether he was asleep (writes an S) or, if awake, the estimated average level of sleepiness using the 1 to 7 level Stanford Sleepiness Scale (24), which is detailed on the form. Coding is also used to note occurrence of specific symptoms or features including sleep attacks (writes SA), naps (N), cataplexy (C), sleep paralysis (SP), vivid hypnagogic hallucinations (HH), sleep drunkenness (SD), and complex behavior with amnesia (CBA). Such a log greatly facilitates the interpretation of the cassette-recorded data and has significant interest in its own right. It will (along with use of the event marker to record the moments of "lights out" and morning awakening) greatly facilitate the later distinction of the night period from the daytime period; this can otherwise be very difficult or virtually impossible, especially in some narcoleptics. It also provides data on temporal aspects of fluctuations in alertness as well as other clinically useful data including timing of the major symptoms mentioned.

After the recorder is attached, the patient then returns to the normal home or work environment. In studies involving withdrawal of medication, and in all patients with significant EDS for any other reason, subjects are driven home by family members, friends, or laboratory staff. They are told to go about their normal activities other than doing those that would jeopardize the equipment such as heavy sports or bathing. The patient returns the next day 24 hr after leaving (the cassette will record some 25 hr of data), and the equipment is removed and the sleep log checked for clarity.

The cassette is then played back for paper writeout at 20 times recording speed using an Elema-Schonander Mingograph apparatus. A 24-hr recording, therefore, takes some 72 min to write out. Once the playback system is functioning, the technologist has but to make sure that the paper is folding properly. Playback at 60 times recording speed is also possible, but the paper comes out so fast that continuous attention must be paid to it. Because the Mingograph uses low viscosity ink, which is jetted at high speed onto the paper from low-inertia oscillographs suspended in an electromagnetic field, the paper record shows differences from normal pen writeouts. The intensity of the ink record is much less, and the extreme high-frequency response of the EEG apparatus leads to much high-frequency activity riding on the usual EEG waveforms. The human eye, however, rapidly attunes to these differences, and sleep scoring becomes equally reliable as for the usual pen recordings. As we have not been satisfied with the reliability of visual scoring from the Medilog system CRT, and as the reliability of the Oxford automatic sleep staging system is not yet adequately assessed, our published results to date involve exclusively visual analysis of paper writeout.

The scoring criteria we use follow traditional Rechtschaffen-Kales manual (25) norms with some additions. The night period is first defined (26) as beginning with the initial 20 min more of consecutive sleep corresponding to the evening sleep onset time in the sleep logs or "lights out" indicated by the event marker. Similarly, its end is defined as the first 30 min of wakefulness in the morning corresponding to the end of the night period as noted on the sleep log or event marker. Definite criteria are important, because, in some patients with very fragmented night sleep, it may be very difficult to ascertain by sleep-wake patterns alone where the nocturnal and diurnal periods begin and end. In the daytime period, we further divide stage 1 of Rechtschaffen-Kales into substages 1A and 1B by published criteria of Valley and Broughton (27), because these substages have striking effects on ability to perform vigilance-type tasks (28). Stage 1A consists of slowing (by 1 Hz or more) and/or anterior diffusion of the alpha rhythm and is often associated with slow pendular eye movements. Stage 1B consists of medium-voltage mixed-frequency activity equivalent to the usual stage 1. These stages are roughly equivalent to the original stages A and B of Loomis et al. (29). In some studies, daytime wakefulness has been separated into "active wakefulness" (presence of EMG and movement artifact superimposed on the EEG channels) and "quiet wakefulness" (easily interpretable EEG, with or without alpha rhythm and searching eye movements), according to the criteria of Volk et al. (30). All other epoch staging follows the Rechtschaffen-Kales guidelines.

Analysis of daytime sleep episodes (whether sleep attacks or voluntary naps) grouped by different durations, and the REM period efficiency measures, are both done according to the criteria of Broughton and Mamelak (26). The epoch-by-epoch visually scored data are entered directly into a computer terminal. The computer calculates all the summary statistics and prints a publishable quality histogram (31,32), examples of which are provided later. Further technical details particular to other applications are provided in context.

NARCOLEPSY-CATAPLEXY

Traditional in-laboratory 24-hr studies of narcoleptics using long wire or cable recordings with ad lib sleep and lack of patient mobility have generally shown fragmented nocturnal sleep patterns with much daytime sleep and no overall increase in total sleep per 24 hr compared with normals (33-35). Our laboratories have documented the sleep-wake patterns in narcoleptics using ambulatory monitoring alone and in combination with wrist actography. The latter was initially introduced to determine whether narcoleptics have greater amounts of restlessness and movement in their efforts to fight off sleepiness, as found in seated subjects completing long-duration (over 11 hr) performance tests by Volk et al. (30). The main results of these projects will be summarized.

Sleep-Wake Patterns

The 24-hr sleep-wake patterns were most recently studied in 10 narcoleptics (six female, four male, mean age 54.3, SD 14.5 years) withdrawn from tricyclic medication for at least 3 weeks and from methylphenidate for 7 or more days compared with controls matched for age, sex, education, and IQ (36,37). Paper writeouts were analyzed visually using 20-sec epochs. Examples of 24-hr histograms in a typical control subject and a typical narcoleptic are provided in Fig. 1.

The *night period* results (Table 1), in general, confirmed findings previously described by usual overnight polysomnography. These included frequent SOREMPs leading to a short mean and highly variable REM latency, reduced sleep-period efficiency, high amounts of wakefulness after sleep onset (WASO), and a more even distribution of slow wave sleep (SWS) across the night (26). We did not, however, observe the low REM period efficiencies described by others and ourselves (26,38). Whether this sole main difference is particular to ambulant monitoring and will be confirmed in future studies remains to be seen.

Another interesting feature in normals and patients (that we have also

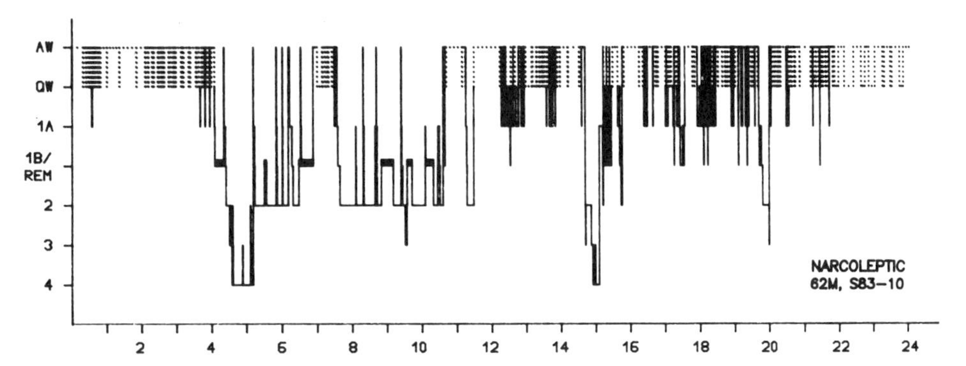

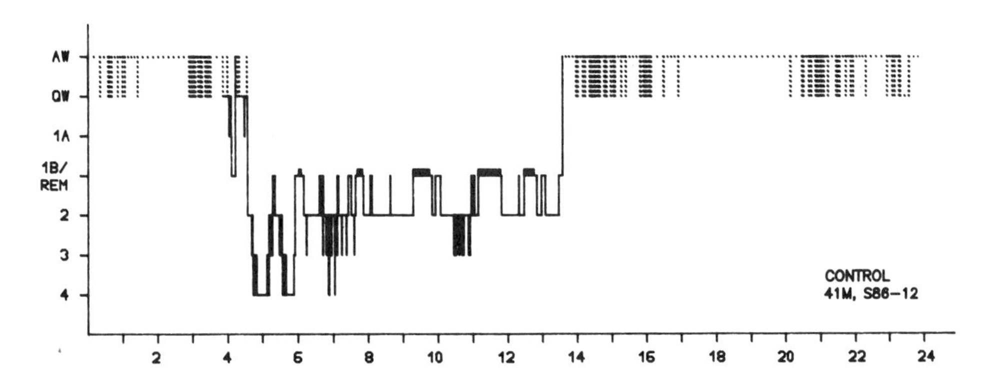

FIG. 1. Histograms of 24-hr ambulant monitoring sleep-wake patterns in a typical patient with narcolepsy-cataplexy **(above)** and matched control **(below).** The narcoleptic shows a nocturnal SOREMP, fragmented night sleep, and high number of stage shifts. In the daytime, there are marked fluctuations of level of alertness, several brief daytime sleep episodes, and two longer ones, the longest being in the midafternoon and containing SWS. The normal control, by comparison, shows a brief episode of late-evening sleepiness followed by well-consolidated normal night sleep patterns and sustained alertness in the daytime. AW, active wakefulness; QW, quiet wakefulness; 1A and 1B, substages 1A and 1B (see text). Other stages following Rechtschaffen-Kales. Time base, hr after recording onset.

TABLE 1. *Night-period sleep-wake patterns in untreated narcoleptics compared with matched controls (N = 10 each group)*

		Narcoleptics		Controls		
		Mean	SD	Mean	SD	*p*
Duration	(min	443.1	147.9	511.3	77.0	ns
TST	(min)	387.2	137.3	475.1	72.6	ns
Sleep eff	(%)	87.3	3.9	93.1	6.3	0.03
WASO	(%)	12.7	3.9	6.9	6.3	0.03
Stage 1	"	12.3	7.1	8.9	7.1	ns
Stage 2	"	32.8	12.2	48.9	7.2	0.002
Stage 3	"	7.1	3.4	5.8	2.1	ns
Stage 4	"	12.9	7.2	9.0	4.6	ns
Stage REM	"	21.0	8.8	18.7	4.7	ns
WASO	(min)	56.0	21.0	36.2	36.9	ns
Stage 1	"	57.5	34.6	44.6	33.6	ns
Stage 2	"	147.7	70.8	248.9	44.1	0.001
Stage 3	"	31.1	16.8	29.3	9.9	ns
Stage 4	"	56.1	34.5	46.8	24.0	ns
Stage REM	"	88.9	39.3	96.6	32.8	ns
Lat. REM	(min)	17.2	33.3	61.7	17.7	0.001
Lat. SWS	"	29.0	17.1	18.8	15.8	ns
REM eff	(%)	89.0	7.7	87.3	10.4	ns
No. Ws > 1 min		9.3	3.0	3.5	2.5	0.0005[a]

All comparisons by ANOVA other than integer (whole-number) data[a], which were by the nonparametric Mann-Whitney U test. ns, Not significant; eff, efficiency; Lat, latency.

repeatedly seen in other studies) is the quite high frequency (about 15–25%) of a short period (usually 10–20 min, sometimes longer) of sleep in the late evening prior to the onset of the consolidated night sleep period. Sleep logs and patient questioning have usually indicated that these sleep episodes occur while reading in a chair or in bed or while watching television. The subject then arouses, goes to bed (if not already there), turns off the light, and enters the true overnight sleep period. These brief evening sleep episodes are entirely missed in routine overnight recordings during which subjects are kept artificially awake until "lights out."

The *daytime* portions indicated, not surprisingly, that narcoleptics obtain much more diurnal sleep than do controls (Table 2). There were significant daytime increases in stages 1A and 1B drowsiness, and in stages 3, 4, and REM sleep. The amount of actual daytime sleep under these real-life conditions is, however, highly variable between patients. We did not find that the amount of actual daytime sleep correlated significantly with objective sleepiness measured by MSLT on a separate day. It seems most likely, therefore, that the amount of daytime sleep obtained is more dependent on the environmental demands and personal choice than on sleep pressure per se. We have found (Table 3) that

TABLE 2. *Day-period sleep-wake patterns in untreated narcoleptics compared with matched controls (N = 10 each group)*

		Narcoleptics		Controls		
		Mean	SD	Mean	SD	p
Duration	(min)	909.0	192.3	924.1	83.1	ns
Total wake	(min)	790.3	203.1	893.4	88.8	ns
Total drowsy/sleep	(min)	133.3	98.0	30.5	46.0	0.008
TST/day period	(%)	18.5	14.0	3.6	5.4	0.006
Active wake	(%)	63.9	13.2	75.8	12.6	0.05
Quiet wake	(%)	19.1	7.8	19.4	8.5	ns
Stage 1A	"	3.3	2.2	1.4	1.3	0.03
Stage 1B	"	3.1	2.0	1.1	1.6	0.02
Stage 2	"	4.8	4.2	1.7	2.8	ns
Stage 3	"	0.8	0.8	0.2	0.4	0.02
Stage 4	"	2.2	3.1	0.2	0.5	ns
Stage REM	"	2.6	2.7	0.2	0.5	0.01
Active wake	(min)	587.3	190.8	702.8	147.4	ns
Quiet wake	"	170.4	67.3	176.9	75.2	ns
Stage 1A	"	32.0	26.9	13.6	13.2	ns
Stage 1B	"	28.0	19.2	10.2	15.5	0.04
Stage 2	"	42.7	39.6	15.8	26.6	ns
Stage 3	"	7.8	6.2	1.5	3.1	0.01
Stage 4	"	18.4	25.4	1.4	4.1	0.05
Stage REM	"	22.0	19.3	1.7	5.3	0.005
SWS interval	(hr)	14.1	3.0	13.6	4.2	ns

All comparisons by ANOVA. ns, Not significant.

TABLE 3. *Daytime nap measures in untreated narcoleptics compared with matched controls (N = 10 each group)*

		Narcoleptics		Controls		
		Mean	SD	Mean	SD	p
No. naps >1 min		2.9	1.2	0.4	0.5	0.0001
No. naps >10 min		2.6	1.1	0.4	0.5	0.0001
Mean nap durn	(min)	46.2	27.9	64.1	59.3	ns[a]
Mean longest nap	(min)	81.0	42.3	64.1	59.3	ns[a]
No. SONREMPs		1.7	1.2	0.4	0.5	0.01
No. SOREMPs		1.2	1.6	0.0	0.0	0.02
No. REMPs		1.6	1.5	0.1	0.3	0.004

All comparisons of data by nonparametric Mann-Whitney U test, other than the noninteger duration measures[a], which were by ANOVA. ns, Not significant; durn, duration.

TABLE 4. *Twenty-four-hr sleep-wake totals in untreated narcoleptics compared with matched controls (N = 10 each group)*

		Narcoleptics		Controls		
		Mean	SD	Mean	SD	*p*
Total wake	(min)	845.6	189.5	917.5	95.6	ns
Total drowsy/sleep	(min)	500.2	148.4	496.8	73.4	ns
Active wake	(%)	44.7	12.4	49.6	9.6	ns
Quiet wake	(%)	13.2	5.2	12.2	6.1	ns
Stage 1A	"	4.3	1.9	2.1	1.6	0.01
Stage 1B	"	6.4	3.3	3.8	3.2	ns
Stage 2	"	14.2	6.4	18.4	3.7	ns
Stage 3	"	2.9	1.5	2.2	0.8	ns
Stage 4	"	5.6	4.3	3.3	1.7	ns
Stage REM	"	8.2	3.9	6.8	2.2	ns
Active wake	(min)	608.4	184.1	712.9	143.4	ns
Quiet wake	"	179.6	70.9	174.4	87.1	ns
Stage 1A	"	57.6	26.2	30.2	23.2	0.02
Stage 1B	"	85.5	44.7	54.8	46.3	ns
Stage 2	"	190.4	86.3	264.6	52.2	0.03
Stage 3	"	38.9	18.2	30.8	11.2	ns
Stage 4	"	74.5	56.1	48.2	23.8	ns
Stage REM	"	110.9	53.4	98.3	31.5	ns

All comparisons by ANOVA. ns, Not significant.

normals not infrequently (about 15% of subjects) obtain daytime sleep, mainly in the form of midafternoon daytime naps, the mean duration being about 0.5 hr.

As well as briefer sleep episodes, most narcoleptics also take one or more prolonged daytime sleeps usually in the midafternoon as voluntary or semi-voluntary naps. The mean duration of these daytime naps in narcoleptics is much longer than expected, being in the order of 80 min, and most contained SWS. The mean interval between the time of onset of SWS (i.e., stage 3) in the night period to the onset of the major daytime peak, when present, was measured in narcoleptics and in controls. It was 14.1 and 13.6 hr, respectively, both being very close to the figure for extended sleep in normals (39,40). Of the average of 2.9 daytime sleep episodes in narcoleptics lasting at least 1 min, only 1.2 contained a SOREMP. These ambulant studies did not confirm the presence of increased amounts of active wakefulness in narcoleptics compared with controls; indeed, a just-significant decrease was found. Finally, outside of overt sleep episodes, narcoleptics showed much "waxing and waning" of alertness compared with controls, rather than so-called microsleeps (20), at least, if one accepts our current laboratory definition of a microsleep as a pattern of definite sleep or sleepiness interrupting sustained waking patterns for 30 sec or less.

The *24-hr totals* (Table 4) of narcoleptics showed somewhat higher amounts of substage 1A mild drowsiness and lesser amounts of stage 2 than in normals.

Otherwise, there were no differences between groups and, specifically, no overall increase of sleep or of sleep plus drowsiness in narcoleptics.

The 24-hr patterns of the main sleep stages have also been graphed for every hour (37) and 2 hr (Fig. 2) in narcoleptics and controls aligning the data for time of evening sleep onset. It can be readily appreciated that sleep is much better sustained across the night of normals and that there is a corresponding marked increase in day sleep in narcoleptics clustering mainly between 15 and 20 hr after sleep onset. In both groups, the maximum amount of REM sleep is in the 7- to 8-hr bin after sleep onset, corresponding well to results in normal greatly extended sleep (40). Both groups show a secondary daytime peak of SWS around 16 to 18 hr after sleep onset and some 14 hr following the first peak after evening sleep onset, again similar to extended sleep (40).

Taken together, these results make a number of important statements about the sleep-wake dysfunction which typifies narcolepsy. The fragmentation of nocturnal sleep is accompanied by a corresponding daytime increase in sleep and sleepiness. Whether the former is primary and the latter a secondary result, or whether both night and day patterns are secondary to an overall 24-hr pathology of sleep-wake regulation is uncertain, but the frequent history of a preceding nocturnal sleep disturbance or of sustained shift work, sleep deprivation, or other altered sleep patterns (6), as well as the therapeutic response to night-sleep consolidating agents such as gamma-hydroxybutyrate (26), both suggest that problems with sustaining the continuity and integration of both NREM and REM sleep are of fundamental importance (41). Because both the main circadian and circasemidian sleep-wake biorhythms are somewhat flattened but otherwise remain relatively normal, the concept of a fundamental and causal circadian biorhythmic disturbance (42) is not strongly supported. There is, however, evidence for considerable disruption of the ultradian REM periodicity during night sleep (35,43,44). The two or more SOREMP criteria of the MSLT cannot be applied to ambulant recordings, as only a mean of 1.2 was found. This number represented, however, an equivalent 41% of sleep episodes over 1 min and 46% of those over 10 min in duration (comparable to the 40% of MSLT naps criterion). Finally, it is evident that narcoleptics have difficulties sustaining daytime alertness that are equivalent to those of sustaining sleep. Both appear to engender the marked difficulties in performance (27).

Movement Measures

The finding of Volk et al. (30) of increasing amounts of daytime "active wakefulness" in narcoleptics compared with matched controls was not confirmed in ambulatory monitoring in the normal home environment. The polygraphic indices of active and passive wakefulness, however, are very indirect measures of motor activity. High-amplitude EMG interferential patterns

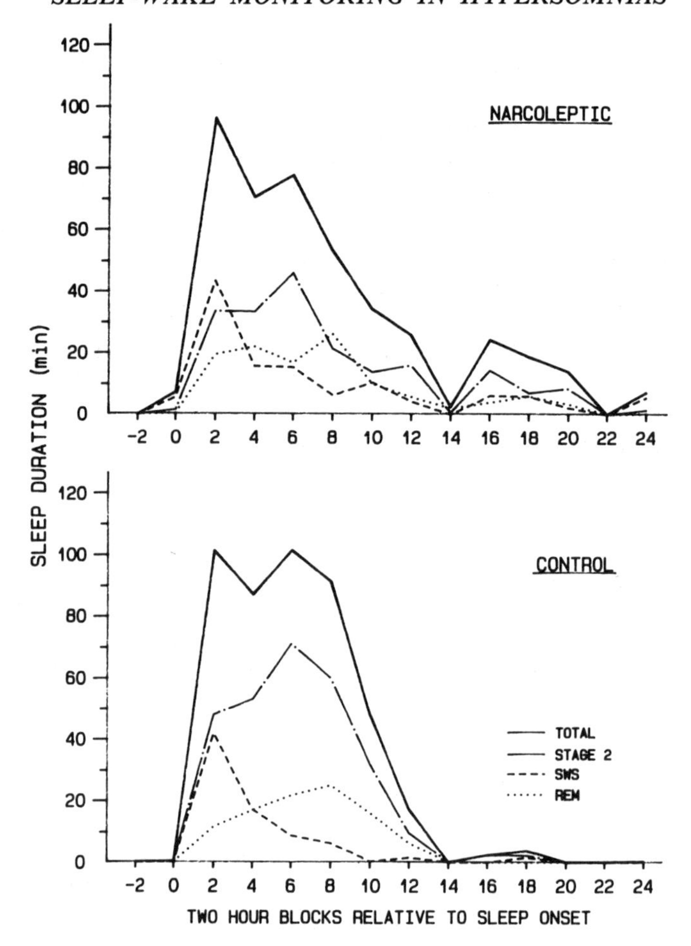

FIG. 2. Histograms of total sleep and individual sleep stages/hr, averaged every 2 hr, in narcoleptics and controls aligning data by hour of sleep onset. In narcoleptics, total sleep is poorly sustained at night, and there is a marked increase of daytime sleep peaking in the 14 to 16- and 16 to 18-hr blocks after sleep onset. In controls, total sleep is well sustained across the night, and there is some sleep in the same blocks after sleep onset corresponding to midafternoon naps in three of the 10 subjects.

obscuring the EEG could, for instance, be due to simple increase in scalp muscle tone rather than to actual movement.

The direct monitoring of movement by actography is an obvious direct measure. Therefore, nondominant wrist actography was performed using the device of Ambulator Monitoring Inc. (New York), combined with 24-hr sleep-wake monitoring by 8-channel Medilog apparatuses. The actograph was programmed to accumulate movement every 20 sec in order to correspond with the sleep-staging epoch. The accuracy of the clocks of both the actograph and Medilog apparatuses permits temporal alignment of the data, and our laboratories are developing software to print combined sleep-wake and movement data. To date, we have analyzed such combined data both to determine whether movement differences exist between narcoleptics and controls and to determine if the actograph data are predictive of the sleep or wake state (45).

We again have found no evidence under normal home conditions that narcoleptics show any overall increase in daytime movement; indeed, the trend is for a decrease. An arbitrary actographic criterion of probable sleep was defined. Sleep was assumed to occur when three or more successive actographic epochs had 20 or fewer activity changes each, and wakefulness was assumed to begin when three or more successive epochs each had 20 or more activity changes. Using these criteria, the actograph had an overall 91% accuracy in predicting sleep or wake state. The actograph confirmed greater nighttime levels of wakefulness (movement) and lower daytime levels (greater apparent sleep) in narcoleptics.

Therefore, it appears that, in normal home conditions, narcoleptics do not fight off drowsiness by increased motor activity. Rather, they have a decrease, which probably relates to actual somnolence or sleep. The results of Volk et al. would suggest that fighting against sleepiness by restlessness may occur only under conditions in which sustained high-performance needs are present. These preliminary results also indicate that wrist actography has promise of becoming a useful tool in the discrimination of sleep and wake states generally.

IDIOPATHIC (CNS) HYPERSOMNIA

Idiopathic hypersomnia is a condition identified by Roth et al. (46) which is characterized by excessively long and deep sleep, increased amounts of daytime sleep, and, in 50% of cases, marked morning sleep drunkenness in which it takes several dozen min or a few hr for the patient to fully awaken. The condition is of CNS origin and is generally familial (although a few sporadic cases have been reported) and in which multiple family members are deep and long sleepers. Patients sometimes sleep for as much as 14 to 18 hr or even more a day.

Our ambulatory experience with this rare cause of referral to the Ottawa General Hospital Sleep Clinic is limited to two patients (female 33 years old; male 51 years old) with a characteristic history and findings. Traditional overnight polysomnography documented long-duration night sleep and ruled out other causes of hypersomnia. Both cases showed prolongation of night sleep being 10.4 hr in one case and 11.4 in the other. Daytime sleepiness and sleep were present in both cases and totaled 1.4 hr in the first patient (Fig. 3) and 3.9 in the other. Sleep stages as a percentage of total sleep time and NREM/REM cyclicity were normal. No sleep-onset REM periods were recorded during the day or night. These findings were similar to those of laboratory-based studies (5,46). Neither patient had significant sleep drunkenness, so that the patterns (19) in this state could not be documented. Both patients showed prolonged

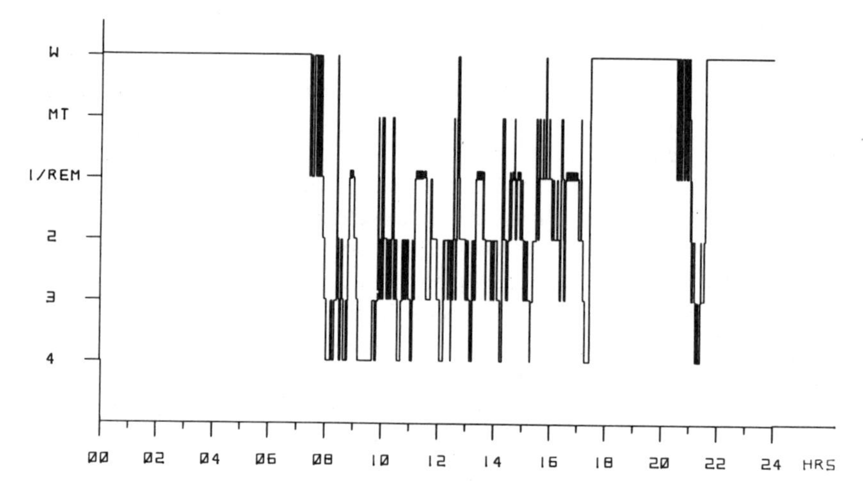

FIG. 3. Idiopathic hypersomnia in a 33-year-old female patient with a strong family history. Night sleep is prolonged (over 10 hr in duration), well sustained across the night with few awakenings, no SOREMP, and with well-defined NREM/REM sleep cyclicity and high amounts of SWS. During the daytime, there was much subjective sleepiness and a single 1.4-hr nap in the midafternoon some 14 hr after onset of night sleep.

midafternoon sleep, supporting the belief that the condition represents a pathological intensification of the sleep systems (5) without significant disruption of the biorhythmic aspects. The main advantage of ambulatory monitoring in idiopathic hypersomnia is one of laboratory convenience for 24-hr studies (after appropriate full overnight polysomnography to exclude other pathologies), plus potential documentation of sleep-wake correlates of sleep drunkenness in patients showing this symptom.

RECURRENT HYPERSOMNIAS

Recurrent hypersomnias are very rare and consist of periods of marked increase in sleep amount between which sleep patterns are essentially normal. The classical example is the Kleine-Levin syndrome (47–49). This condition mainly afflicts adolescent males, although a number of cases involving females or older males have been reported. During the hypersomnic periods the patients characteristically show a marked increase in eating (megaphagia), which often becomes compulsive, associated at times with sexual disturbances (hypersexuality, inappropriate sexual behavior), personality changes, and even feelings of depersonalization or actual hallucinations.

We have had the opportunity to study a single female patient with this syndrome during and outside a hypersomnic period.

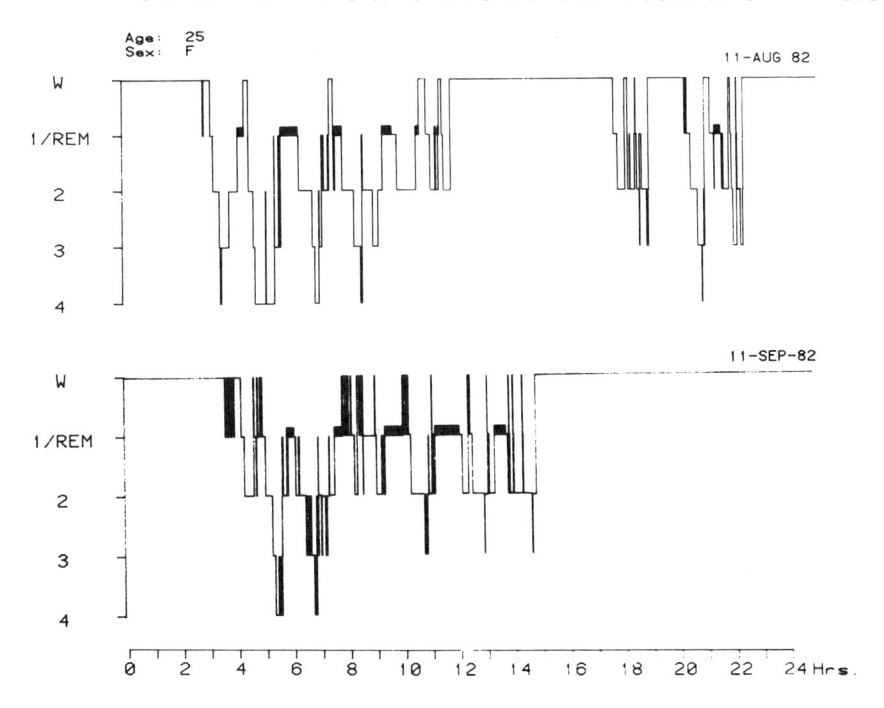

FIG. 4. Kleine-Levin syndrome in a 25-year-old female patient with episodes of increased sleep and sleepiness associated with megaphagia. The **top** histogram represents sleep recorded toward the end of an episode. The **bottom** histogram was 1 month later, when the patient was asymptomatic.

Case Report

The patient was a 24-year-old, who, since the age of 8 years, had experienced recurrent bouts about yearly and lasting 7 to 30 days that consisted of marked increase in sleep and sleepiness. During these periods she slept "all day long" and would only get up for food. She also ate excessively, at least twice the normal amount, and at their peak would sleep 18 to 20 hr/24 hr rather than her habitual somewhat long 9- to 10-hr single (monophasic) night sleep pattern. She and others noted personality changes with depression during hypersomnic bouts. There was, however, no unusual sexual behavior at these times. A family history of such a disorder was lacking, and there was no personal history of cataplexy, sleep paralysis, or vivid hypnagogic hallucinations to suggest narcolepsy. The episodes were serious and had led to job loss on two occasions. Physical examination was normal. An overnight polysomnogram ruled out sleep apnea, periodic movements in sleep, and other sleep pathologies. The patient was asked to phone when a hypersomnia period started. She did this some months later toward the end of a bout, when its intensity was declining. Ambulatory monitoring plus the sleep log with SSS was immediately done and

TABLE 5. *Sleep measures in a patient with Kleine-Levin syndrome studied by 24-hr ambulatory monitoring during a symptomatic hypersomnic episode and during an asymptomatic period*[a]

		Symptomatic				Asymptomatic	
		Night		Daytime	Total 24 hr	Night period	
TSP	(min)	484		—	—	640	
TST with stage 1		450		237	687	606	
TST without stage 1		397		166	563	489	
Sleep eff. with S1	(%)	92.4				95.4	
Sleep eff. without S1	(%)	85.5		—	—	77.1	
WASO	min + (%)	37	(7.6)	—	—	34	(5.4)
Stage 1	"	53	(10.9)	71	124	117	(19.3)
Stage 2	"	208	(42.6)	117	325	306	(47.7)
Stage 3	"	77	(15.2)	35	109	29	(4.6)
Stage 4	"	44	(0.0)	1	45	15	(2.4)
Stage REM	"	63	(12.9)	13	76	136	(21.1)
Movement time	"	8	(1.8)	0	8	3	(0.4)

[a]No daytime sleep occurred when in the asymptomatic period. TSP, total sleep period; TST, total sleep time; eff, efficiency.

then repeated some weeks later, when the bout was entirely over. The sleep histograms and sleep statistics during and outside the period of hypersomnia are provided in Fig. 4 and Table 5, respectively.

It can be seen from the results that outside of a hypersomnic bout the patient was indeed a relatively long sleeper with, however, normal sleep statistics for her age. The period of hypersomnia was characterized by a reduction in duration and a curious increase in depth of night sleep and the appearance of much sleep and great subjective daytime sleepiness (mean SSS of 5.4 versus 1.3 outside of periods of hypersomnia). The overall 24-hr increase in actual sleep in this patient during the period of hypersomnia was only of the order of 1 hr. However, there was impressive redistribution of sleep around the nycthemeron. The patient was later successfully treated with lithium carbonate.

We have not yet studied cases with menstrual hypersomnia or the subgroup of manic-depressive bipolar patients who present mainly with repeated hypersomnia and depression but without mania and insomnia. But this case demonstrates the particular usefulness of ambulatory monitoring in patients with recurrent hypersomnia. The results were similar to those reported in other Kleine-Levin syndrome patients using 24-hr in-laboratory polysomnography (50).

MULTIPLE SLEEP LATENCY TEST

A further area of application of ambulatory monitoring in the hypersomnias in which our laboratory has experience concerns ambulatory MSLT testing. The five-nap MSLT (11,51) provides an objective measure of daytime sleepiness or, more specifically, what Carskadon and Dement (52) have more appropriately called "physiological sleep tendency." Patients with sleep disorders associated with excessive daytime sleepiness generally show an abnormally short mean sleep latency (usually below 5 min), whereas non–sleep-deprived alert controls exhibit a mean sleep latency of greater than 15 min. Such shortened sleep latencies have been well documented for narcolepsy-cataplexy (11,12,53) and sleep apnea (53,54). As mentioned earlier, it has also been stated that two or more SOREMPs are essential for the diagnosis of narcolepsy-cataplexy (12). However, some narcoleptics on repeated testing have, in our experience, shown only one or no SOREMP. SOREMPs are not exclusive to narcolepsy, having been described in sleep apnea, drug-withdrawal states, endogenous depression, and even in very irregular sleep habits in normals. Moreover, there is some degree of overlap of groups (55). Occasionally, one encounters untreated narcoleptics who may have much cataplexy but are quite alert and have sleep latencies in the normal range. Some nonsleepy normals exhibit sleep latencies in the pathological range, most likely due to an ability to facilitate sleep onset ("easy napper") rather than from sleep pressure per se (55).

Nevertheless, the MSLT remains the most sensitive measure of sleepiness yet devised and is of considerable clinical utility. A main disadvantage, however, is its considerable cost and the fact that it ties up a sleep lab for some 10 hr for a single main measure, i.e., mean sleep latency. In order to minimize these drawbacks, we have attempted to introduce ambulant home MSLT tests.

The subjects come to the laboratories at 0800 hr, an 8-channel Medilog recorder with event button is attached using the already described montage, the nature of the test is carefully explained, and a typed test schedule plus a commercially available 100-min timer are provided. The patient is then taken home and follows the schedule. At 1000 hr, the subject goes to bed, sets the alarm for 20 min, presses the event button on the recorder to place a signal on the tape (for the sleep-latency measure), immediately turns out the light, and attempts to go to sleep. When the alarm sounds, the first scheduled nap is finished. The alarm is immediately set for 100 min, which will be the start of the scheduled 1200-hr nap; the cycle is then repeated through to the end of the 1800-hr nap. It is essential to use such a self-timed routine rather than awakening the subject by a telephone call from the laboratory. The dependent measures are, of course, the traditional individual and overall mean sleep

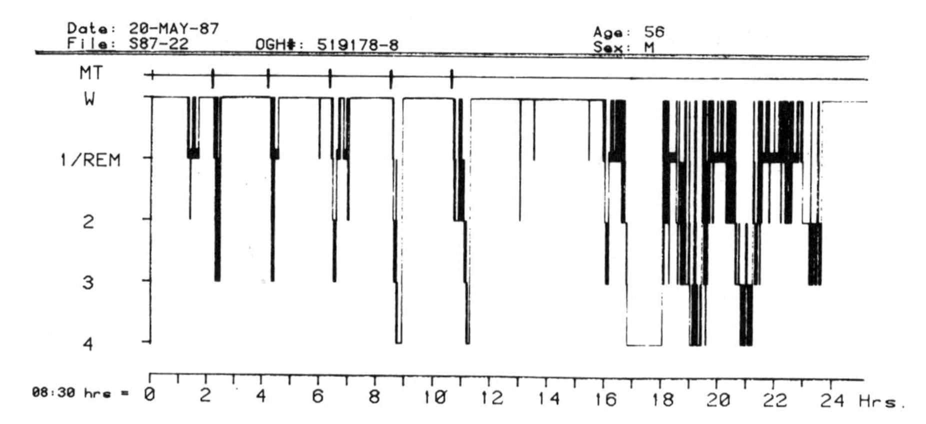

FIG. 5. Multiple sleep latency test and 24-hr sleep-wake patterns in a patient with narcolepsy-cataplexy. The recording was begun at 0800 hr. An 18-min sleep attack (mainly in REM) precedes the five scheduled 20-min naps at 1000, 1200, 1400, 1600, and 1800 hr, the moment of lights out being indicated by the long vertical lines at the top. The mean sleep latency of these five naps was 4.5 min; the second and third had SOREMPs. These data corresponded well to an in-laboratory traditional MSLT. Subsequent nocturnal sleep showed a SOREMP and much sleep fragmentation, especially of REM sleep.

latencies from the button signal to 1 or more min of sleep, the number of sleep-onset REM periods, and also the latencies and amounts of sleep stages from sleep onset to the end of the naps. Because the sleep-wake status is not available until tape playback, a protocol that terminates the nap after three consecutive epochs of sleep (56) cannot be done by this technique.

We have employed this approach and, to date, compared it to traditional laboratory-based studies in six patients with narcolepsy-cataplexy. Therefore, we have only preliminary data to report. In five patients, the protocol was well followed and the mean sleep latencies and number of SOREMPs were quite similar (Fig. 5; Table 6). In the sixth patient, there were great difficulties at home in having peaceful nap periods. During the first nap, the patient was jumped on by his dog; during the second nap, the telephone rang shortly after the nap onset and again aborted sleep; and, during the third nap, his wife came noisily home from shopping. Needless to say, the test was rescheduled and a successful ambulant MSLT was performed a week later.

Our current overall assessment of ambulatory MSLT may be summarized as follows. It is important to attempt ambulatory MSLT only in cooperative and intelligent subjects able to follow the protocol. It is essential that a quiet, undisturbed sleeping environment be available. Given these prerequisites, positive data of abnormally short sleep latencies are reliable indicators of sleepiness similar to those found with in-laboratory MSLT studies. Such data are then obtained with considerable savings in technician time (reduced to about 1 hr) and in laboratory overhead. However, negative results in the presence of a history of excessive daytime sleepiness, even in instances where the protocol has

TABLE 6. *Comparison of Multiple Sleep Latency Test results in six untreated narcolepsy-cataplexy patients by ambulatory monitoring and by in-laboratory techniques*

			In-laboratory		Ambulatory	
Subject	Age	Sex	Lat.	SOREMPs	Lat.	SOREMPs
1	24	m	3.4	3	3.9	2
2	33	m	2.6	2	3.5	2
3	66	f	5.6	4	4.7	4
4[a]	44	m	5.1	2	5.9	3
5	55	f	4.2	2	4.0	2
6	36	f	2.9	5	3.1	4

[a]Rescheduled test because of technical problems with the first home recording.

been carefully followed, are suspect and should be checked by the traditional laboratory approach.

SUMMARY

The usefulness of ambulatory monitoring in the hypersomnias is currently being actively assessed. The potential advantages and disadvantages that were mentioned in the introduction have been confirmed by experience. With technical care, high-quality recordings can be achieved. We currently have a less than 5% repeat rate due to technical problems; we doubt that this can be significantly lowered, due to unforeseeable problems with batteries, electrodes occasionally coming off, and other problems of recordings in the field. It is our experience that a sleep log and use of an event marker are of great help in this group of patients (and others such as sleep-wake–schedule disorders) in both the analysis and interpretation of the cassette-tape data. We recommend that sleep logs always be employed, as should the event marker, where available. We have not found that technologist visits or telephone calls to the home provide cost-effective help. In the small proportion of studies in which technical problems have occurred, it is best simply to reschedule the test.

All patients should have a traditional overnight polysomnogram prior to ambulatory monitoring, as sleep pathologies such as sleep apnea and periodic movements in sleep may be totally occult and not be suggested by patient history. Of course, this need may change in the future, with such technological progress as a larger number of channels and less-fragile (e.g., digital) recorders. To what extent 24-hr ambulant sleep-wake patterns may be actually diagnostic of a particular clinical form of hypersomnia is still uncertain and will require investigation of a much larger variety of hypersomnic conditions. Finally, technically satisfactory MSLT tests appear to be possible, but these require judicious interpretation.

ACKNOWLEDGMENTS

Many research assistants, graduate students, research associates, and visiting scientists have been involved in the initiation and/or assessment of ambulatory monitoring techniques over the years. Their help is gratefully acknowledged. Included are David Barker, Bernardo da Costa, Pierre Duchesne, Wayne Dunham, Tom Healey, Steven Liddiard, Kathy Lutley, Jagdish Maru, Janet Mullington, Janice Newman, Martin Rivers, Janet Roberts, Claudio Stampi, and Wlodeck Suwalski. The author also thanks the Medical Research Council of Canada, which has supported the laboratory's research in this area.

REFERENCES

1. Association of Sleep Disorders Centers. *Diagnostic classification of sleep and arousal disorders,* first ed, prepared by the Sleep Disorders Classification Committee, Roffwarg HP, Chairman. *Sleep* 1979;2:1–137.
2. Coleman RM, Roffwarg HP, et al. Sleep-wake disorders based on a polysomnographic diagnosis: a national cooperative study. *JAMA* 1982;247:997–1003.
3. Dement WC, Carskadon M, Ley R. The prevalence of narcolepsy II. *Sleep Res,* 1973;2:147.
4. Billiard M. Narcolepsy. In: Nicholson AN, Welbers IB, eds. *Sleep and wakefulness.* Ingelheim: Postgraduate Medical Series, Boehringer, 1986;31–54.
5. Roth B. *Narcolepsy and the hypersomnias.* Basel: Karger, 1980.
6. Broughton R, Ghanem Q, Hishikawa Y, et al. Life effects of narcolepsy in 180 patients from North America, Asia and Europe. *Can Neurol Sci* 1981;8:299–304.
7. Broughton R, Nevsimalova S, Roth B. The socioeconomic effects of idiopathic hypersomnia—comparison with controls and with compound narcoleptics. In: Popoviciu L, Asgian B, Badiu G, eds. *Sleep 1978.* Basel: Karger, 1980;103–111.
8. Broughton R, Guberman A, Roberts J. Comparison of the socioeconomic effects of epilepsy and narcolepsy-cataplexy. *Can J Neurol Sci* 1984;25:423–433.
9. Guilleminault C, Dement WC. Pathologies of excessive sleepiness. In: Drucker-Colin RR, McGaugh JL, eds. *Neurobiology of sleep and memory.* New York: Academic, 1977;439–456.
10. Broughton R, Mamelak M. The treatment of narcolepsy-cataplexy with nocturnal gamma-hydroxybutyrate. *Can J Neurol Sci* 1979;6:1–6.
11. Richardson GS, Carskadon MA, Flagg W, et al. Excessive daytime sleepiness in man: multiple sleep latency measurements in narcoleptic and control subjects. *Electroencephalogr Clin Neurophysiol* 1978;46:621–627.
12. Mitler MM, van den Hoed J, Carskadon MA, et al. REM sleep episodes during the Multiple Sleep Latency Test in narcoleptic patients. *Electroencephalogr Clin Neurophysiol* 1979;46:479–481.
13. Aschoff J. Freerunning and entrained circadian rhythms. In: Aschoff J, ed. *Handbook in behavioral neurobiology,* vol. 4, *Biological rhythms.* New York: Plenum, 1981;81–94.
14. Wever RA. *The circadian system of man.* New York/Heidelberg/Berlin: Springer-Verlag; 1979.
15. Broughton R. Biorhythmic fluctuations in consciousness and psychological functions. *Can Psychol Rev* 1975;16:217–230.
16. Zulley J, Campbell S. Napping behavior during "spontaneous internal desynchronization": sleep remains in synchrony with body temperature. *Hum Neurobiol* 1985;4:123–126.
17. Lavie P. Ultradian rhythms in human sleep and wakefulness. In: Webb WB, ed. *Biological rhythms, sleep and performance.* Chichester: Wiley, 1982;239–272.
18. Manseau C, Broughton R. Bilaterally synchronous ultradian EEG rhythms in awake adult humans. *Psychophysiology* 1984;21:265–273.
19. Roth B, Nevsimalova S, Sagova V, et al. Neurological, psychological and polygraphic findings in sleep drunkenness. *Arch Suisse Neurol Neurochir Psychiat* 1981;129:209–222.
20. Guilleminault C, Billiard M, Montplaisir J, et al. Altered states of consciousness in disorders of

daytime sleepiness. *J Neurol Sci* 1975;26:377–393.
21. Healey T, Maru J, Broughton R. A 4-channel portable recording system. *Sleep Res* 1975;4:254.
22. Broughton R. Polysomnography: principles and applications in sleep and arousal disorders. In: Niedermeyer E, Lopes da Silva F, eds. *Electroencephalography: basic principles, clinical applications and related fields,* 2nd ed. Baltimore/Munich: Urban and Schwarzenberg, 1987;687–724.
23. Jasper HH. The ten-twenty system of the International Federation. *Electroencephalogr Clin Neurophysiol* 1958;10:371–375.
24. Rechtschaffen A, Kales A, eds. *A manual of standardized terminology, techniques and scoring system for sleep stages in human subjects.* Washington: US Govt Printing Office, Department of Health, Education and Welfare, 1968.
25. Hoddes E, Zarcone V, Smyth H, et al. Quantification of sleepiness—a new approach. *Psychophysiology* 1973;1:431–436.
26. Broughton R, Mamelak M. Effects of gamma-hydroxybutyrate on sleep/waking patterns in narcolepsy-cataplexy. *Can J Neurol Sci* 1980;7:23–31.
27. Valley V, Broughton R. The physiological (EEG) nature of drowsiness and its relation to performance deficits in narcoleptics and normals. *Electroencephalogr Clin Neurophysiol* 1983;55:243–251.
28. Valley V, Broughton R. Daytime performance deficits and physiological vigilance in untreated patients with narcolepsy-cataplexy compared to controls. *Rev EEG Neurophysiol (Paris)* 1981;11:133–139.
29. Loomis AL, Harvey AN, Hobart GA. Cerebral states during sleep as studied by human brain potentials. *J Exp Psychol* 1937;21:127–144.
30. Volk S, Simon O, Schulz H, et al. The structure of wakefulness and its relation to daytime sleepiness in narcoleptic patients. *Electroencephalogr Clin Neurophysiol* 1984;57:119–128.
31. Broughton R, Barker D, Roberts J. A computer generated sleep histogram. *Sleep Res* 1984;134:197.
32. Broughton R, Lutley K, Duchesne P, et al. Computer (IBM-PC) assisted polysomnogram, MSLT and ambulant monitoring reports. *Sleep Res* 1988,17:328.
33. Berti-Ceroni G, Coccagna G, Lugaresi E. Twenty-four hour polygraphic recordings in narcoleptics. In: Gastaut H, Lugaresi E, Berti-Ceroni G, et al., eds. *The abnormalities of sleep in man.* Bologna: Aulo Gaggi, 1968;235–238.
34. Billiard M, Quera Salva M, De Koninck J, et al. Daytime sleep characteristics and their relationships with night sleep in the narcoleptic patient. *Sleep* 1986;9:167–174.
35. Hishikawa Y, Wakamatsu H, et al. Sleep satiation in narcoleptic patients. *Electroencephalogr Clin Neurophysiol* 1976;41:1–18.
36. Broughton R, Dunham W, Suwalski W, et al. Ambulant 24-hour sleep/wake recordings in narcolepsy-cataplexy. *Sleep Res* 1986;15:109.
37. Broughton R, Dunham W, Newman J, et al. Ambulatory 24-hour sleep-wake monitoring in narcolepsy-cataplexy compared to matched controls. *Electroencephalogr Clin Neurophysiol* 1988:70:473–481.
38. Montplaisir J, Billiard M, Takahashi S, et al. 24-hour polygraphic recordings in narcoleptics with special reference to nocturnal sleep disturbance. *Biol Psychiat* 1978;13:73–89.
39. Gagnon P, De Koninck J. Reappearance of EEG slow waves in extended sleep. *Electroencephalogr Clin Neurophysiol* 1984;58:155–157.
40. Broughton R, De Koninck J, Gagnon P, et al. Chronobiological aspects of SWS and REM sleep in extended sleep of normals. *Sleep Res* 1988;17:361.
41. Broughton R, Valley V, Aguirre M, et al. Excessive daytime sleepiness and the pathophysiology of narcolepsy. *Sleep* 1986;9:205–215.
42. Kripke DF. Biological rhythm disturbance might cause narcolepsy. In: Guilleminault C, Dement WC, Passouant P, eds. *Narcolepsy.* New York: Spectrum, 1976.
43. Meier-Ewert K, Schopfer B, Ruther R. Drei narkoleptische Syndrome. *Nervenarz* 1975;46:624–635.
44. Montplaisir J. Disturbed nocturnal sleep. In: Guilleminault C, Dement WC, Passouant P, eds. *Narcolepsy.* New York: Spectrum, 1976;43–56.
45. Newman J, Stampi C, Dunham W, et al. Does wrist actigraphy approximate polysomnographic detection of sleep and wakefulness in narcolepsy-cataplexy? *Sleep Res* 1988;17:343.
46. Roth B, Nevsimalova S, Rechtschaffen A. Hypersomnia with "sleep drunkenness." *Arch Gen*

Psychiat 1972;26:456–462.
47. Kleine W. Periodische Schlaftsucht. *Monatschr Psychiat Neurol* 1925;57:285–320.
48. Levin M. Periodic somnolence and morbid hunger: a new syndrome. *Brain* 1936;59:494–515.
49. Critchley M. Periodic hunger and megaphagia in adolescent males. *Brain* 1962;85:627-656.
50. Billiard M. Recurring hypersomnias. In: Popoviciu L, Asgian B, Badiu G, eds. *Sleep 1979.* Basel: Karger, 1980;233–238.
51. Carskadon MA, Dement WC. Sleep tendency: an objective measure of sleep loss. *Sleep Res* 1977;6:20.
52. Carskadon MA, Dement WC. The multiple sleep latency test: what does it measure? *Sleep* 1982;5(suppl):67–72.
53. Walsh JK, Smitson SA, Kramer M. Sleep-onset REM sleep: comparison of narcoleptic and obstructive sleep apnea patients. *Clin Electroencephalogr* 1982;13:57–60.
54. Roth T, Harste KM, Zorick F, et al. Multiple naps and the evaluation of daytime sleepiness in patients with upper airway sleep apnea. *Sleep* 1980;3:425–439.
55. Broughton R, Aguirre M, Dunham W. A comparison of multiple and single sleep latency and cerebral evoked potential (P300) measures in the assessment of excessive daytime sleepiness in narcolepsy-cataplexy. *Sleep* 1988;11:537–545.
56. Carskadon M, Dement WC, Mitler MM, et al. Guidelines for the Multiple Sleep Latency Test (MSLT): a standard measure of sleepiness. *Sleep* 1986;9:519–524.

Ambulatory EEG Monitoring,
edited by John S. Ebersole.
Raven Press, Ltd., New York © 1989

19

Ambulatory Cassette Recording of Sleep Apnea

Sonia Ancoli-Israel

Department of Psychiatry, University of California, San Diego 92093; and Veterans Administration Medical Center, San Diego, CA 92161

The medical community now recognizes the importance of sleep apnea, a disorder characterized by cessation of respiration during sleep. Sleep apnea is diagnosed when there are at least five apneas (complete cessation of respiration) and/or hypopneas (partial cessation of respiration) per hour of sleep, each lasting a minimum of 10 sec. The apneic event is usually followed by an awakening or arousal. Patients seen at sleep disorders centers, however, may have over 70 apneas per hour of sleep (i.e., more than 1/min), lasting from 30 sec to over 2 min. Thus, sleep apnea can be life-threatening, as some apnea patients cannot breathe and sleep at the same time.

There are three types of sleep apnea (1–3). Obstructive apnea usually involves partial or complete blockage of air flow due to changes in the anatomy of the pharynx and hypopharynx. The obstruction is caused by excessive relaxation of the throat muscles and is related to an anatomically small airway. Central sleep apnea is caused by the central nervous system's failing to stimulate the diaphragm and intercostal muscles, the muscles of respiration. This can be caused by many factors including neurological disorders, impairment of respiratory feedback regulation, or by excessive sedation. Mixed sleep apnea is a combination of central and obstructive apneas.

There are many side effects of sleep apneas. Blood oxygen saturation levels drop, ventricular irritability develops, and, at times, asystoles are seen (4–7). Hypertension is more common in apnea patients (8,9), as is loud snoring (10–12). Other symptoms include excessive daytime sleepiness [caused by multiple arousals during the night (13,14) and by multiple episodes of hypoxia (15)], nighttime confusion, and neuropsychological impairment (16,17). Apneas are also often accompanied by leg jerks. These leg jerks, when seen without apneas, are also a separate sleep disorder called periodic leg movements in sleep (PLMS) (see Chapter 17).

The traditional methodology for objectively evaluating sleep apnea is the nocturnal polysomnogram. Patients are brought into the laboratory or clinic to sleep for 1 or more nights. Electroencephalography (EEG), electrooculography (EOG), and chin electromyography (EMG) are recorded to determine the different stages of sleep (18). Respiration is recorded by one of many techniques including strain gauges or plethysmography. Tibialis EMG is recorded, as are the electrocardiogram (EKG) and blood oxygen saturation levels. A technician must watch over the patient and the polygraph all night. The product of 8 hr of sleep monitoring is approximately a quarter of a mile of paper, which then needs to be read and scored. While this is the gold standard, it is a very expensive and cumbersome technique.

Over the past decade, ambulatory monitors have been used more and more frequently for evaluating sleep disorders, particularly sleep apnea and PLMS. The first cassette recorders were able to record four channels of information. More recently, cassette recorders have been expanded to eight channels, allowing recording of many of the same variables recorded in the laboratory.

Our experience has been with the 4-channel cassette recorder. We have recorded and evaluated over 1000 people in the past 8 years, both clinically and for research purposes, with a system called the modified Respitrace/Medilog recording system.

MODIFIED RESPITRACE/MEDILOG SYSTEM

Figure 1 shows the modified Respitrace/Medilog system. Two channels of respiratory plethysmography, one channel of tibialis EMG, and one channel of wrist activity are recorded onto a 4-channel Medilog cassette recorder. Although standard 120-min cassettes are used, the extremely slow speed of the tape drive (2 mm/sec) allows over 24 hr of recording time. Once the recording is complete, the tape is played onto a polygraph (at 60$\times$ real time) via a special playback unit, and a hard paper copy is obtained, which can then be scored.

Respiration is recorded with Respitrace bands (Ambulatory Monitoring, Inc.) placed around the thorax and abdomen. These transducer bands respond to inductance changes caused by chest and abdominal expansion (19). Leg jerks are measured by recording tibialis EMG with standard electrodes. The techniques for recording respiration and leg jerks are similar to those used for polysomnography. The technique for distinguishing wake from sleep, however, is different in that, rather than recording EEG, EOG, and chin EMG, we record wrist activity.

Wrist-activity scoring has been shown to correlate highly with EEG scoring for determining wake from sleep (20,21). The wrist actigraph transducer consists of a small weight soldered off-center onto a springlike wire. The other end of the wire is clamped against a piezoceramic element, which is excited whenever the transducer is moved in any direction (20). The transducer is inside a small acrylic box (about the size of a matchbox), which is worn on the wrist with a watchband (see Fig. 1). Scoring criteria have been established (22–24) for determining wake and sleep with the wrist actigraph. Basically, when we are awake, we move, and when we are asleep, we do not move. Wake is, therefore, scored when activity is seen, often accompanied by movement artifact in the other three channels. Sleep is scored when there are no signals in the wrist actigraph and no movement artifacts in the respiration or EMG channels. The amount of time scored asleep is dependent on the previous amount of wake time. For example, after 4 min of wake, the first minute that looks like sleep is still scored as wake; after 10 min of wake, the first 3 min that look like sleep are still scored as wake, etc. Figure 2 shows a sample of a normal individual's wake and sleep recording as recorded by the wrist actigraph.

Mullaney et al. (21) compared the wrist actigraph to traditional EEG in 102 recordings. On a minute-by-minute basis, there was agreement for 94.5% of the minutes. The correlation between wrist activity and EEG was 0.98 ($p < 0.0001$) for total sleep time and 0.97 ($p < 50.0001$) for wake time.

Figures 3 through 7 show samples of sleep apneas recorded with the modified Respitrace/Medilog system. Note that a third channel of respiration, labeled SUM, appears in each figure. This is the sum of the thoracic and abdominal

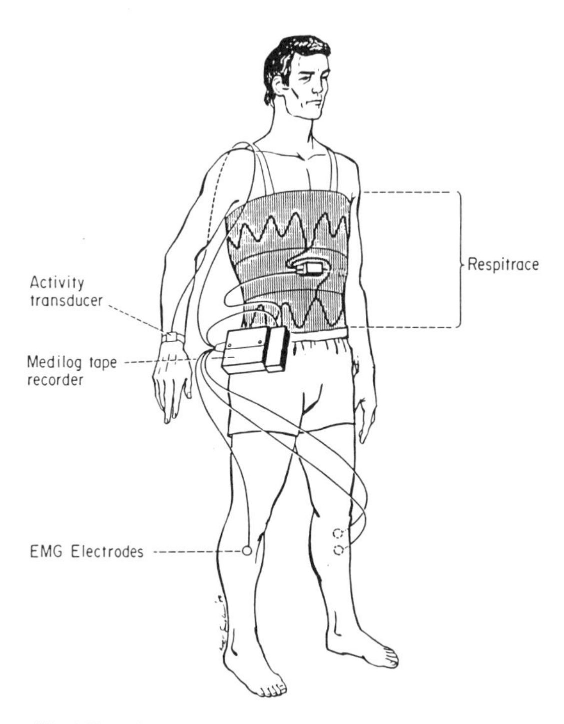

FIG. 1. The modified Respitrace/Medilog system. Reprinted with permission from ref. 24.

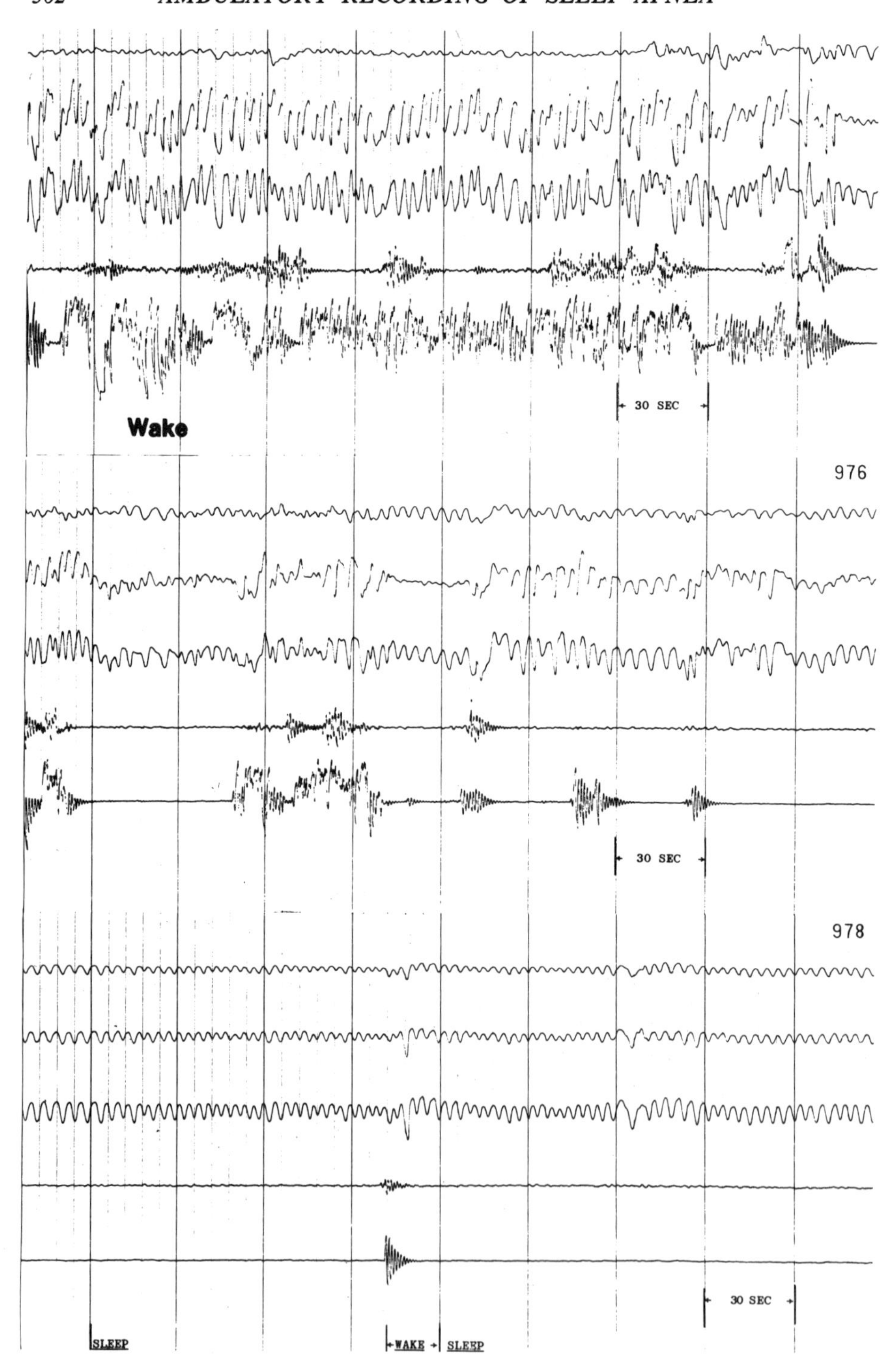
Wake
30 SEC
976
30 SEC
978
30 SEC
SLEEP
WAKE
SLEEP

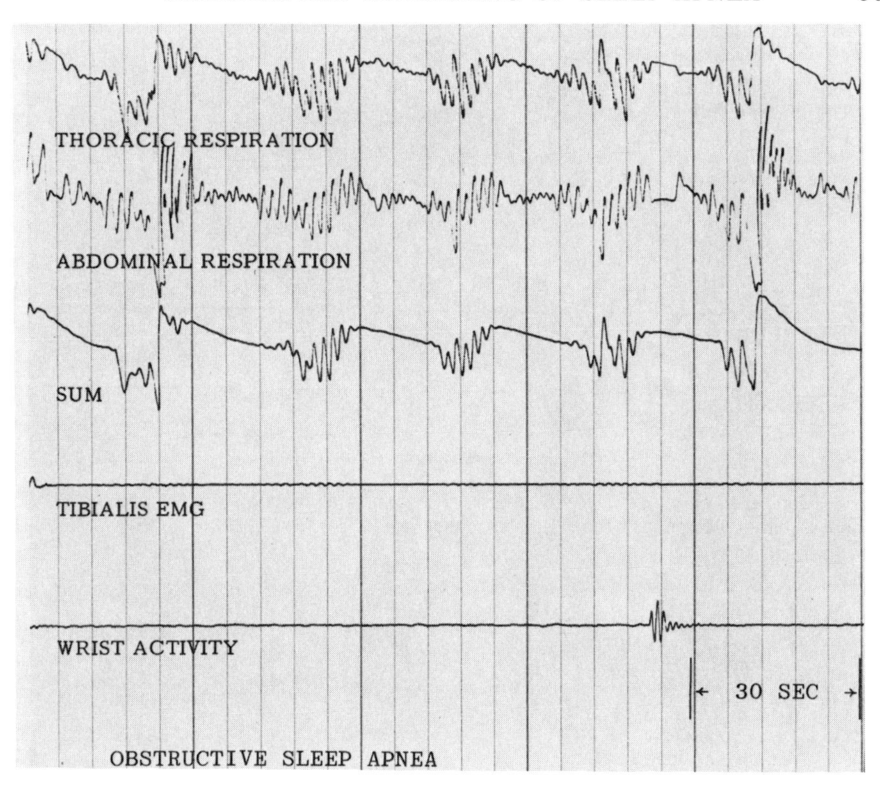

FIG. 3. Obstructive sleep apnea. Note the thorax and abdominal channels are 180° out of phase and the SUM channel is either flat or less than 10% of baseline.

channels and is representative of tidal volume. The data of the sum channel are determined electronically by a Respitrace calibration unit. In obstructive apnea (Fig. 3), the thorax and abdominal channels are 180° out of phase, and the sum channel is flat or less than 10% of the baseline respiration. Central apnea (Fig. 4) is represented by flat thorax and abdominal channels and a flat sum channel (or less than 10% of baseline). Mixed apneas (Fig. 5) begin with a central component followed by the thorax and abdomen moving 180° out of phase (obstructive component).

Hypopneas can also be identified with this modified Respitrace/Medilog recording method. During an obstructive hypopnea (Fig. 6), the thoracic and

FIG. 2. Wake and sleep scored from a wrist actigraph. Note that the pages are nonconsecutive. Page 975 had 5 min of wake; therefore, page 976 is also scored as wake. Page 977 had only 1 min of wake scored in the first minute of the page. The rest of the page had no activity; therefore, sleep is scored as beginning 5 min after the end of the last movement.

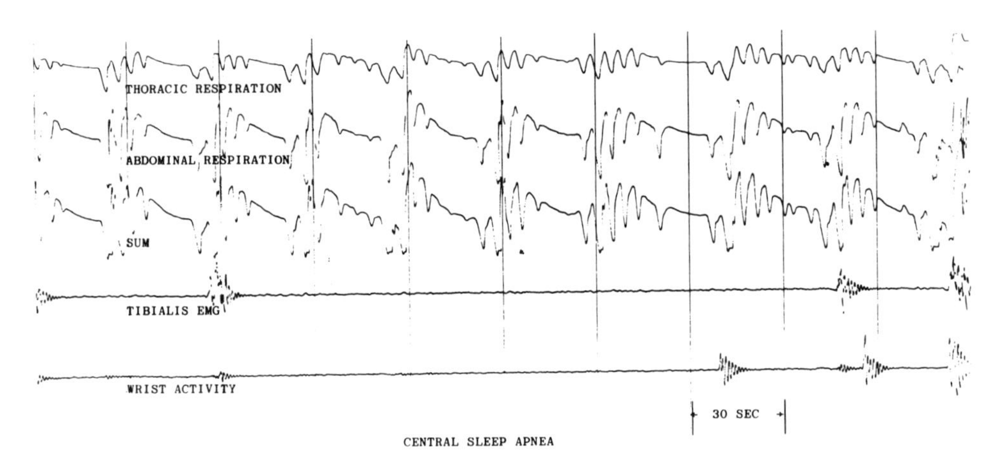

FIG. 4. Central sleep apnea. Note the thorax and abdominal channels are flat and the SUM channel is either flat or less than 10% of baseline.

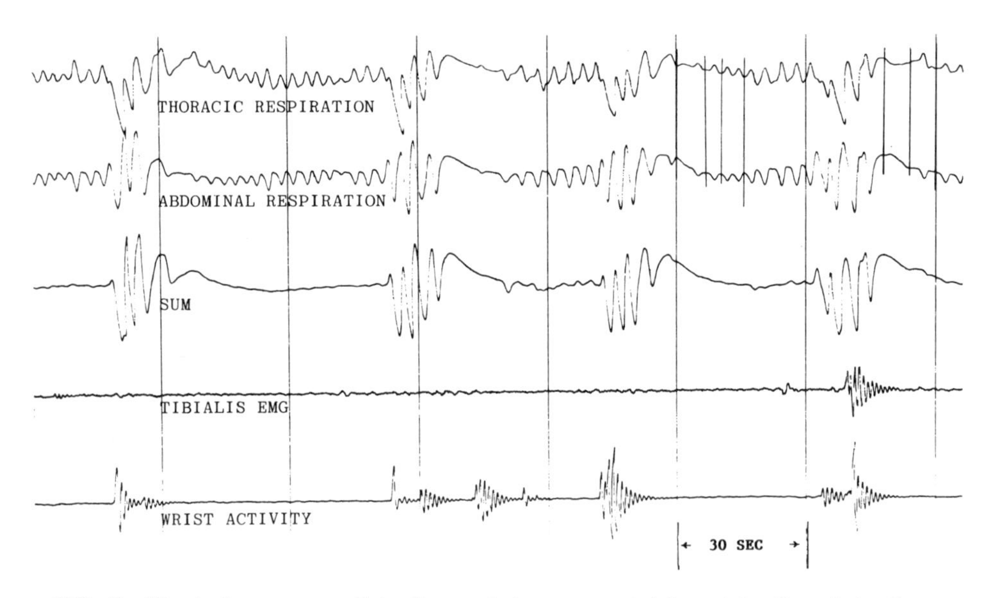

FIG. 5. Mixed sleep apnea. Note the central component followed by the obstructive component.

abdominal channels are 180° out of phase, the the sum is less than 50% but greater than 10% of resting. During a central hypopnea (Fig. 7), the thoracic, abdominal, and sum channels are in phase and are less than 50% but greater than 10% of resting.

The reliability of the modified Respitrace/Medilog recording system has been compared to the traditional polysomnogram (25). Subjects with and without

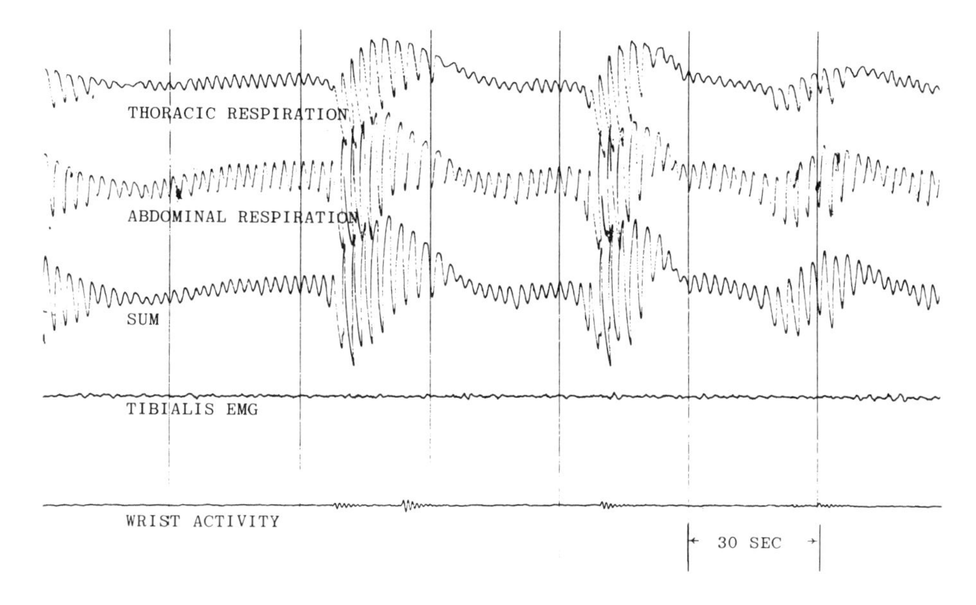

FIG. 6. Obstructive hypopnea. Note the thorax and abdominal channels are 180° out of phase and the SUM channel is less than 50% but greater than 10% of baseline.

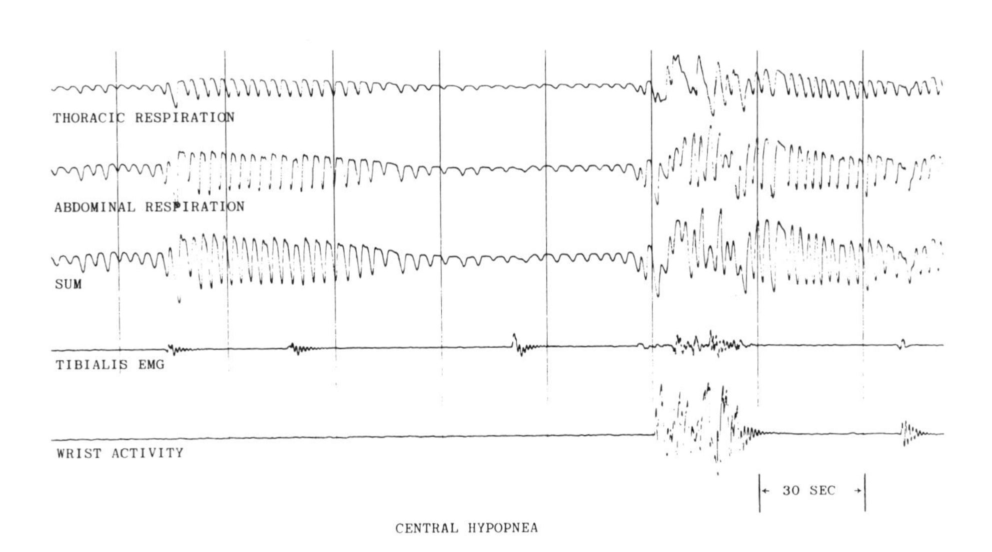

FIG. 7. Central hypopnea. Note the thorax, abdominal, and SUM channels are all in phase and are less than 50% but greater than 10% of baseline.

TABLE 1. *Reliability of modified Respitrace/Medilog system compared to traditional polysomnography*[a]

	r	p
Number of apneas	.80	< 0.01
Number of leg jerks	.64	< 0.005
Total sleep period	.82	< 0.01
Total sleep time	.69	< 0.01
Wake time	.61	< 0.01

[a]From Ancoli-Israel et al. (25).

sleep apnea were recorded with both techniques on the same night. The resulting reliabilities are shown in Table 1. These correlations compare well with the reliabilities of different scorers of the same EEG recording (26). The sensitivity of the portable system (i.e, the ability to detect sleep apnea) was 100%, with one false positive. The intermethod agreements were, therefore, highly significant for the diagnoses of sleep apnea and for sleep parameters. When a portable recording is negative, we can feel confident that there is no sleep apnea. A positive result is also likely to be correct, but, depending on the severity, a second recording may be indicated.

There are obvious advantages and disadvantages in using this system. The main advantages include the capacity to record for 24 hr and the possibility of studying the patients in their natural environment. Since the system can record for 24 hr, patients' nighttime and daytime behavior can be monitored. For example, with sleep apnea patients who complain of excessive daytime sleepiness, both napping behavior and presence of apneas during naps can be documented. Since patients' sleep can be further disrupted by sleeping in a strange laboratory, allowing them to sleep in their own beds provides for a more accurate picture of their characteristic sleep. Using the actigraph instead of additional wires (EEG, EOG, EMG) also makes it comfortable for the patient. The system allows for recording patients in their hospital-ward bed, intensive-care-unit bed, or nursing-home bed, when it might be difficult to move them or bring them into the sleep laboratory. Allowing patients this flexibility also increases the compliance rate.

Another advantage is the cost-effectiveness of the portable system. While the price of a clinical polysomnogram can run over $1000, the portable recording is analogous to that of Holter monitoring, i.e., about one-third the cost of the polysomnogram. The reduced cost and increased comfort make it easier to perform multiple recordings and to do follow-up recordings to evaluate treatment effects.

The main disadvantage of the system is the restriction of the number of available channels. Now that an 8-channel recorder is available, however, other measures can be recorded. Since EEG is not recorded with our system, it is not possible to distinguish rapid eye movement (REM) sleep from non-REM (NREM) sleep. Although it is useful to show when apneas are occurring during REM, the clinical reality is that a diagnosis of sleep apnea and a determination of severity of apnea can be accomplished without sleep-stage information.

Another disadvantage of the cassette recorder is that equipment failures are not detected until the record is played back. In our experience, using new batteries for each recording, using tape surgerflex material and Velcro to hold the equipment in place, and checking all wires with an ohm-meter before sending the patient home increase the likelihood of a good recording (24). In the event that there is still an equipment malfunction, the procedure is easy to repeat. The advantages of the convenience and low cost still outweigh the disadvantage of possible lost recordings.

CLINICAL EXPERIENCE WITH THE MODIFIED RESPITRACE/MEDILOG SYSTEM

The modified Respitrace/Medilog system has been used in our Veterans Administration (VA) Sleep Disorders Clinic since 1981. Since 1984, portable recordings have been done on 97% of the patients. In only 2% were recordings lost due to equipment problems. Between 1981 and 1984, 23% of the patients had a laboratory polysomnogram, 61% were evaluated by portable recordings alone, 5% had a portable recording followed by a laboratory polysomnogram, and 1% had a laboratory polysomnogram followed by a portable recording. In 10%, the history did not indicate a need for a recording.

Of the five patients who had the portable recording followed by the laboratory polysomnogram, three were given a laboratory polysomnogram because the portable recording had indicated severe apnea, and EKG and oximetry were desired before treatment was selected. In all three cases, the results of the polysomnogram confirmed those of the portable recordings.

For the remaining two patients, the laboratory recordings were ordered because the portable recordings were of poor quality. One alcoholic patient was unable to comply with the instructions for home recording. The patient repeatedly disconnected the equipment during the night, despite multiple telephone contacts. During the few hours that were recorded, as many as 100 leg jerks were counted. It was not possible to count apneas. Since the patient could not cooperate with the home recording, a polysomnogram was scheduled. The results indicated 199 leg jerks and no sleep apnea.

The second patient with a poor-quality record used a heating pad during the night, which interfered with the electronics of the portable recorder. The recording was suggestive of mild sleep apnea and no leg jerks, so a polysomnogram was scheduled to obtain a clearer picture. The laboratory polysomnogram confirmed the diagnosis of mild sleep apnea and no leg jerks.

One patient presented with a history of sleep apnea, but no apnea was recorded in the laboratory. This patient felt that his laboratory night was not representative of his sleep, so an additional portable recording was ordered. The portable recording confirmed the laboratory result.

Some of the patients had multiple portable recordings for follow-up purposes. For example, several patients with sleep apnea who lost weight or had uvulapalatopharyngoplasty surgery were rerecorded to confirm the treatment effect.

In summary, in our clinical experience, a home cassette recording can be an excellent screening device for sleep apnea.

RESEARCH EXPERIENCE WITH THE MODIFIED RESPITRACE/MEDILOG SYSTEM

We have been studying sleep apnea in three populations of elderly: (a) independently living elderly, (b) hospitalized medical inpatients, and (c) nursing-home patients.

Independently Living Elderly

In the study of independently living elderly (27,28), volunteers were randomly selected from a reverse telephone directory (i.e., a directory in which entries are ordered by telephone number rather than by name). Each individual who agreed to participate and was 65 or older had a brief telephone interview, a more extensive home interview, and one modified Respitrace/Medilog sleep recording.

Using this procedure, we identified 1865 elderly from whom 1526 (82%) agreed to a telephone interview. Of these 1526, 615 (40%) agreed to a home interview. Of the 615, 427 (69%) agreed to a sleep recording. The greatest difficulty, therefore, was getting a home interview scheduled; however, once we were in their homes, the majority of the volunteers did not object to wearing the recording equipment.

The equipment was usually attached in the late afternoon or early evening (mean time, 1656 hr) in the subject's home. The following morning, the technician returned to the home to remove the equipment (mean time, 0825 hr). The average duration of recordings was 15 hr. Each recording was scored, minute by minute, for total minutes asleep; total minutes awake; number, type, and duration of apneas; and number of leg jerks. Hypopneas were not scored, for, at the time this study began in 1981, there was no precedent or any criteria for scoring hypopneas. For similar reasons, the records at that time were not calibrated.

Using this methodology and technology, 427 randomly selected elderly were recorded (28,29). The overall results indicated that 24% of these elderly (28% males and 19.5% females) had an apnea index (AI) ≥ 5 (i.e., number of apneas per hour of sleep), and 44% (46% males and 43% females) had a myoclonus index (MI) ≥ 5 (i.e., number of leg jerks per hour of sleep) (28).

As mentioned, at the time of this study, it was not possible to score hypopneas or to calibrate the Respitrace. In further improving the reliability of the portable modified Respitrace/Medilog system, we examined the issue of calibration. Ten records were blindly scored, calibrated and uncalibrated. Correlations for type of apnea (obstructive, $r_s = .87$; central, $r_s = .71$; mixed, $r_s = .68$), total apneas ($r_s = .84$), total hypopneas ($r_s = .95$), and total events ($r_s = .88$) were all significant, indicating a high association between the calibrated and uncalibrated records. We found that, in the uncalibrated records, apneas tended to be underscored, while hypopneas were overscored. There was essentially no difference in scoring of total events. Therefore, the portable modified Respitrace/Medilog recording technique, when used uncalibrated, may actually give a conservative estimate of apneas. Whenever possible, we recommend calibrating portable recordings as well as counting hypopneas. In situations where calibration is just not possible (such as with frail elderly or demented patients), a respiratory disturbance index (RDI or number of apneas *plus* hypopneas, i.e., respiratory events, per hour of sleep) should be used rather than just an apnea index.

Stability of Sleep Apnea and PLMS

In order to examine the stability of sleep apnea and PLMS over time, 61 elderly were recontacted and 20 were rerecorded 4 to 5 years after their initial recording (30). Each initial record was rescored for apneas, hypopneas, and leg jerks, and each follow-up record was scored for apneas, hypopneas, and leg jerks. Spearman Rank Order Correlations were computed for apnea index, RDI, and MI. The resulting correlations were: AI, $r_s = .58$ ($p < 0.05$); RDI, $r_s = .83$ ($p < 0.001$); MI, $r_s = .47$ ($p < 0.05$).

Wilcoxin Matched Pair Signed Ranks tests were also done to examine changes over time. There were no significant differences in AI or RDI nor were there any significant differences in weight; however, there was a significant increase in MI from 9.5 to 18.6 ($p < 0.02$). These results indicated that apneas and hypopneas, as recorded by our portable system, are rather stable over time in elderly whose weights are stable. Leg jerks, on the other hand, seemed to increase with age. These data also indicate that single-night measurements with the modified Respitrace/Medilog system reflect long-term traits in apnea, but perhaps less reliable traits in PLMS.

Sleep Disorders in Younger Females

As part of this larger study of prevalence of apnea and PLMS in the elderly, we became interested in the prevalence of these disorders in younger adults.

Eighteen females, between the ages of 30 and 40 years (mean age, 33.5), were randomly selected using the same methodology described above and from the same geographic area as 88 older females (mean age, 73.3) in the original sample (31). All 18 younger females were premenopausal, while all 88 older females were postmenopausal.

The prevalence of sleep apnea (i.e., AI $\geq$ 45) was significantly lower among the younger females ($p < 0.05$). In fact, none (0%) of the premenopausal females compared with 12 (14%) of the postmenopausal females had an AI $\geq$ 5. The mean AI for the younger group was 0.6, while for the older group the mean AI was 2.2. It has been known that premenopausal women rarely present with sleep apnea (32,33), but this study was the first to confirm the paucity of sleep apnea among premenopausal females in a representative survey. These results are consistent with the theory that hormones such as progesterone protect females from sleep apnea (34). Studies of subjects around the time of menopause are still needed to distinguish specific endocrine effects from other aspects of aging.

Leg jerks were also compared among the pre- and postmenopausal women. There was no significant difference in the prevalence of MI $\geq$ 5 in the two samples. Four (23.5%) of the premenopausal females (MI = 7.8; range = 5.4–12.7) and 39 (45%) of the postmenopausal females (MI = 25.2; range = 5.9–104.9) had an MI $\geq$ 5. The postmenopausal group had significantly more leg jerks ($p < 0.05$) and a higher MI ($p < 0.05$) than the premenopausal group, indicating that the severity of leg jerks seems to increase with age.

Sleep timing was also compared between the two groups. The postmenopausal group had more wake time (88 min) than the premenopausal group (47 min) ($p < 0.001$). There were no significant differences, however, in total sleep time. More of these types of studies are needed, and portable cassette systems make it more feasible to conduct them.

Portable Recordings in Medical-Ward Patients

In the ongoing VA Medical Ward Study, we are examining the relationship between sleep apnea and mortality. Patients aged 60 and over are randomly selected from each day's new admissions to the VA medical ward. Each patient who agrees to participate is interviewed about his sleep, his medical records are abstracted, and EKG and chest X-rays are reviewed. Each patient is then recorded with the modified Respitrace/Medilog system. Whenever possible, 2 nights are recorded. In addition, portable finger pulse oximetry is recorded on one of the nights.

To date, 812 patients have been asked to participate, and 300 (37%) have agreed. Of these, all had at least 1 night recorded and 50% had 2 nights recorded. Each Respitrace/Medilog recording was scored for total sleep time; wake time; number of awakenings; number, type, and duration of apneas and hypopneas; AI; hypopnea index [(HI) number of hypopneas per hour of sleep)];

TABLE 2. *Night-to-night Spearman Rank Order Correlations with modified Respitrace/Medilog system (N = 110)*

	r_s	p
Number of apneas	.77	< 0.001
Number of hypopneas	.66	< 0.001
Apnea index	.76	< 0.001
Hypopnea index	.65	< 0.001
Respiratory disturbance index	.79	< 0.001
Longest apnea	.62	< 0.001
Longest hypopnea	.23	< 0.005
Number of obstructive apneas	.56	< 0.001
Number of obstructive hypopneas	.51	< 0.001
Number of central apneas	.77	< 0.001
Number of central hypopneas	.70	< 0.001
Number of mixed apneas	.67	< 0.001
Number of mixed hypopneas	.63	< 0.001
Number of leg jerks	.70	< 0.001
Myoclonus index	.72	< 0.001

RDI; number of leg jerks; and MI. The night-to-night correlations of the first 110 patients are presented in Table 2. The correlations confirm that AI varies from night to night. Wittig et al. (35) and Bliwise et al. (36) have also shown that the number of apneas varies from night to night. Therefore, if it is desirable to record multiple nights, it is much easier to do so with a portable system.

Apnea indices were also correlated with oxygen saturation levels (37). The correlation of apneas plus hypopneas (i.e., number of respiratory disturbances) with the number of oxygen desaturations ($>4\%$) per night was 0.97 ($p < 0.001$). These data indicate that the measurement of respiratory disturbances with portable modified Respitrace/Medilog systems and the measurement of desaturations with oximetry are remarkably equivalent, further validating the modified Respitrace/Medilog system.

Nursing-Home Study

We have also been exploring the prevalence of sleep apnea and the relationship of apnea to dementia in a skilled nursing-home population (38). Patients aged 65 and over were once again randomly selected from all new admissions to the nursing home. Each patient had a sleep interview, medical records were abstracted, a dementia rating scale was administered, and, whenever possible, 2 nights of sleep were recorded with the modified Respitrace/Medilog system. In this population, due to their frail condition, it was not possible to calibrate the Respitrace, but total sleep time; wake time; and type, duration, and number of apneas and hypopneas were scored. AI, HI, and RDI could still be computed.

In this population, 473 patients were asked and 293 (62%) agreed to participate. Of the first 200 subjects, all had at least one recording, and 63% had two recordings. Therefore, even in a very sick and frail population, the compliance rate for being recorded with the portable system was high.

The prevalence of sleep apnea in this sample was also very high, with 41% having an AI ≥ 5 (mean AI = 16.3; SD = 11.8) and 68% having an RDI ≥ 5 (mean RDI = 25.6; SD = 17.4) (39,40). Since sleep/wake activity was recorded for an average of 15 hr in the sample, we have also been able to look at the architecture of sleep. Remarkably fragmented sleep was seen with some sleep occurring in almost every hour, but patients were *never* asleep for an entire hour (40,41). These results emphasize the importance of 24-hr monitoring of sleep/wake states, something that can only be accomplished with ambulatory monitoring.

SUMMARY

Our experience with the modified Respitrace/Medilog system suggests that portable recording techniques are very effective for screening sleep apnea and PLMS. The portable recording is more cost-effective than a full-night polysomnogram, and, in some cases, such as with inpatients or frail elderly, it is the only option for obtaining sleep recordings. In addition, with portable recorders, it is easier to do multiple recordings, follow-up studies, and studies of treatment efficacy. As mentioned above, data are now available that show that the number of apneas and number of leg jerks vary from night to night, especially in mild cases (35,36). With the portable recorder, it is very easy to record 2 or 3 nights without too much inconvenience to the patient. Patients do not have to disrupt their routines, as they can still sleep in their own beds (whether at home or on the ward).

There is some controversy whether sleep apnea can properly be treated on the basis of portable recording alone (42). In our opinion, this decision should be individualized for each patient (43). As sleep apnea becomes more widely recognized by the public, patients who have no substantial subjective symptoms of disturbed sleep at night or daytime sleepiness are being seen because bed partners observe apneas. If portable recording reveals too few apneas to justify a diagnosis of sleep apnea or if the condition appears quite mild, we think the patient could be reassured without a laboratory polysomnogram. Obese subjects could benefit from a recommendation of weight loss based on portable recording, and all patients with any sleep apnea should be advised to avoid alcoholic beverages and other sedatives at bedtime. If the portable recording shows central apnea or if the severity of an obstructive apnea syndrome is not sufficiently serious to motivate the patient toward surgical correction, we believe the patients can also be given specific medical treatment such as acetazolamide, theophylline, or protriptyline without laboratory polysomnography. Nevertheless, in most cases, we would be reluctant to initiate continuous positive airway pressure treatment or advise surgical treatments, such as rhinoplasty, uvulapalatopharyngoplasty, or tracheostomy, for obstructive sleep apnea without a laboratory polysomnogram.

Large epidemiological research studies such as ours could never be done without the use of portable recorders. These types of studies have never before been done by any research group. Our compliance rates of 37 to 69% could never have been accomplished without portable recording systems. The continuation of research examining the effect of sleep apnea on daytime and nighttime functioning is dependent on portable recorders, which allow the greatest flexibility. With the advancement of expanded recording capacity, the ambulatory recorder should become a necessity for both the clinician and the researcher interested in sleep and sleep disorders.

ACKNOWLEDGMENTS

The work described here was part of a large collaborative effort with Dr. Daniel F. Kripke, William Mason, Linda Parker, Jennifer Bloomquist, and Beth George. This work was supported by NIA AGO2711, NIA TNH AGO3990, and by the Veterans Administration.

REFERENCES

1. Guilleminault C, Dement WC. *Sleep apnea syndromes.* New York: Alan R Liss, 1978.
2. Phillipson EA. Control of breathing during sleep. *Am Rev Respir Dis* 1978;118:909–939.
3. Weitzman ED, Pollak C, Borowiecki B, et al. The hypersomnia sleep-apnea syndrome: site and mechanism of upper airway obstruction. *Trans Am Neurol Assoc* 1977;102:1–3.
4. Guilleminault C, Connolly SJ, Winkle RA. Cardiac arrhythmia and conduction disturbances during sleep in 400 patients with sleep apnea syndrome. *Am J Cardiol* 1983;52:490–494.
5. Guilleminault C, Eldridge FL, Simmons FB, et al. Sleep apnea syndrome. Can it induce hemodynamic changes? *West J Med* 1975;123:7–16.
6. Guilleminault C, Motta J, Mihm F, et al. Obstructive sleep apnea and cardiac index. *Chest* 1986;89:331–334.
7. Romaker AM, Ancoli-Israel S. The diagnosis of sleep-related breathing disorders. *Clin Chest Med* 1987;8:105–117.
8. Lavie P, Ben-Yosef R, Rubin AE. Prevalence of sleep apnea syndrome among patients with essential hypertension. *Am Heart J* 1984;108:373.
9. Pollak CP, Bradlow HG, Spielman AJ, et al. A pilot survey of the symptoms of hypersomnia-sleep apnea syndrome as possible prediction factors for hypertension. *Sleep Res* 1979;8:210.
10. Lugaresi E, Coccagna G, Cirignotta F. Snoring and its clinical implications. In: Guilleminault C, Dement WC, eds. *Sleep apnea syndromes.* New York: Alan R Liss, 1978;13–22.
11. Lugaresi E, Coccagna G, Mantovani M. Hypersomnia with periodic apneas. In: Weitzman ED, ed. *Advances in sleep research,* vol 4. New York: Spectrum, 1978, pp. 1–151.
12. Mondini S, Zucconi M, Cirignotta F, et al. Snoring as a risk factor for cardiac and circulatory problems: an epidemiological study. In: Guilleminault C, Lugaresi E, eds. *Sleep/wake disorders: natural history, epidemiology, and long-term evolution.* New York: Raven Press, 1983;99–106.
13. Phillipson EA, Bowes G, Sullivan CE, et al. The influence of sleep fragmentation on arousal

and ventilatory responses to respiratory stimuli. *Sleep* 1980;3:281–288.

14. Stepanski E, Lamphere J, Badia P, et al. Sleep fragmentation and daytime sleepiness. *Sleep* 1984;7:18–26.
15. Orr WC, Martin RJ, Imes NK, et al. Hypersomnolent and nonhypersomnolent patients with upper airway obstruction during sleep. *Chest* 1979;75:418–422.
16. Moldofsky H, Goldstein R, McNicholas WT, et al. Disordered breathing during sleep and overnight intellectual deterioration in patients with pathological aging. In: Guilleminault C, Lugaresi E, eds. *Sleep/wake disorders: natural history, epidemiology, and long-term evolution.* New York: Raven Press, 1983;143–150.
17. Yesavage J, Bliwise D, Guilleminault C, et al. Preliminary communication: intellectual deficit and sleep-related respiratory disturbance in the elderly. *Sleep* 1985;8:30–33.
18. Rechtschaffen A, Kales A. *A manual of standardized terminology, techniques and scoring system for sleep stages of human subjects,* 3rd ed. Los Angeles: Brain Information Service, 1973.
19. Cohn M. Weisshaut R, Scott F, et al. A transducer for non-invasive monitoring of respiration. In: Scott FD, Raftery EB, Sleight P, et al., eds. *International symposium on ambulatory monitoring.* London: Academic Press, 1978;119–128.
20. Kripke DF, Mullaney DJ, Messin S, et al. Wrist actigraphic measures of sleep and rhythms. *Electroencephalogr Clin Neurophysiol* 1978;44:674–676.
21. Mullaney DJ, Kripke DF, Messin S. Wrist-actigraphic estimation of sleep time. *Sleep* 1980;3:83–92.
22. Webster JB, Kripke DF, Messin S, et al. An activity-based sleep monitor system for ambulatory use. *Sleep* 1982;5:389–399.
23. Webster JB, Messin S, Mullaney DJ, et al. Transducer design and placement for activity recording. *Med Biol Eng Comput* 1982;20:741–744.
24. Mason WJ, Kripke DF, Messin S, et al. The application and utilization of an ambulatory recording system for the screening of sleep disorders. *Am J EEG Technol* 1986;26:145–146.
25. Ancoli-Israel S, Kripke DF, Mason W, et al. Comparisons of home sleep recordings and polysomnograms in older adults with sleep disorders. *Sleep* 1981;4:283–291.
26. Bliwise D, Gourash-Bliwise N, Chmura-Kraemer H, et al. Measurement error in visually scored electrophysiological data: respiration during sleep. *J Neurosci Meth* 1984;12:49–56.
27. Ancoli-Israel S, Kripke DF, Mason W, et al. Sleep apnea and periodic movements in an aging sample. *J Gerontol* 1985;40:419–425.
28. Ancoli-Israel S, Kripke DF, Mason WJ, et al. Sleep apnea and periodic movements in sleep in a randomly selected elderly population: final prevalence results. *Sleep Res* 1986;15:101.
29. Ancoli-Israel S, Kripke DF, Mason W. Characteristics of obstructive and central sleep apnea in the elderly: an interim report. *Biol Psychiatry* 1987;22:741–750.
30. Ancoli-Israel S, Mason W, Kaplan O, et al. Stability of apneas and leg jerks in the elderly. *Sleep Res* 1987;16:297.
31. George B, Ancoli-Israel S, Kripke DF. Comparison of sleep apnea and periodic movements in sleep in two age groups of females. *Sleep Res* 1985;14:156.
32. Guilleminault C, van den Hoed J, Mitler MM. Clinical overview of sleep apnea syndromes. In: Guilleminault C, Dement WC, eds. *Sleep apnea syndromes.* New York: Alan R Liss, 1978;1–12.
33. Block AJ, Wynne JW, Boysen PG. Sleep-disordered breathing and nocturnal oxygen desaturation in postmenopausal women. *Am J Med* 1980;69:75–79.
34. Block AJ, Wynne JW, Boysen PG, et al. Menopause, medroxyprogesterone and breathing during sleep. *Am J Med* 1981;70:506–510.
35. Wittig RM, Romaker A, Zorick FJ, et al. Night-to-night consistency of apneas during sleep. *Am Rev Respir Dis* 1984;129:244–246.
36. Bliwise DL, Carey E, Dement W. Nightly variation in sleep-related respiratory disturbance in older adults. *Exp Aging Res* 1983;9:77–81.
37. Kripke DF, Mason WJ, Bloomquist J, et al. Relationship of respitrace apnea-hypopnea counts and 4% desaturations. *Sleep Res* 1988, *17*:208.
38. Ancoli-Israel S, Parker L, Butters N, et al. Respiratory disturbances during sleep and mental status: preliminary results from a TNH. *Gerontologist* 1985;25:6.
39. Ancoli-Israel S, Parker L, Kripke DF. Preliminary comparison of nursing home patients with and without sleep apnea: differences in sleep and reported daytime sleepiness. *Sleep Res* 1985;14:141.
40. Ancoli-Israel S, Parker L, Sinaee R, et al. Sleep in a nursing home population. *Sleep Res*

1987;16:298.

41. Ancoli-Israel S, Parker L, Sinaee R, et al. Sleep fragmentation from a nursing home. *J Geront Med Sci* 1989;41:M18–21.
42. Overfield WD. Letter to the editor. *West J Med* 1983;139:714.
43. Kreis P, Kripke DF, Ancoli-Israel S. Letter to the editor. *West J Med* 1983;139:714.

Ambulatory EEG Monitoring,
edited by John S. Ebersole.
Raven Press, Ltd., New York © 1989

20

Ambulatory Evaluation of Periodic Movements of Sleep

Rodney A. Radtke*, Timothy J. Hoelscher*, and Andrew C. Bragdon*,**

**Duke Sleep Disorders Center, Duke University Medical Center, Durham, North Carolina 27710; and **Neurodiagnostic Center, Veterans Administration Medical Center, Durham, North Carolina 27705*

Periodic movements of sleep (PMS) are stereotyped, repetitive movements of the legs that occur during sleep and are capable of disrupting sleep (1–4). Over the past 20 years, PMS have come to be recognized as an important source of sleep disturbance causing insomnia in some patients and excessive daytime somnolence in others. As the clinical history is only occasionally suggestive of PMS, polysomnography (PSG) is essential for definitive diagnosis. Recently, some sleep disorders centers, including our own, have begun to use ambulatory monitoring equipment to perform PSG evaluations of PMS for clinical or research purposes. This chapter reviews the clinical characteristics, pathophysiology, and treatment of PMS and describes the procedures for PSG evaluation of PMS with an ambulatory monitoring system.

DESCRIPTION

The typical movement of PMS consists of dorsiflexion of the ankle plus extension of the great toe lasting for a period of 0.5 to 4.0 sec. The movement may be a sustained tonic contraction or a series of briefer contractions. The degree of movement can vary from subtle dorsiflexion of the ankle or toes to prominent dorsiflexion of the ankle accompanied by partial flexion of the knee and hip. The latter is reminiscent of the "triple flexion response"—an exaggerated form of Babinski's sign that is elicited in some patients with upper motor neuron lesions (5). Rarely, the arm may also flex at the elbow as part of the periodic movement complex. The movements can occur in one or both legs, or even alternate between legs.

PMS are easily distinguished from most other movements by both their stereotypic pattern and remarkable periodicity. In most patients, the movements occur with monotonous regularity every 20 to 40 sec, although intervals as short as 10 sec and as long as 90 sec do occur. Movements that induce some degree of arousal are considered clinically significant. PMS are most prominent during non-REM (NREM) sleep, but can also be seen during REM sleep. In some cases, PMS may emerge during quiet wakefulness as the patient is attempting to fall asleep (4).

PMS were previously called "nocturnal myoclonus," but that name was replaced with PMS because the movements are not true myoclonic jerks, which typically last less than 250 msec (3). In addition, there are other conditions that may accurately be called nocturnal myoclonus—conditions in which true myoclonic jerks appear during sleep and can lead to sleep disruption (6–9). The term nocturnal myoclonus was first used by Symonds, who described involuntary clonic movements, which prevented or disrupted sleep in five patients (6). The characterization of these movements was largely subjective and no polysomnographic (PSG) monitoring was performed. Symonds thought his patients had epileptic variants, but one may have had PMS. It was not until Lugaresi's polysomnographic studies of nocturnal myoclonus in the 1960s that PMS was recognized as a common disorder distinct from these other sleep-related movement disorders (1,2).

RELATION TO RESTLESS LEGS SYNDROME

Lugaresi's initial observations were made in PSG recordings from patients with restless legs syndrome (RLS). RLS is a condition characterized by deep, ill-described paresthesias in the lower extremities that arise primarily during periods of muscular inactivity and induce a profound compulsion to move the legs to gain relief (4,10,11). RLS is an important cause of insomnia. Patients with RLS often state that their symptoms are most severe when attempting to fall asleep at night. Many report that getting out of bed and walking do ease the sensations, but often only transiently.

An association with RLS has been reported for anemia, especially from iron or folate deficiency (10–13), pregnancy (10,11), uremia (14), vitamin deficiency (11), frostbite damage (10,11), peripheral neuropathy (4,15), myelopathy (4,15), Parkinson's syndrome (16), hyperexplexia (startle disease) (17), chronic pulmonary disease (18), and excess consumption of methylxanthines (e.g., caffeine) (19) or tobacco (20). RLS is familial in about one-third of the cases (21), and autosomal dominant transmission has been reported in one pedigree (22).

There is a strong association between RLS and PMS. Since Lugaresi's reports, it has been found that virtually all patients with RLS have PMS; also, in familial

RLS, some family members without RLS symptoms have been found to have PMS. However, subsequent experience has revealed that RLS patients account for only a portion of all patients with PMS. For example, at the Duke Sleep Disorders Center, approximately one-half of the patients with PMS also have RLS.

PMS AND SLEEP DISORDERS

Since their initial recognition, PMS have been found in a variety of circumstances. First, it is important to point out that PMS may be present in asymptomatic individuals, particularly with increasing age. In a PSG study of 100 asymptomatic subjects with ages ranging from 18 to 74 years, Bixler and colleagues found PMS in 11% (23). The prevalence of PMS was slightly higher in males and increased markedly with age. PMS was found in none of the subjects under 30, 5% of those between 30 and 49, and 29% of those over 50 years of age. Among affected individuals, the mean number of movements per night was 171 ($>$20 movements/hr of sleep), but only 12% were associated with arousals ($<$ 5 arousals/hr of sleep). Thus, it appears that the important factor determining whether patients will be symptomatic from PMS is not the frequency of the movements, but, rather, the frequency of movement-related arousals. Patients who have PMS, but less than five movement-related arousals per hour, are considered to have clinically insignificant PMS, which is then classified as a parasomnia.

A substantial portion of patients with sleep complaints have clinically significant PMS. In some of these cases, PMS appears to be the primary cause of sleep disruption, whereas, in other cases, a different primary cause is identified, and the PMS appear to be secondary or incidental. In a national survey of sleep disorders centers, PMS was reported as the primary diagnosis in 2.8 to 26.3% (mean, 12.2%) of patients presenting with a disorder of initiating and maintaining sleep [(DIMS) insomnia] and in 0 to 13.7% (mean, 3.5%) of patients with a disorder of excessive somnolence [(DOES) hypersomnolence] (24). Our experience at Duke has been similar (Table 1). Among patients presenting with insomnia, 23.5% have received a primary diagnosis of PMS. These patients exhibited a mean of 49.5 movements and 23.0 movement-related arousals per hour of NREM sleep. As with the asymptomatic subjects, the prevalence of PMS as the primary cause of insomnia increased with age (Table 2). Among Duke patients presenting with hypersomnolence, only 3% received PMS as a primary diagnosis.

Why some patients with a primary diagnosis of PMS present with insomnia, whereas others present with hypersomnolence, is not understood. Rosenthal and colleagues found that patients with PMS/insomnia had significantly fewer and longer awakenings, whereas patients with PMS/hypersomnolence had more and briefer awakenings, as well as more partial arousals to stage 1 sleep (25).

TABLE 1. *Percentage of patients given a primary diagnosis of PMS*

	Duke	1982 ASDC[a] Data	
Patient type	%	%	Range[b]
DIMS	23.5[c]	12.2	2.8–26.3
DOES	3.0[d]	3.5	0.0–13.7

[a]Association of Sleep Disorders Centers.
[b]Range among sleep disorders centers.
[c]Based on 85 DIMS patients.
[d]Based on 100 DOES patients.

TABLE 2. *Percentage of DIMS patients with a primary diagnosis of PMS* by decade[a]

Age group	% PMS[b]
20–29	6.6
30–39	10.5
40–49	26.7
50–59	26.7
60–69	35.7
70–79	66.7

[a]Based on 20 PMS patients out of a total sample of 85 consecutive DIMS patients.
[b]Represents the percentage of DIMS patients in each group given a final diagnosis of PMS.

PMS are often found in patients with other primary sleep disorder diagnoses (3). Among the Duke patients with DIMS, in addition to the 12% with a primary diagnosis of PMS, an additional 7% had a significant number of PMS with arousals, but other conditions (e.g., depression) were considered to be primary causes of their sleep complaints. Similarly, about 20% of the DOES patients had a significant number of PMS with arousals, but received primary diagnoses of sleep apnea or narcolepsy.

Interestingly, among patients with both sleep apnea and PMS, we have often noted that the leg movements persist with only minimal sleep disruption after effective treatment of the sleep apnea, and, in many cases, the movements eventually disappeared completely. Coleman et al. have reported the prevalence of PMS to be similar in sleep apnea, insomnia, narcolepsy, and other sleep disorders (3). Observations such as these raise the question as to whether PMS are simply epiphenomena that appear in chronic sleep disruption of any cause, or whether they are capable of disrupting sleep themselves. However, in many patients, the movements do appear responsible for the sleep disruption, and treatments that produce symptomatic improvement also reduce the number or severity of movements. In such cases, PMS certainly appear responsible for the patients' symptoms.

PATHOPHYSIOLOGY

What little is known of the pathophysiological mechanisms underlying PMS suggests that it has a central, suprasegmental basis. The similarity of the leg movement to the triple flexion response is at least suggestive of this possibility (5). An electrophysiological study of six patients with PMS has provided objective support for this hypothesis (26). This study demonstrated disinhibition of the blink reflex in all six patients and of some spinal reflexes in four. None of the six patients had a peripheral neuropathy or myopathy. In contrast to these abnormal motor responses, somatosensory and brainstem auditory-evoked responses were normal in another study of 10 patients with RLS and moderate-to-severe PMS (27). Overall, these data suggest that patients with PMS have impaired suprasegmental control of brainstem and spinal reflexes and that the level of the abnormality is at or rostral to the pons. The absence of neuropathy in some patients with PMS suggests that when PMS and neuropathy are found together, as in uremia, the two may be independent effects of a common underlying condition.

TREATMENT

The first point with regard to treatment is that asymptomatic or nonarousing PMS should not be treated. The second, emphasized in the RLS literature, is that reversible underlying causes should be identified and corrected when possible. For example, iron-replacement therapy is reported to relieve the symptoms of RLS resulting from iron deficiency, and folate has been claimed to benefit pregnant women with RLS who presumably were folate deficient. The remaining patients, who are the majority, must rely on symptomatic medical treatment.

A note of caution is required in discussing medical treatment of PMS, as the literature on this subject is diverse in both quality and scope. Double-blind, placebo-controlled studies are rare, and many reports are anecdotal. Some studies focus only on RLS symptoms, whereas others address PMS-induced insomnia or hypersomnolence independent of RLS. Surprisingly few studies have used PSG monitoring of periodic movements and arousals. This is a deficiency that will likely be corrected with the advent of ambulatory monitoring.

A variety of treatments have been claimed to relieve different PMS-related symptoms, including restless legs, insomnia, or hypersomnolence. Among these, there is fairly convincing evidence that clonazepam and similar benzodiazepines (28–30), a variety of opiates (31), L-DOPA or bromocriptine (32–35), carbamazepine (36,37), and baclofen (38) may benefit some some patients. In those studies in which PSG monitoring was performed, clonazepam and opiates reduced the total number of movements and movement-related arousals per night. In contrast, baclofen increased the frequency (and total number) of movements but decreased their amplitudes and associated arousals, and improved sleep symptomatology overall. The effects of dopaminergic agents and carbamazepine on movements remain to be clarified.

Other proposed, but unproved, treatments for RLS include red wine, vitamin E, vasodilators, 5-hydroxytryptophan, clonidine, propranolol, and phenoxybenzamine.

CLINICAL ASSESSMENT OF PMS

PMS should be considered in the differential diagnosis of every patient with a sleep complaint, because the historical information about possible PMS is notoriously unreliable (unless there is a history of RLS). Although PMS can occasionally be seen in quiet wakefulness, they are usually subtle enough that neither patients nor their bed partners are able to identify their presence. Patients who do report movements usually describe "hypnic jerks" [isolated focal or generalized jerks that occur at sleep onset and awaken the patient (7)]. In contrast, PMS are usually subtle enough to go unnoticed by both patient and bed partner.

To determine the accuracy of clinical evaluation without PSG, we retrospectively examined the case records of 20 DIMS patients given a final primary diagnosis of PMS after a PSG study. The clinical history alone correctly predicted only 11 of the 20 PMS patients (55%). These correct predictions were due to descriptions of RLS in 10 of these cases and a strong family history of RLS in the 11th. Reports of possible PMS by the patient or bed partner identified no additional cases correctly. We have also encountered a substantial number of false-positive errors in attempting to predict PMS from the history. These data suggest that clinical assessment of PMS without PSG is generally unreliable, except when a history of RLS is obtained.

POLYSOMNOGRAPHIC EVALUATION OF PMS

Objective evaluations of PMS are usually obtained with an overnight PSG performed in a sleep laboratory (39). Two channels of the PSG are dedicated to recording EMG activity from the left and right tibialis anterior muscles to detect PMS. At least four channels are used to record EEG, EOG, and chin (submental) EMG. These are not only for monitoring sleep stages; they are critical for detecting movement-related arousals and awakenings to determine whether the PMS are clinically significant. Additional channels are used for monitoring respirations (thoracic and abdominal movements, oral and nasal airflow) (40) to detect and characterize apneic events. Apneas and hypopneas can occur fairly regularly, and motor activity often accompanies the end of each episode. Thus, leg movements occurring only with termination of respiratory events are interpreted to be part of a generalized arousal response and not true PMS. Many sleep centers also videotape patient behavior during PSG performed in the laboratory. When available, these recordings can provide further assistance in determining the nature of a patient's movements.

AMBULATORY MONITORING OF PMS

With the introduction of ambulatory sleep monitoring systems, it is now possible to evaluate for PMS in the patient's home (41). Advantages of this approach are that the study is performed in the patient's normal sleep environment, which appears to limit the first-night effect (42), and that the study does not require a standard sleep laboratory and constant attendance by a technician. The disadvantage is that no qualified person is present to intervene should technical problems arise during the study, or to observe the patient for behavior typical of PMS or other sleep disorders.

While several ambulatory systems are capable of monitoring PMS, little information is available regarding the diagnostic reliability of such systems. Ancoli-Israel and colleagues have reported on the use of a modified Medilog-Respitrace system to screen for PMS as well as for sleep apnea (43,44). The four channels of this system were used to monitor thoracic movements, abdominal movements, tibialis anterior EMG summed from both legs, and one channel of wrist activity used roughly to distinguish wakefulness from sleep. In one study, they compared results from 36 patients, each studied for 1 night using this system and conventional PSG simultaneously (43). Counts of the total number of leg movements obtained using the two systems correlated at $r = 0.64$ ($p < 0.005$). Using more than 40 periodic leg movements as the diagnostic criterion of PMS, the portable system had a diagnostic sensitivity of 100% with one false positive. These data suggest this is a cost-effective system for the screening of PMS. However, the principal disadvantage of this system is that, due to the lack of EEG recording, the polysomnographer cannot determine the extent to which leg movements are associated with EEG arousal.

Our laboratory is currently using an Oxford Medilog 9000 ambulatory cassette recording system to evaluate DIMS of various etiologies, including PMS. This system can record eight channels of physiological data for 24 hr. Additional features include an event marker and a digital record of the time at 1-sec intervals. Based on our first 339 ambulatory studies, we have found that the system is well tolerated by patients and produces technically acceptable recordings over 90% of the time (45).

To evaluate PMS with this system, we use two channels for EEG (C_3-M_2 and O_z-C_z), two channels for EOG (left outer canthus to M_2 and right outer canthus to M_1), one channel for submental EMG, two channels for left and right tibialis anterior EMG, and one channel for airflow (summed signals from oral and nasal thermistors). This montage allows us to evaluate PMS fully, including standard sleep staging, checking for PMS-associated arousals, and checking for apnea-associated movements. It is important to point out that, whereas this system is adequate for screening for apneic events, it is not sufficient for the accurate assessment of the character and severity of sleep apnea.

The placement of the tibialis anterior electrodes is shown in Fig. 1. The technologist can easily locate the muscle by instructing the patient to dorsiflex the ankle against resistance applied by pushing down on the toes. With ambulatory monitoring, it is imperative to attach electrodes securely. Our laboratory uses standard Grass gold disk electrodes secured with electrode collars and reinforced with tape as shown.

Records obtained with this system are scored on a Medilog 9000 scanner, which displays the record on a video screen. A previous study from our laboratory demonstrated that sleep stages (46) can be scored reliably and accurately directly on the scanner (47). We have not yet compared the recording and scoring of PMS on the Medilog 9000 system with conventional PSG conducted on the same night. Scoring PMS on the Medilog scanner has both

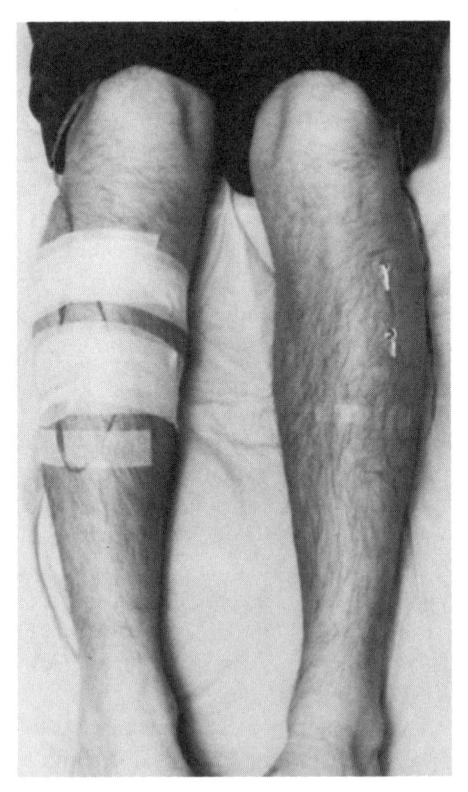

FIG. 1. Electrode attachment for monitoring tibialis anterior EMG. The left leg illustrates electrode placement. The right leg illustrates a taping method for securing the electrodes to prevent loss of quality EMG recording.

advantages and disadvantages. The principal disadvantage is that frequent stopping and starting of the playback mechanism is required to examine the record for the presence of an arousal coincident with a periodic movement. On the other hand, a significant advantage of the Medilog scanner is its ability to display the data on screen in either 16- or 8-sec epochs, which correspond to paper speeds of 15 and 30 mm/sec respectively. Thus, while scoring in 16-sec epochs, the reader has the option of switching to an 8-sec epoch to examine the EEG in greater detail for EEG evidence of arousal. Figure 2 shows a typical periodic movement, as observed on the Medilog scanner. Guidelines for scoring PMS directly on the Medilog scanner are identical to those used for scoring conventional paper records.

GUIDELINES FOR SCORING PMS

Although scoring criteria for PMS vary among authors (3,4,23,48), the criteria outlined by Coleman (39) are the most widely accepted and are a reasonable integration of our present understanding of PMS. A *movement* is defined as a distinct increase in one or both tibialis anterior EMG signals, which

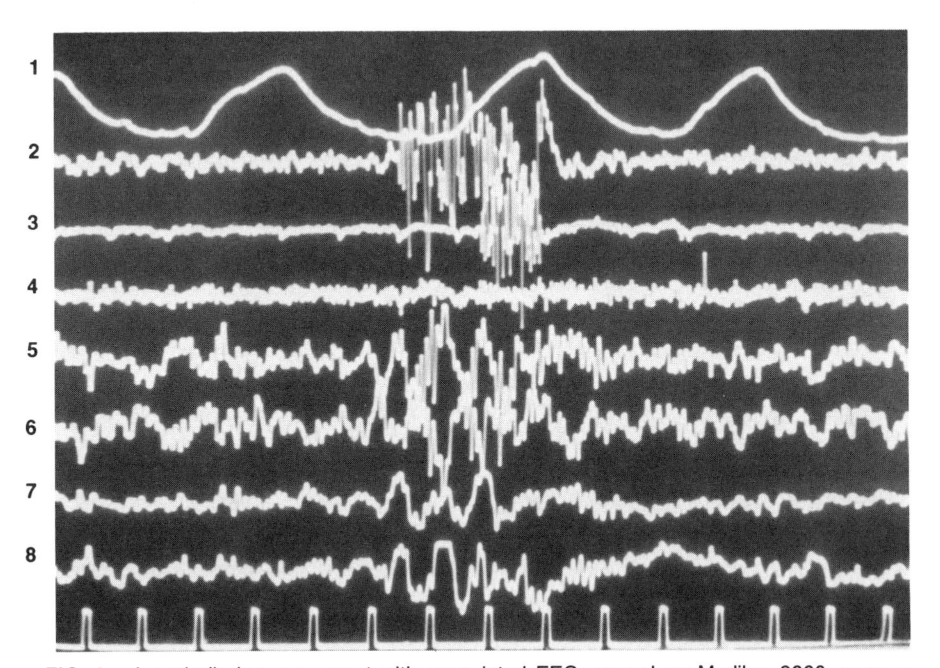

FIG. 2. A periodic leg movement with associated EEG arousal on Medilog 9000 scanner. Note left tibialis anterior EMG activity in channel 2, with accompanying EEG arousal manifested by rhythmic slow waves with superimposed fast activity in channels 5 and 6. Channel 1, nasal-oral thermistor; 2, left tibialis anterior EMG; 3, right tibialis anterior EMG; 4, submental chin EMG; 5, C_3-M_2 EEG; 6, O_z-C_z EEG; 7, left EOG; 8, right EOG. *Cursor* on bottom of screen depicts 1-sec markings across the 16-sec screen display.

lasts at least 0.5 sec (and usually less than 4 sec) and occurs as one of a series of at least four consecutive movements with an intermovement interval of between 4 and 90 sec (usually between 20 and 40 sec). Coleman also recommends that, in order to be scored, a movement's amplitude must be at least 50% of the amplitude of a baseline voluntary movement obtained prior to sleep. We have not found this criterion useful, probably in part because the degree of effort in dorsiflexion of the foot is not standardized. Moreover, we have encountered numerous instances in which movements with amplitudes distinctly below 50% of baseline are clearly and consistently associated with arousal in symptomatic patients. Therefore, we require only that each leg movement be represented by a distinct burst of EMG activity lasting at least 0.5 sec. We do not score unsustained EMG activity lasting less than 0.5 sec, or extremely low amplitude (< 30–50 μV) EMG discharges.

Criteria for scoring *arousals* are even more variable than those for the movements themselves (3,23,48). The appearance of 2 or more sec of either low-voltage fast activity or background alpha activity is often required for scoring an arousal. We also score an arousal when the EEG demonstrates a sustained period of rhythmic, high-amplitude slow activity or repetitive vertex waves in association with chin or scalp EMG changes. As isolated K-complexes are not generally scored as arousals, we do not score movement-associated K-complexes as arousals.

Whereas most arousals in PMS immediately follow leg movements, it is common in the course of a record to see some arousals occur either synchronous with or just before the periodic movements. As these arousals are likely not triggered by the subsequent movements, one hypothesis holds that both may be triggered by a common pacemaker or generator (4). The term "movement-associated" avoids the implication that the movement causes the arousal in every instance. In scoring, therefore, an arousal is scored as *movement-associated* if the onset of the arousal occurs within 2 sec before or after the onset of the movement. Note, however, that, when arousals *consistently* precede movement discharges, one should look for an etiology other than PMS.

Finally, the movement index (MI) and movement arousal index (MAI) are calculated by dividing the number of scored movements and of movement-associated arousals, respectively, by the number of hours of sleep (39). Alternatively, some authors think that division by the number of hours of NREM sleep provides a more accurate measure of the severity of the disorder, as PMS rarely occur during REM sleep. The MAI is the measure of primary importance in determining the clinical significance of PMS.

CLINICAL INTERPRETATION OF PSG RESULTS

For a diagnosis of clinically significant PMS, the Diagnostic Classification of Sleep and Arousal Disorders (48) requires three distinct periods of PMS, each containing a minimum of 30 movements "consistently followed by a partial arousal or awakening." However, the MAI has gained greater acceptance as a measure of movement severity and associated sleep disruption. Coleman has proposed that a MAI of five or more movement-associated arousals per hour of sleep is sufficient for a diagnosis of clinically significant PMS (39), and this criterion is generally used today. However, the exact number, character, timing, and temporal distribution of the movements that are clinically significant remain open to question, and a broader normal range may be appropriate, especially in elderly patients. In terms of reliability, a single overnight PSG study is usually adequate to characterize the presence and severity of PMS. The limited data available suggest that PMS is a stable phenomenon when studied night to night for a short interval (49).

Two notes of caution are appropriate in regard to diagnosing PMS. First, one should be very cautious about assigning a primary diagnosis of PMS in the presence of an additional accompanying sleep disorder. Second, PSG evaluations for PMS should be performed only at a time when there have been no recent drug manipulations and preferably when the patient has been drug free for at least 2 weeks. Treatment with tricyclic antidepressants and withdrawal from benzodiazepines, barbiturates, or anticonvulsants are known to exacerbate PMS. Thus, a complete knowledge of the patient's medication history is important for proper interpretation of PSG studies of PMS.

CONCLUSION

Ambulatory monitoring, incorporating EEG and simultaneous or prior assessment of sleep apnea, is sufficient for diagnostic assessment of PMS. Ambulatory monitoring without accompanying EEG is of limited utility and may even be clinically misleading. Major advantages of ambulatory monitoring over other means of sleep evaluation include a reduced first-night effect and the relatively limited requirements for technical support, both of which are beneficial for performing serial studies and clinical trials. Major disadvantages are the lack of behavioral observation and the potential for loss of an entire study from electrode displacement. Final acceptance of ambulatory monitoring for PMS awaits validation studies comparing this approach with PSG performed in a sleep laboratory.

REFERENCES

1. Lugaresi E, Tassinari CA, Coccagna G, et al. Relievi poligrafici soi fenomeni motori nella syndrome della Gambe Senze Riposo. *Rev Neurol (Paris)* 1965;35:550–561.
2. Lugaresi E, Coccagna G, Gambi D, et al. A propos de quelques manifestations nocturnes myocloniques (Nocturnal Myoclonus de Symonds). *Rev Neurol (Paris)* 1966;115:547–555.
3. Coleman RM, Pollak C, Weitzman ED. Periodic movements in sleep (nocturnal myoclonus): relation to sleep-wake disorders. *Ann Neurol* 1980;8:416–421.

4. Lugaresi E, Cirginotta F, Coccagna G, et al. Nocturnal myoclonus and restless legs syndrome. In: Fahn S, et al., eds. *Advances in neurology,* vol 43: Myoclonus. New York: Raven Press, 1986;295–307.
5. Smith RC. Relationship of periodic movements in sleep (nocturnal myoclonus) and the Babinski sign. *Sleep* 1985;8:239–243.
6. Symonds CP. Nocturnal myoclonus. *J Neurol Neurosurg Psychiatry* 1953;16:166–171.
7. Oswald I. Sudden bodily jerks on falling asleep. *Brain* 1959;82:93–103.
8. Lugaresi E, Coccagna G, Mantovani M, et al. The evolution of different types of myoclonus during sleep. *Eur Neurol* 1970;4:321–331.
9. Broughton R, Tolentino MA, Krelina M. Excessive fragmentary myoclonus in NREM sleep: a report of 38 cases. *Electroencephalogr Clin Neurophysiol* 1985;61:123–133.
10. Ekbom KA. Restless legs. *Acta Med Scand (suppl)* 1945;158:1–123.
11. Ekbom KA. Restless legs syndrome. *Neurology* 1960;10:868–873.
12. Behrman S. Disturbed relaxation of the limbs. *Br Med J* 1958;1:1454–1457.
13. Nordlander NB. Therapy in restless legs. *Acta Med Scand* 1953;145:453–457.
14. Callaghan N. Restless legs syndrome in uremic neuropathy. *Neurology* 1966;16:359–361.
15. Lugaresi E, Coccagna G, Berti Ceroni G, et al. Mioclonie notturne sintomatiche. *Sist Nerv* 1967;19:71–80.
16. Strang RR. The symptom of restless legs. *Med J Aust* 1967;1:1211–1213.
17. DeGroen JHM, Kamphuisen HAC. Periodic nocturnal myoclonus in a patient with hyperexplexia (startle disease). *J Neurol Sci* 1978;38:207–213.
18. Spillane JD. Restless legs syndrome in chronic pulmonary disease. *Br Med J* 1970;4:796–798.
19. Lutz EG. Restless legs, anxiety and caffeinism. *J Clin Psychiat* 1978;39:693–698.
20. Montifield JA. Restless leg syndrome relieved by cessation of smoking. *Can Med Assoc J* 1985;133:426–427.
21. Montagna P, Coccagna G, Cirignotta F, et al. Familial restless legs syndrome: long-term follow-up. In: Guilleminault C, Lugaresi E, eds. *Sleep/wake disorders: natural history, epidemiology, and long-term evolution.* New York: Raven Press, 1983;231–235.
22. Boghen D, Peyronnard JM. Myoclonus in familial restless legs syndrome. *Arch Neurol* 1976;33:368–370.
23. Bixler EO, Kales A, Vela-Bueno A, et al. Nocturnal myoclonus and nocturnal myoclonic activity in a normal population. *Res Commun Chem Pathol Pharmacol* 1982;36:129–140.
24. Coleman RM, Roffwarg HP, Kennedy SJ, et al. Sleep-wake disorders based on a polysomnographic diagnosis: a national cooperative study. *JAMA* 1982;247:997–1003.
25. Rosenthal L, Roehrs T, Sicklesteel J, et al. Periodic movements during sleep, sleep fragmentation, and sleep-wake complaints. *Sleep* 1984;7:326–330.
26. Wechsler LR, Stakes JW, Shahani BT, et al. Periodic leg movements of sleep (nocturnal myoclonus): an electrophysiological study. *Ann Neurol* 1986;19:168–173.
27. Mosko SS, Nudleman KL. Somatosensory and brainstem auditory evoked responses in sleep-related periodic leg movements. *Sleep* 1986;9:399–404.
28. Ohanna N, Peled R, Rubin A-HE, et al. Periodic leg movements in sleep: effect of clonazepam treatment. *Neurology* 1985;35:408–411.
29. Moldofsky H, Tullis C, Quance G, et al. Nitrazepam for periodic movements in sleep (sleep-related myoclonus). *Can J Neurol Sci* 1986;13:52–54.
30. Mitler MM, Browman CP, Menn SJ, et al. Nocturnal myoclonus: treatment efficacy of clonazepam and temazepam. *Sleep* 1986;9:385–392.
31. Hening WA, Walters A, Kavey N, et al. Dyskinesias while awake and periodic movements in sleep in restless legs syndrome: treatment with opioids. *Neurology* 1986;36:1363–1366.
32. von Scheele C. Levodopa in restless legs. *Lancet* 1986;2:426–427.
33. Montplaisir J, Godbout R, Poirier G, et al. Restless legs syndrome and periodic movements in sleep: physiopathology and treatment with L-DOPA. *Clin Neuropharmacol* 1986;9:456–463.
34. Guilleminault C, Mondini S, Montplaisir J, et al. Period leg movement, L-DOPA, 5-hydroxytryptophan, and L-tryptophan. *Sleep* 1987;10:393–397.
35. Akpinar S. Restless legs syndrome treatment with dopaminergic drugs. *Clin Neuropharmacol* 1986;9:456–463.
36. Lundvall O, Abom P-E, Holm R. Carbamazepine in restless legs: a controlled pilot study. *Eur J Clin Pharmacol* 1983;25:323–324.
37. Telstad W, Sorensen O, Larsen S, et al. Treatment of the restless legs syndrome with

carbamazepine: a double blind study. *Br Med J* 1984;288:444–446.
38. Guilleminault C, Flagg W. Effect of baclofen on sleep-related periodic leg movements. *Ann Neurol* 1984;15:234–239.
39. Coleman RM. Periodic movements in sleep (nocturnal myoclonus) and the restless legs syndrome. In: Guilleminault C, ed. *Sleeping and waking disorders: indications and techniques.* Menlo Park: Addison-Wesley, 1982;265–295.
40. Bornstein SK. Respiratory monitoring during sleep: polysomnography. In: Guilleminault C, ed. *Sleeping and waking disorders: indications and techniques.* Menlo Park: Addison-Wesley, 1982;155–183.
41. Sewitch DE, Kupfer DJ. Polysomnographic telemetry using Telediagnostic and Oxford Medilog 9000 systems. *Sleep* 1985;8:288–293.
42. Sharpley AL, Solomon R, Cowen P. First night effect on sleep using ambulatory cassette recording, analysed by automatic sleep stager. *Sleep Res* 1987;16:579.
43. Ancoli-Israel S, Kripke DF, Mason W, et al. Comparisons of home sleep recordings and polysomnograms in older adults with sleep disorders. *Sleep* 1981;4:283–291.
44. Mason WJ, Kripke DF, Messin S, et al. The application and utilization of an ambulatory recording system for the screening of sleep disorders. *Am J EEG Technol* 1986;26:145–156.
45. Hoelscher TJ, Erwin CW, Marsh GR, et al. Ambulatory sleep monitoring with the Oxford-Medilog 9000: technical acceptability, patient acceptance, and clinical indications. *Sleep* 1987;10:606–607.
46. Rechtschaffen A, Kales A, eds. *A manual of standardized terminology, techniques, and scoring system for sleep stages of human subjects.* Los Angeles: UCLA Brain Information Service/Brain Research Institute, 1968.
47. Hoelscher TJ, McCall WV, Powell J, et al. Sleep scoring with the Oxford Medilog 9000: comparison to conventional paper scoring. *Sleep* (in press).
48. Association of Sleep Disorders Centers. Diagnostic classification of sleep and arousal disorders, 1st ed. Prepared by the Sleep Disorders Classification Committee, Roffwarg HP, chairman. *Sleep* 1979;2:1–137.
49. Coleman RM, Bliwise DL, Sajben N, et al. Epidemiology of periodic movements during sleep. In: Guilleminault C, Lugaresi E, eds. *Sleep/wake disorders: natural history, epidemiology, and long-term evolution.* New York: Raven Press, 1983;217–229.

Ambulatory EEG Monitoring,
edited by John S. Ebersole.
Raven Press, Ltd., New York © 1989

21

Sleep Disturbances in Psychiatric Disease

Gail R. Marsh and W. Vaughn McCall

Department of Psychiatry, Duke University Medical Center,
Durham, North Carolina 27710

Sleep disturbance is often encountered in psychiatric disorders and can be part of the criteria for diagnosis. Undoubtedly, the most prominent example is that of the affective disorders. Patients with mania may go without sleep for a day or more, and poor sleep and early-morning awakening of patients with depression have been known for centuries (1) and have become part of the diagnostic criteria (2,3).

Despite numerous studies, there are still a number of findings about the relationship of sleep to the psychiatric categorization of disease that remain in contention. For instance, there are well-controlled studies that show schizophrenics both do and do not have rapid eye movement (REM) sleep early in the sleeping period (4,5). This chapter will review how sleep disturbance has been related to psychiatric disorders.

Ambulatory recording can be an aid in assessing sleep in several ways. One of the problems of recording sleep in the laboratory has been that sleepers usually do not sleep as well in a new environment, and, thus, the first night of sleep, in a laboratory setting, is typically not analyzed because it has been somewhat disrupted by the unfamiliar environment. Of course, habituation to the environment is not complete in 1 night, and the habituation rate may be different among different patient and normal groups (different ages, for instance). Using ambulatory methods and allowing subjects to sleep in their usual environments thus may give better results with a much reduced "first-night effect." Of course, even ambulatory equipment requires some habituation time but may be significantly reduced by placing the equipment on the subject in the afternoon, and not just before bedtime. This allows the subject to habituate to the equipment well before entering bed.

In a sleep laboratory with a technician monitoring all recording, the loss of an electrode or other malfunction can often be overcome without severe loss of data (although waking the subject to replace a malfunctioning electrode must be seen as a significant intrusion into the subject's sleep). With ambulatory methods, the application of electrodes or other monitoring devices must be secure enough to weather a full night of sleep without on-site attention. One can also plan for the possible loss of some channels by building in redundancy, so that loss of a channel is not devastating to the entire night's data analysis.

MEASURES OF SLEEP

Sleep requires several physiological inputs for adequate categorization of its several stages; thus, the term "polysomnogram" is used to describe the record of data from a sleeper. The minimum amount of data is at least one channel of EEG, usually obtained from a site near the central portion of the scalp (C_3 or C_4), recorded with a reference on the opposite mastoid. Two channels are devoted to recording eye movements. The usual montage is an electrode below the outer canthus of the left eye and above the outer canthus of the right eye, each referenced to the opposite mastoid. The fourth and last of the basic channels is of chin EMG to measure the reduction in muscle tension when the person enters REM sleep.

These channels of input are used to categorize sleep into five stages: stages 1 through 4 of non-REM (NREM) sleep and REM sleep (6). The stages from 1 through 4 are increasingly deeper stages of NREM. Stage 1 is very light, more drowsy wakefulness than sleep. Stage 2 is a light stage of sleep. Stages 3 and 4 are characterized by large slow waves and are often lumped together as delta or slow-wave sleep (SWS).

On entering sleep, the typical sleeper progresses from wakefulness to stage 1, staying there only briefly before passing into stage 2. SWS sleep follows and is sustained, especially in children and young adults, until entry into a brief REM period. This completes the first cycle of sleep, which is then repeated several times during the night, with the SWS rapidly diminishing in the ensuing cycles and REM steadily growing. Despite the attention given to SWS and REM, stage 2 makes up about 50% of a night's sleep. It should be thought of as a light stage of SWS, since it does contain some slow waves, but may have other properties that remain unexplored.

In assessing sleep disturbance, clinicians routinely rely on the patient's report of insomnia. His report, however, is often in significant error (7). Polysomnography allows objective verification of sleep disturbance and, further, has found specific perturbations of sleep parameters in psychiatric patients (8), which suggests that the polysomnogram would be a valuable laboratory test in diagnosis. Acceptance of the polysomnogram as a diagnostic test should depend on its power to identify the diagnostic groups, the relative ease of obtaining the data, and superiority over other data sources such as patient interview.

Polysomnographic Abnormalities in Depression

Persistent sleep disturbance is a hallmark symptom of depression. Reduction of total sleep time (TST) during a night is an important sign of depression. Three factors contribute to this loss of sleep: long sleep onset latency, multiple awakenings after sleep onset, and early-morning awakening (EMA) with an inability to fall back to sleep. However, this shortening of sleep is not universally found in all depressed patients (9). In addition to short sleep, there are four other disturbances of sleep that are revealed only by a polysomnogram. REM latency (the time from sleep onset to the beginning of REM sleep) tends to be short in depressed patients compared with control patients of similar ages (10,11). Importantly, REM latency is abnormally short, even if the depressed patient's total sleep time is normal or hypersomniac, as may be found in some depressed and manic-depressive patients (12). This short latency to REM is one marker of a general tendency for all REM sleep to shift earlier in the night. Another is that the first REM period shows an increase in the intensity of REM per minute of REM sleep (REM density). Another way of saying that REM latency is short is to say that the amount of NREM preceding the first REM is short. It is not surprising, therefore, that the first NREM period contains little or no SWS. Depressed patients often will have fewer slow waves across the entire night, reflecting a tendency for lighter sleep.

The REM latency in normal individuals ranges from 70 to about 100 min in young normal adults (13). There are some differences between laboratories in how sleep onset and REM onset should be defined (14). Thus, there is more variation than one might expect in the reported data on sleep latency and REM latency due to variation not only among sleepers, but also among laboratories. For comparison to the young normal persons given above, Kupfer et al. (8) found their primary depressed patients to have an average REM latency of 38 min using a strict definition of sleep onset (about 10 min of continuous stage 2 sleep), while another study (15) found 49 min using a more lenient definition (3 min of stage 2 sleep).

REM sleep is normally found in recurring bouts throughout the night at about 80- to 90-min separations (16). The initial REM period is short (about 10–20 min) with each REM period growing longer. For depressed patients, all the REM periods are about the same duration, thus making the first longer than normal (25–30 min) (17–20). Also, the intensity of these periods (as measured by the number of eye movements per minute—REM density) is higher (11,17,18). Unfortunately, eye movement has been measured differently in each laboratory, and there are no universally accepted scoring criteria, which makes comparison across studies difficult.

Lack of SWS has been noted in the sleep of depressives, both as a general lack of delta sleep and also as a reduced number of delta waves in the record as counted by computer (21,22). In general, the sleep level of the depressed person is lighter. Another expression of this is an increased number of awakenings after sleep onset (WASO), which gives rise to a lower efficiency of sleep (the percentage of time spent asleep while in bed). Since the sleep of normal older adults tends to show some of these same tendencies—lighter sleep, more awakenings, and less SWS—it was necessary to test if depressives, matched for age, could be distinguished from normals. It has been shown that depressives across the adult age range can be distinguished from normals on this and other important parameters of sleep (11).

Age changes in sleep have been described in numerous studies, which have pointed out what was just mentioned above: lighter sleep, more awakenings, less SWS, smaller amounts of sleep accumulated across a night, and lowered sleep efficiency. However, there has been some controversy over whether there is a shorter REM latency in the elderly. One report found shorter REM latency (11), but others have reported relatively unchanged REM latency (15). In depressed patients, there may be a significantly greater reduction in REM latency in older subjects than in young, but this is not entirely clear, since the studies addressing this question seem to have found the greater reduction only in quite severely depressed patients (23) but not in more moderately depressed outpatients (24). Even on the question of SWS there seems to be some controversy, since one study has shown a startling interaction of age and depression with delta wave counts *higher* in depressed than normal elderly persons (25) when frequencies from 2–4 Hz are included.

The question of whether the alterations seen in the sleep variables covary with the extent of the depth of depression has been addressed (15). The patients with primary depression had much shorter REM latencies (< 70 min) than normal persons, those with depression secondary to other psychiatric problems, or those with psychiatric problems that were not disturbances of mood. All the latter categories fell within the normal range.

Several recent studies have shown that the categorization into endogenous/nonendogenous may provide a better fit to those depressed patients with altered REM parameters than does the older categorization into primary/secondary (24,26,27). However, no categorization scheme has yet been shown to be ideal. It seems likely that the strength of the depression, and even the evolving processes during the course of a depressive bout, may determine some of the parameters being measured in both sleep and behavioral variables (28).

Since there are a number of parameters of sleep that have been shown to be involved in the correlation of sleep with depression, it seems natural that studies would explore the possibility of whether multiple parameters could be used in conjunction with one another to achieve better prediction. Only a few such studies have been performed.

Gillin et al. (29) compared 41 normal volunteers, 56 primary depressed patients, and 18 primary insomniacs. The depressed patients were moderately to severely depressed. The primary insomniacs were not mentally ill, and none was depressed. All three groups averaged about 45 years in age, had adequate representation of men and women in all groups, and were drug-free for at least 2 weeks. While the depressed subjects and the insomniacs shared several characteristics that distinguished them from normal controls, such as decreased total sleep, decreased SWS, and decreased sleep efficiency, only decreased REM latency, increased REM density, and EMA time distinguished depressed patients from insomniacs. The average REM latency in depressed patients was about 45 min, while both the insomniacs and normals had REM latencies of 70 to 80 min.

Since both these groups also were tested against a normal group, variables other than REM variables provided the best discrimination among all three groups. The best combination of sleep variables was total sleep time, time in bed, sleep efficiency, sleep latency, time awake, EMA, REM time, and REM percent (the percentage of sleep spent in REM).

To measure how adequately a categorization method works, some specific measures have been generally agreed on: *Sensitivity* is the percentage of the depressed group correctly identified by the procedure. *Specificity* is the percentage of the control group correctly identified. The discriminant analysis in the above study provided 84% correct classification with a sensitivity of 70% and a specificity of 100% (16,29). Replication using a second group of patients obtained a sensitivity of 83% and a specificity of 100%. While these figures indicate good success at distinguishing depressed patients from normals by sleep variables, it was hypothesized that even better separation could have been achieved if identification of insomniacs were not also part of the study. That is, depressed patients were identified less well, since some variables had to be included in the discriminant analysis to permit separating insomniacs from normal sleepers.

Thus, a study was conducted that reanalyzed the data from the above study leaving out the insomniac group (30). The discriminant function correctly identified 86% of the subjects; sensitivity was 77% and specificity 98%, and needed only five variables: REM latency, sleep efficiency, awake time, EMA, and time in bed. REM density did not seem to be an important variable in this constellation. Using a discriminant function based only on REM latency and density produced only 73% correctly classified (as compared with 86% using all five measures); sensitivity was also reduced to 71% and specificity was 76%. A new group of depressed subjects was developed not only with an interest in replicating the former results, but to also test the difference in sleep between endogenous and nonendogenous depressive patients. The nonendogenously depressed group was considered to be normal for the purposes of developing sleep variables. Replication of the five-variable discrimination on this new group of depressed patients showed 55% sensitivity and 82% specificity. Using only REM latency and REM density in combination on this new group of patients offered the best separation with markedly increased sensitivity (73%) and somewhat decreased specificity (71%). This may have been because of the mix of patients. The continuity measures did well on unipolar, but poorly on bipolar, patients who made up about half the replication sample (the number of bipolar patients in the first study is not given). The REM measures did equally well on each type.

The generalizability of inpatient data to an outpatient population was investigated in about an equal number of endogenous and nonendogenous moderately depressed patients who had been medication-free for at least 10 days before testing (24). Endogenous patients had a significantly faster average REM latency (56 min) than nonendogenous patients (73 min). Sleep onset was defined as starting with stage 1. Using a REM latency cutoff of 62 min yielded a sensitivity of 66% and a specificity of 79% in separating endogenous from nonendogenous patients, which is very similar to the findings with inpatients.

In summary, these studies provide strong evidence that polysomnography can distinguish endogenous patients from nonendogenous patients, nondepressed insomniacs, and normals in both inpatient and outpatient populations with acceptable sensitivity (60–80%) and specificity (70–100%). Sensitivity and specificity may be enhanced by examining combinations of REM and sleep-continuity parameters; considering REM latency alone is probably inadequate to judge whether a polysomnogram is consistent with depression (31).

The polysomnogram may have application in further subdividing groups of depressed patients according to the presence or absence of significant medical illness contributing to depressive symptoms, presence or absence of psychosis, and severity of illness. Abnormally short REM latency and increased REM density mark those with primary, but not secondary, depression. They both share other aspects of disturbed sleep such as lighter and fragmented sleep. Among patients with secondary depression, coexisting medical illness is associated with a decrease in REM density as compared with controls and depressed patients without medical illness (17,32). Sleep efficiency and REM latency have been found to vary inversely with severity as measured by Hamilton scores in primary depression (33).

Reduced REM latency may also be a marker for some minor affective disturbances in patients who do not merit a diagnosis of major affective disorder. Polysomnographic abnormalities have been reported as characteristic of patients with borderline personality disorder who have prominent affective symptoms (34). Looking at REM latencies alone, an abnormally short REM latency identified a subset of patients with borderline personality disorder and a prior history of minor affective illness such as dysthymia or cyclothymia. Shortened REM latency typically was not seen in the more schizoid borderline patients. Other aspects of sleep such as SWS or sleep continuity, which form the rest of the picture of the depressive patient, were not discussed.

Those patients that suffer from psychotic depression initially show long sleep-onset latency, increased amounts of stage 1, and a long REM latency (35,36). In patients who have endured the disease for several years, the REM latency becomes very short (< 20 min). Psychotic depressives are also different from primary depressive patients in that the psychotically depressed have a REM percent that is below normal and a decreased density of REM during REM periods. Both of these are the reverse of the findings for primary depressives. Other measures such as amount of SWS or continuity of sleep are apparently not different if age, severity of illness, and agitation are controlled (36).

In summary, the evidence is best in supporting the polysomnogram as a laboratory test to separate depressed from nondepressed patients. Several studies also suggest the polysomnogram is useful in identifying some subtypes of depressed patients as long as other factors such as age and duration of illness are taken into account. Identifying affective disturbance in patients not suffering from major affective disorder may also be possible, but more work is needed to confirm these early impressions.

Specificity of the Polysomnogram

While the polysomnogram separates depressives from normals with a high degree of specificity, recent challenges to the notion of characteristic polysomnogram patterns in depression have come from authors describing depression-like changes in the sleep studies of other psychiatric and nonpsychiatric conditions. Schulz and Lund (37) catalog sedative withdrawal, narcolepsy, infancy, time-zone shifts, and experimental free-running sleep-wake cycles as potential conditions under which REM latencies of less than 20 min may be seen. These conditions would not usually be confused with depression.

A more serious objection was raised by a recent study (38). Sleep-deprived young normal males were assessed before and after partial sleep deprivation for 17 days (retiring at midnight and rising at 5 a.m.) to mimic depressive sleep patterns. Mean REM latencies at baseline were 78.8 min as compared with sleep-deprivation REM latencies of 55.9 min. The authors argued that reduced REM latency was an epiphenomenon of partial sleep deprivation rather than specific to depression.

This conclusion has been challenged (39) for examining REM latency carefully while ignoring and not reporting other crucial variables. Sleep efficiency, REM density, REM distribution, and slow-wave sleep must also be considered. In fact, an earlier study performed a similar experiment in which four graduate-student couples underwent gradual partial sleep reduction (40). Three couples slept an average of 8 hr per night while the fourth couple routinely slept 6.5 hr. All subjects succeeded in reducing their sleep period to 5.5 hr. Comparison of baseline data to the fully restricted sleep period revealed that subjects fell asleep more quickly and experienced few awakenings, with overall improved sleep efficiency. SWS increased significantly in percent and total time at the expense of stage 2 during sleep deprivation. Mean REM latency also fell from 89 min to 60 min with no change in REM percent. Other REM parameters such as REM density received no comment. Aside from the change in REM latency, the increases in SWS and sleep efficiency in these sleep-deprived normal subjects are exactly opposite the findings in depressives.

SCHIZOPHRENIA

While it is reasonably clear that the characteristic polysomnographic changes of depression are not merely an epiphenomenon of sleep loss, the specificity of these changes to depression has been contested by comparative studies in patients with schizophrenia or schizoaffective disorders. The findings on psychotic depression, which were reviewed in the previous section, show that, as aspects of schizophrenic behavior are added to the depressive picture, parts of the typical depressive sleep syndrome begin to disappear. The question then becomes what features of sleep are shared by patients who are clearly depressed or clearly schizophrenic, and what features clearly differentiate these groups? A number of studies in the late 1960s and early 1970s gave conflicting conclusions and were based on patient selection criteria and sleep measures that are not totally acceptable by today's standards. However, the conflicting results still persist, as reflected in two recent studies.

One study (4) contrasted 18 normal volunteers with 12 patients with schizophrenia, eight with schizoaffective disorder, and 12 with major depression. All patients met research diagnostic criteria (RDC) criteria for their diagnosis and were moderately ill. All groups were about 30 years old except the depressed group, which had an average age of 40. After a minimum of 2 weeks off medication, subjects were studied for 2 nights in the lab after 1 adaptation night. These investigators did not report REM density, REM distribution, or sleep efficiency (although there appears to be a difference in amount of WASO). Median REM latencies for the normal, depressed, schizoaffective, and schizophrenic groups were 70, 44, 55, and 56 min, respectively. Only the normal group was different from the other groups. There were also no differences in percentage of REM sleep or total amount of SWS except between the normal group and the others. Amount of SWS in just the first NREM period or counts of slow waves per minute of SWS, which some investigators believe differentiate between these groups (31), were not given.

These findings are countered by a second study (5), which examined eight never-medicated patients with schizophrenia, eight subjects with delusional depression, 16 with nondelusional depression, and 16 healthy controls. The average age varied from 22 to 26 years across groups, except for the delusional depressive group, which had an average age of 41 years. All diagnoses met RDC criteria. The patients with schizophrenia were "mild to moderately" ill, while the depressed patients were severely ill. The schizophrenic subjects were never medicated, which may be important, since treatment with neuroleptics may alter the brain long after medication has been discontinued. The alterations seen in this group of depressed young adults were very similar to findings in another study of young depressed patients (22) and typical of depressed patients in general. Sleep architecture for the schizophrenics and controls was not different with the exception of reduced sleep continuity in the schizophrenics. The two groups of depressed patients, however, showed reduced REM latency (< 50 min) and SWS percent (< 6%), while schizophrenics and normals were indistinguishable, on the whole, based on REM latency (> 80 min) and SWS percent (> 13%). REM density was also higher in the depressed group. Within the schizophrenic group, there was a strong correlation between decreased SWS and presence of the so-called negative symptoms of schizophrenia. To take into account possible differences due to age, an analysis of covariance was conducted to adjust for age differences. These results were not materially different from the original findings. The remaining difficulty, the severity of illness difference between the depressed and schizophrenic patients, cannot be easily or directly overcome. However, the principal finding, that schizophrenics do not share the characteristic sleep changes seen in similarly aged depressed patients, does not seem to depend on this minor difference. Further, the first study seems to have used schizophrenic patients of about this same level of illness.

Both these studies on schizophrenia are methodologically sound, the main difference being the medication history of the schizophrenics in the two studies. A coexisting affective component in some schizophrenic subjects may also be the basis of some components of the depressive polysomnographic features showing up in some studies. More work is needed to resolve the controversy on this issue.

ANXIETY DISORDERS

The anxiety disorders (generalized anxiety, panic disorder, agoraphobia, obsessive-compulsive disorder) can occur by themselves or in combination with depression, which raises the question of whether these disorders by themselves, or in combination with depression, have specific identifying characteristics in sleep. It appears that long sleep-onset latency, fragmented sleep, and diminished amounts of SWS are seen in both generalized anxiety and depression (41). There are some sleep characteristics that are unique to patients with depression. In general, patients with anxiety disorders do not have short REM latency, prolonged first REM periods, heightened eye movements during the first REM period, an increase in REM percentage, or as great a loss of SWS (i.e., loss of stage 4) as do patients suffering from major depression (41,42). Based on the preceding criteria, the depressed patients could be distinguished from a normal control group. Patients with anxiety disorders could not be differentiated from a normal control group using a mixture of measures. Moreover, patients with both anxiety and depression concomitantly show less intense shifts in the sleep variables (42), making identification of these patients as depressed, based on sleep variables, less likely.

Panic attacks, when they do occur during sleep, likely arise out of SWS and do not appear to have any warning indications in the polysomnogram (43). Thus, there seems to be no additional information that can be given to the patient from nighttime recordings that could not be obtained from daytime recordings with regard to panic attacks.

Obsessive-compulsive disorder shares several clinical features in common with depression and often responds to treatment with antidepressants. An examination of the sleep of these patients showed a number of common elements (44). In comparison with normal subjects, the obsessive-compulsive patients showed shortened REM latency, less SWS, a decreased amount of total sleep time, and more fragmented sleep. Depressed patients were different in several subtle ways: the depressed patients had more REM density, had more REM in the early part of the night, and, perhaps most striking, had short REM latency on each of the test nights, while the obsessive patients showed a first-night effect of having a normal REM latency on the first night.

In conclusion, short REM latencies are not specific to depression but are also seen in sleep-deprived normals, possibly in schizophrenics, and other conditions. It is the constellation of reduced REM latency, SWS, sleep efficiency, and increased REM density, with a shift forward in the night of REM sleep, that appears to be characteristic of depression. This constellation of findings has yet to be reported in a condition other than depression, except in laboratory studies of normals given prolonged bed rest (45). The polysomnogram, when assessed for the proper set of variables, therefore, remains a reliable laboratory test for depression and can be helpful in assessing other psychiatric disorders.

Neurobiological Bases for Polysomnographic Findings in Depression

If there is, indeed, a characteristic polysomnogram of major depression, it is tempting to integrate this information with theoretical etiologies of depression. An early model was that the alterations seen in depression represented REM deprivation (46). This model has been abandoned, since the evidence is that there is no loss of REM sleep before the onset of the characteristic depressive REM alterations (47,48) and continuation of short REM latency during unmedicated, spontaneous remission, which was accompanied by the normalization of both REM percent and REM density (49).

Several authors (50–52) have proposed sensitivities or interactions among specific neuronal groups that are active in sleep and employing neurotransmitters altered by antidepressants. One model (53) proposes muscarinic cholinergic supersensitivity as driving the alterations seen in REM sleep in depression. A number of studies have shown that REM sleep can be induced in normal persons with treatments of muscarinic agonists or by the withdrawal of muscarinic antagonists (54).

A competing model has presented a comparison between neurotransmitter regulation of sleep architecture and mood as a means of understanding the phenomenon of short REM latency in depression. Brainstem monoaminergic systems exert an inhibitory effect on the pontine reticular formation cholinergic neurons, which may generate many of the phenomena of REM sleep. As depletion of CNS monoamines has been imputed in the etiology of depression, critical loss of CNS norepinephrine or serotonin could precipitate low mood *and* disinhibition of cholinergic systems, resulting in reduced REM latency.

Other models of sleep alteration in depression may have a basis in neurotransmitters or neuronal interactions, but they are not as thoroughly worked through. One early model suggested that the early REM latency, increased REM density, and other features of the depressive syndrome were found in normal persons given extended periods of sleep: they had achieved sleep satiety (55,56). Working from this finding would predict that sleep deprivation would aid depressed patients, which is what has been found (57). In many ways, such changes cannot be differentiated from an increased level of arousal, and experiments at the neurobiological level support such an interpretation with induction of REM and arousal with a cholinergic agonist (58). Also, normal persons subjected to such extended rest tend to show changes in circadian rhythms. These changes form the basis of another model and are discussed below.

Reduced REM latency can be the product of interactions among the circadian rhythms in normal REM physiology. Many studies (59–63) have demonstrated that the propensity toward REM sleep as measured by REM latency and REM percent varies within a 24-hr cycle in normals. The methods of measuring circadian variation in REM drive include polysomnographic recording during daytime naps, during shifting of the entire sleep period from night to day, or during sleep periods broken into 1-hr bits distributed throughout the day. Regardless of method, the results are consistent across the studies. REM latency is longest when sleep is initiated around the usual bedtime of 11 p.m. or midnight and gets progressively shorter when sleep is initiated during early-morning hours, reaching a nadir around 10 or 11 a.m. From this point, REM latency progressively lengthens until bedtime.

REM sleep shares a common circadian rhythm with other biological events such as cortisol secretion and core body temperature. REM latency and body temperature vary in an inverse relationship throughout the day: when body temperature is lowest, REM propensity is at its maximum and vice versa (64).

It has been proposed that reduced REM latency in depression is a result of a phase shift forward in circadian REM rhythms, e.g., as if the patient who retires at midnight had retired later in the night when REM propensity is higher (65). Many depressed patients show such alterations in those functions, which are highly correlated with body temperature (66). Alternatively, it has been argued that depressed patients have a lower amplitude swing in their circadian cycle with flattening of REM drive and body temperature across the 24-hr period. Consequently, nocturnal REM latency is reduced as it approaches values of daytime REM latency (36,67,68).

Studies of manic-depressive patients who cycle rapidly (especially those on a 48-hr schedule) have shown the clearest relationships among circadian rhythms, sleep, and affective illness (69). At present, it is impossible to say whether changes in sleep architecture or in any circadian rhythm precede or follow the onset of affective illness. Although intriguing, therefore, etiologic implications remain speculative.

Another approach to determining relationships between depression and sleep has been to examine the relationships between particular aspects of sleep and particular aspects of depression. For instance, the question was posed if a specific type of patient would emerge if the cutoff for "short REM latency" was made increasingly short. What emerged was a patient with increasingly strong genetic ties to immediate family members with depressive symptoms and an increasing tendency to be endogenous (70). Interestingly, many of the symptoms used to identify an endogenous patient did not correlate with REM latency. Only terminal insomnia, appetite loss, distinct quality of mood, and unreactive mood (in decreasing order) were related to REM latency. This may constitute the basis of a specific subtype of depression with a set of biologically based alterations of function (i.e., "markers"). Such a concept is also backed by the finding that reduced REM latency is often coincident with failure to regulate cortisol normally, as evidenced by a failure to suppress cortisol output after a challenge with dexamethasone (24). This nonsupression has become a useful marker for endogenous depression.

Limitations of the Polysomnogram in Depression

Although the polysomnogram has acceptable sensitivity (60–80%) and specificity (70–100%) for a diagnostic laboratory test, like other laboratory tests there are clinical situations in which it is difficult to make a meaningful interpretation of the polysomnogram. These situations include the extremes of age and the effects of psychotropic medications.

There are fewer studies in depressed adolescents than in adults, but available information suggests that depressed adolescents do not develop the usual polysomnographic findings until they reach their early to mid-20s. One study compared sleep in 49 patients meeting RDC criteria for depression, who were younger than 18 years old, with 40 age-matched normal controls (71). The depressed and normal groups were indistinguishable from each other on the basis of REM latency, REM density, sleep efficiency, or slow-wave sleep. The only difference found was longer sleep latency in depressed adolescents compared with controls (33 versus 24 min, respectively).

Conversely, healthy elderly subjects develop some polysomnographic changes reminiscent of depression as a part of normal aging. One study looked at 69 hospitalized patients with primary depression and 37 normals ranging in age from 15 to 65 years old (11). Normal subjects showed a progressive decline in REM latency, slow-wave sleep, and sleep efficiency with age so that the record of elderly normals resembled that of younger depressives. In other words, the polysomnograms of young depressed patients appear "older than stated age." For example, REM latency in a 65-year-old normal may be about the same as a 25-year-old depressive—approximately 60 min. Despite these physiological age-related changes, it may still be possible to separate depressed from normal polysomnograms in the elderly by using age-adjusted criteria (23). Also, interpretation of an elderly depressed patient's polysomnogram can rely relatively more heavily on measures other than REM latency.

Most psychotropic drugs have significant effects on polysomnographic variables during both administration and withdrawal. Antidepressant and sedative drugs decrease REM sleep percent and total number of eye movements, and increase the number of delta waves (31). Withdrawal of these drugs produces changes similar to alcohol withdrawal, with increased amounts of REM activity. The period of drug withdrawal required before the polysomnogram is free of drug effects is unknown, but, in research settings, a period of 2 weeks is often used. Urgent clinical considerations may not allow for such a lengthy drug-free period, but a meaningful interpretation of the polysomnogram depends on a delay long enough to reduce substantially drug effects.

Fortunately, the issue of the patient's acclimation to the recording situation is not a limiting factor in most polysomnographic interpretations. Although there is some night-to-night variability in REM latency, other sleep parameters are relatively consistent over nights. One study performed polysomnograms across four consecutive nights in 92 depressives and found the mean REM latency varied within a narrow range—48, 51, 44, and 47 min on the respective nights (72). Moreover, depressed patients do not show a first-night acclimation effect on sleep parameters, thereby obviating the necessity of multiple recordings for clinical purposes.

A second night of polysomnography does not materially enhance sensitivity and specificity in the separation of primary and secondary depressives and controls using only REM latency (cutoff at 70 min) (15). The first night yielded a sensitivity of 59% and specificity of 81%. Obtaining a second study and using the lowest REM latency of the 2 nights increased sensitivity by only 3% and specificity by 7%. In most instances, therefore, a single night of polysomnography is sufficient.

Perhaps the greatest limitation in the acceptability of the polysomnogram as a laboratory test for depression is the cost and difficulty in procuring laboratory space, polygraphs, and trained technicians, and obtaining patient acceptance of the procedure. A step toward overcoming some of these obstacles may have been realized in the Telediagnostic and Medilog recording systems. Both systems allow recording in the home environment (73). The Telediagnostic system interfaces with the phone system, and the subject sends his polysomnogram over the phone lines to a technician in the sleep laboratory. The Medilog system is similar to the Holter cardiac monitor. The necessary electrode attachments are made in the afternoon prior to the polysomnogram. A small tape recorder is worn on a belt or shoulder strap and records the polysomnographic data. The following day, the polysomnographic data are played back off the tape on a telemonitor at high speed for scoring. Advantages of this system are that one technician can outfit several patients in a single day, the technician's services are not required at night, and data are rapidly scored and easily stored on the cassette tape. These home recording systems may offer the features required to evolve more routine clinical use of the polysomnogram.

Polysomnographic Changes Before and After Treatment

During treatment, as the patient shows recovery in his behavior, is there a concomitant alteration in his sleep? The REM suppressant effect of antidepressant drugs complicates the use of serial polysomnograms to monitor drug treatment of depression. Patients have been examined before and after treatment, however, to explore if alterations of sleep are a marker of depression itself ("state") or if they are more a marker of persons likely to experience depression ("trait"). One study examined 13 subjects with major depression by RDC criteria (nine endogenous, four nonendogenous) (28). Mean age was 37, and, at the time of initial study, subjects were moderately depressed. Each subject was studied in the laboratory for 2 consecutive nights during the active phase of his illness and again 6 months later during remission after at least 2 weeks of discontinuation of antidepressants. During the active phase of illness, subjects had abnormally low REM latencies (mean of 52 min) and unusually low percentage of stage 4. No polysomnographic variable showed significant change during the remitted phase of illness. This suggests abnormal sleep-study parameters may be trait markers in depressed patients.

Prior studies tend to confirm this view, although previous studies had not been able to follow their patients in such a complete longitudinal manner. However, there is some evidence that patients with symptoms of depression show greater changes in their sleep than those in remission (74,75). Thus, REM and sleep continuity parameters may have both state and trait characteristics in depressed patients: during the progression from active illness to resolution of symptoms, sleep variables start to approach normal values but still remain abnormal (28,76). This might form an ever-worsening spiral if the patient undergoes several bouts of depression. It is unknown if these markers could identify patients before the first episode of depression or if they signal vulnerability to relapse.

CONCLUSION

The distinctive pattern of depressive polysomnograms has acceptable sensitivity (60–80%) and specificity (70–100%) in separating patients with major depression from normal controls. No single polysomnographic abnormality is pathognomonic for depression; instead, a profile of several abnormal parameters supports the diagnosis. While isolated sleep abnormalities such as shortened REM latency may be seen in other conditions, it is the profile that is characteristic of depression. Use of the polysomnogram in corroborating the clinical diagnosis of depression is best limited to patients over 25 years old who have been drug-free at least 5 to 7 days, although a longer drug washout is preferable. Polysomnographic data must be corrected for age in the geriatric population. Using the polysomnogram to follow a somatic treatment course is complicated by the direct effects of antidepressant drugs. During the course of treatment and at remission, REM latency tends toward normalization, but rarely fully normalizes, suggesting both state and trait influences on REM latency.

RECOMMENDATIONS FOR CLINICAL USE

Each patient with depression does not require polysomnography to make a definitive diagnosis of depression. An accurate history and examination remain the cornerstones of diagnosis. As with other diagnostic tests, a polysomnogram is not necessary when the history and examination are clear, and it is meaningless when used as a screening test when clinical suspicion is low. Its utility and promise lie chiefly in those indecisive histories and examinations suggestive of, but not conclusive for, major depression. Familiar examples would include the patient who appears depressed but fails to respond to initial antidepressant treatment. A polysomnogram at this point to confirm the initial impression could aid in the decision to pursue more vigorous treatment. Also consider the depressed patient with significant cardiovascular disease. A polysomnogram to confirm the clinical impression would help justify the decision to undertake aggressive somatic treatment with its attendant risks. In these cases, a polysomnogram characteristic of depression may tip the balance, but a polysomnogram alone should never be used to make a diagnosis or rule it out.

The polysomnogram may be used to predict whether an antidepressant is likely to prove effective. Rather than wait the 1 to 3 weeks required to evaluate a clinical trial of antidepressant medication, marked REM suppression on the first night of amitriptyline administration predicted a good response to this drug in one study (31).

As a final aside, it should be noted that, if a clinician elects to obtain a polysomnogram in the assessment of depression, it is convenient to rule out sleep apnea and periodic leg movements at the same time. While sleep apnea and periodic leg movements of sleep are no more common in depressed patients than age-matched controls, these sleep disorders can mimic or exacerbate depressive symptoms (77). Moreover, routine use of a benzodiazapine as an adjunctive treatment in an anxious depressed patient with unrecognized sleep apnea could dramatically exacerbate the sleep apnea (78).

In summary, the polysomnogram has sufficient diagnostic power and precision to serve as a clinical aid in the diagnosis of depression when applied to the right cases with good judgment. It provides information that cannot be elicited any other way, and the means of obtaining that information are becoming accessible enough, especially with ambulatory monitoring, to justify development of the polysomnogram as a diagnostic test in psychiatry.

REFERENCES

1. Adams F. *The genuine works of Hippocrates.* Baltimore: Williams & Wilkins, 1939.
2. Spitzer RL, Endicott J, Robins E. Research diagnostic criteria. *Arch Gen Psychiatry* 1978;34:773–782.
3. American Psychiatric Association Committee on Nomenclature and Statistics. *Diagnostic and statistical manual of mental disorders,* 3rd ed. Washington: American Psychiatric Association, 1980.
4. Zarcone VP, Benson KL, Berger PA. Abnormal rapid eye movement latencies in schizophrenia. *Arch Gen Psychiatry* 1987;44:45–48.
5. Ganguli R, Reynolds III CF, Kupfer DJ. Electroencephalographic sleep in young, never-medicated schizophrenics. *Arch Gen Psychiatry* 1987;44:36–44.
6. Rechtschaffen A, Kales AA. *A manual of standardized terminology, techniques and scoring system for sleep stages of human subjects.* Bethesda: National Institute of Neurological Diseases and Blindness, 1968.
7. Carskadon MA, Dement WC, Mitler MM, et al. Self reports versus sleep laboratory findings in 122 drug-free subjects with complaints of chronic insomnia. *Am J Psychiatry* 1976;133:1382–1388.
8. Kupfer DJ. REM latency: a psychobiologic marker for primary depressive disease. *Biol Psychiatry* 1976;11:159–174.
9. Kupfer DJ, Foster FG, Detre TP. Sleep continuity changes in depression. *Dis Nerv Syst* 1973;34:192–195.
10. Kupfer DJ, Spiker DG, Coble PA, et al. Electroencephalographic sleep recordings and depression in the elderly. *J Am Geriatr Soc* 1978;26:53–57.
11. Gillin JC, Duncan W, Murphy DL, et al. Age-related changes in sleep in depressed and normal subjects. *Psychiatr Res* 1981;4:73–78.
12. Kupfer DJ, Himmelhoch J, Schwartzburg M, et al. Hypersomnia in manic-depressive disease. *Dis Nerv Syst* 1972;33:720–724.
13. Williams RL, Karacan I, Hursch CJ. *Electroencephalography of human sleep: clinical applications.* New York: John Wiley and Sons, 1974.
14. Knowles JB, MacLean AW, Cairns J. Definitions of REM latency: some comparisons with particular reference to depression. *Biol Psychiatry* 1982;17:993–1002.
15. Akiskal HS, Lemmi M, Yerevanian B, et al. The utility of the REM latency test in psychiatric diagnosis: a study of 81 depressed outpatients. *Psychiatry Res* 1982;7:101–110.
16. Gillin JC, Sitaram N, Wehr T, et al. Sleep and affective illness. In: Post RM, Ballenger JC, eds. *Neurobiology of mood disorders.* Baltimore: Williams & Wilkins, 1984;157–189.
17. Foster FG, Kupfer DJ, Coble P, et al. Rapid eye movement sleep density: an objective indicator in severe medical-depressive syndromes. *Arch Gen Psychiatry* 1976;33:1119-1123.
18. Duncan WC, Pettigrew KA, Gillin JC. REM architecture changes in bipolar and unipolar patients. *Am J Psychiatry* 1979;136:1424–1427.
19. Kupfer DJ, Broudy D, Spiker DG, et al. EEG sleep and affective psychoses. I. Schizoaffective disorders. *Psychiatry Res* 1979;1:173–178.
20. Kupfer DJ, Broudy D, Coble PA, et al. EEG sleep and affective psychosis. *J Affect Dis* 1980;2:17–25.
21. Kupfer DJ, Ulrich RF, Coble PA, et al. Application of automated REM and slow wave sleep analysis: II. Testing the assumptions of the two-process model of sleep regulation in normal and depressed subjects. *Psychiatry Res* 1984;13:335–343.
22. Kupfer DJ, Ulrich RF, Coble PA, et al. EEG sleep of younger depressives: comparison to normals. *Arch Gen Psychiatry* 1985;42:806–810.

23. Ulrich RF, Shaw DH, Kupfer DJ. Effects of aging on sleep in depression. *Sleep* 1980;3:31–40.
24. Rush AJ, Giles DE, Roffwarg HP, et al. Sleep EEG and dexamethasone suppression test findings in outpatients with unipolar major depressive disorders. *Biol Psychiatry* 1982;17:327–341.
25. Reynolds III CF, Kupfer DJ, Taska LS, et al. Slow wave sleep in elderly depressed, demented, and healthy subjects. *Sleep* 1985;8:155–159.
26. Kupfer DJ, Thase ME. The use of the sleep laboratory in the diagnosis of affective disorders. *Psychiatr Clin N A* 1983;6:3–25.
27. Thase ME, Kupfer DJ, Spiker DG. Electroencephalographic sleep in a secondary depression: a revisit. *Biol Psychiatry* 1984;19:805–814.
28. Rush AJ, Erman MK, Giles DE, et al. Polysomnographic findings in recently drug-free and clinically remitted depressed patients. *Arch Gen Psychiatry* 1986;43:878–884.
29. Gillin JC, Duncan W, Pettigrew KD, et al. Successful separation of depressed, normal, and insomniac subjects by EEG sleep data. *Arch Gen Psychiatry* 1979;36:85–90.
30. Feinberg M, Gillin JC, Carroll BJ, et al. EEG studies of sleep in the diagnosis of depression. *Biol Psychiatry* 1982;17:305–316.
31. Kupfer DJ. The sleep EEG in diagnosis and treatment of depression. In: Rush AJ, Altshuler KZ, eds. *Depression: basic mechanisms, diagnosis, and treatment.* New York: Guilford Press, 1986;102–125.
32. King D, Akiskal HS, Lemmi H, et al. REM density in the differential diagnosis of psychiatric from medical-neurological disorders: a replication. *Psychiatry Res* 1981;5:267–276.
33. Spiker DG, Coble P, Cofsky J, et al. EEG sleep and severity of depression. *Biol Psychiatry* 1978;13:485–488.
34. Akiskal HS, Yerevanian BI, Davis GC, et al. The nosologic status of borderline personality: clinical and polysomnographic study. *Am J Psychiatry* 1985;142:192–198.
35. Feinberg M, Carroll BJ. Biological "markers" for endogenous depression: effects of age, severity of illness, weight loss, and polarity. *Arch Gen Psychiatry* 1984;41:1080–1085.
36. Thase ME, Kupfer DJ, Ulrich MA. Electroencephalographic sleep in psychotic depression: a valid subtype? *Arch Gen Psychiatry* 1986;43:886–893.
37. Schulz M, Lund R. On the origin of early REM episodes in the sleep of depressed patients: a comparison of three hypotheses. *Psychiatry Res* 1985;16:65–77.
38. Mullen PE, Linsell CR, Parker D. Influence of sleep disruption and calorie restriction on biological markers for depression. *Lancet* 1986;8:1051–1055.
39. Carroll BJ. Sleep disruption, calorie restriction, and biological markers for depression. *Lancet* 1986;13:1390.
40. Mullaney DJ, Johnson LC. Sleep during and after gradual sleep reduction. *Psychophysiology* 1977;14:237–243.
41. Reynolds III CF, Shaw DH, Newton TF, et al. EEG sleep in outpatients with generalized anxiety: a preliminary comparison with depressed outpatients. *Psychiatry Res* 1983;8:81–89.
42. Dube S, Jones DA, Bell J, et al. Interface of panic and depression: clinical and sleep EEG correlates. *Psychiatry Res* 1986;19:119-133.
43. Lesser IM, Poland RE, Holcomb C, et al. Electroencephalographic study of nighttime panic attacks. *J Nerv Ment Dis* 1985;173:744–746.
44. Insel TR, Gillin JC, Moore A, et al. The sleep of patients with obsessive-compulsive disorder. *Arch Gen Psychiatry* 1982;39:1370–1377.
45. Campbell SS, Zulley J. Induction of depressive-like sleep patterns in healthy young adults. In: Halaris A, ed. *Chronobiology and neuropsychiatric disorders.* New York: Elsevier, 1987.
46. Snyder F. Dynamic aspects of sleep disturbance in relation to mental illness. *Biol Psychiatry* 1969;1:119–130.
47. Cairns J, Waldron J, MacLean AW, et al. Sleep and depression: a case study of EEG sleep prior to relapse. *Am J Psychiatry* 1980;25:259–263.
48. Knowles J, Waldron J, Cairns J. Sleep preceding the onset of a manic episode. *Biol Psychiatry* 1979;14:671–675.
49. Coble PA, Kupfer DJ, Spiker DG, et al. EEG sleep in primary depression: a longitudinal placebo study. *J Affect Disord* 1979;1:131–138.
50. Karczmar AG, Longo VG, Carolis S. A pharmacological model of paradoxical sleep: the role of cholinergic and monoamine systems. *Physiol Behav* 1970;5:175–182.
51. Hobson JA, McCarley RW, McKenna TM. Cellular bearing on the pontine brain stem hypothesis of desynchronized sleep control. In: Steriade M, Hobson M, eds. Neuronal activity

during the sleep-waking cycle. *Prog Neurobiol* 1976;6:279–376.
52. McCarley RW. REM sleep and depression: common neurobiological control mechanisms. *Am J Psychiatry* 1982;139:565–570.
53. Gillin JC, Sitaram N, Duncan WC. Muscarinic supersensitivity: a possible model for the sleep disturbance of primary depression? *Psychiatry Res* 1979;1:17–22.
54. Sitaram N, Moore AJ, Gillin JC. Scopolamine induced muscarinic supersensitivity in man: changes in sleep. *Psychiatry Res* 1979;1:9–16.
55. Aserinsky E. The maximal capacity for sleep: rapid eye movement density as an index of sleep satiety. *Biol Psychiatry* 1969;1:147–159.
56. Feinberg I, Fein G, Floyd TC. EEG patterns during and following extended sleep in young adults. *Electroencephalogr Clin Neurophysiol* 1980;50:467–476.
57. Vogel GW, Vogel F, McAbee RS, et al. Improvement of depression by REM sleep deprivation. *Arch Gen Psychiatry* 1980;37:247–253.
58. Sitaram N, Mendelson WB, Wyatt RJ, et al. Time-dependent induction of REM sleep and arousal by physostigmine infusion during human sleep. *Brain Res* 1977;122:562–567.
59. Webb WB, Agnew HW. Sleep cycling within twenty-four hour periods. *J Exp Psychology* 1967;74:158–160.
60. Karacan I, Finley WW, Williams RL, et al. Changes in stage 1-REM and stage 4 sleep during naps. *Biol Psychiatry* 1970;2:261–265.
61. Webb WB, Agnew HW, Williams RL. Effect on sleep of a sleep period time displacement. *Aerospace Med* 1971;42:152–155.
62. Weitzman ED, Nogeire C, Perlow M, et al. Effects of a prolonged 3-hour sleep-wake cycle on sleep stages, plasma cortisol, growth hormone and body temperature in man. *J Clin Endocrinol Metab* 1974;38:1018–1030.
63. Knauth P, Kiesswetter E, Bruder S, et al. Day sleep during the morning and during the afternoon between experimental night shifts. In: Koella WP, ed. *Sleep 1980.* Paris: Karger, 1980;198–202.
64. Czeisler CA, Weitzman ED, Moore-Ede MC, et al. Human sleep: its duration and organization depend on its circadian phase. *Science* 1980;210:1264–1267.
65. Papousek M. Chronobiologische aspekete der Zyklothymie. *Fortschr Neurol Psychiatr* 1975;43:381–440.
66. Wehr TA, Gillin JC, Goodwin FK. Sleep and circadian rhythms in depression. In: Chase MH, Weitzman ED, eds. *Sleep disorders: basic and clinical research.* New York: Spectrum Publications, 1983;195–225.
67. Kupfer DJ, Gillin JC, Coble PA, et al. REM sleep, naps, and depression. *Psychiatry Res* 1981;5:195–203.
68. Schulz H, Lund R. Sleep onset REM episodes are associated with circadian parameters of body temperature. *Biol Psychiatry* 1983;18:1411–1426.
69. Sitaram N, Gillin JC, Bunney Jr WE. Circadian effects on the time of switch, clinical ratings and sleep in bipolar patients. *Acta Psychiatr Scand* 1978;58:267–278.
70. Giles DE, Roffwarg HP, Schlesser MA, et al. Which endogenous depressive symptoms relate to REM latency reduction? *Biol Psychiatry* 1986;21:473–482.
71. Goetz RR, Puig-Antich J, Ryan N, et al. Electroencephalographic sleep of adolescents with major depression and normal controls. *Arch Gen Psychiatry* 1987;44:61–68.
72. Ansseau M, Kupfer DJ, Reynolds III CF. Internight variability of REM latency in major depression: implications for the use of REM latency as a biological correlate. *Biol Psychiatry* 1985;20:489–505.
73. Sewitch DE, Kupfer DJ. A comparison of the Telediagnostic and Medilog systems for recording normal sleep in the home environment. *Psychophysiology* 1985;22:718–726.
74. Schulz H, Lund R, Cording C, et al. Bimodal distribution of REM sleep latencies in depression. *Biol Psychiatry,* 1979;14:595–600.
75. Cartwright RD. Rapid eye movement sleep characteristics during and after mood-disturbing events. *Arch Gen Psychiatry,* 1983;40:197–201.
76. Kupfer DJ. EEG sleep as a biological marker in depression. In: Hanin I, Usdin E, eds. *Biological markers in psychiatry and neurology.* New York: Pergamon Press, 1982;387–396.
77. Reynolds III CF, Coble PA, Spiker DG, et al. Prevalence of sleep apnea and nocturnal myoclonus in major affective disorders. *J Nerv Ment Dis* 1982;170:565–567.
78. Mendelson WB, Garnett D, Gillin JC. Flurazepam-induced sleep apnea syndrome in a patient with insomnia and mild sleep related respiratory changes. *J Nerv Ment Dis* 1981;169:261–264.

Subject Index

B